HASHIMOTO'S
FOOD
PHARMACOLOGY

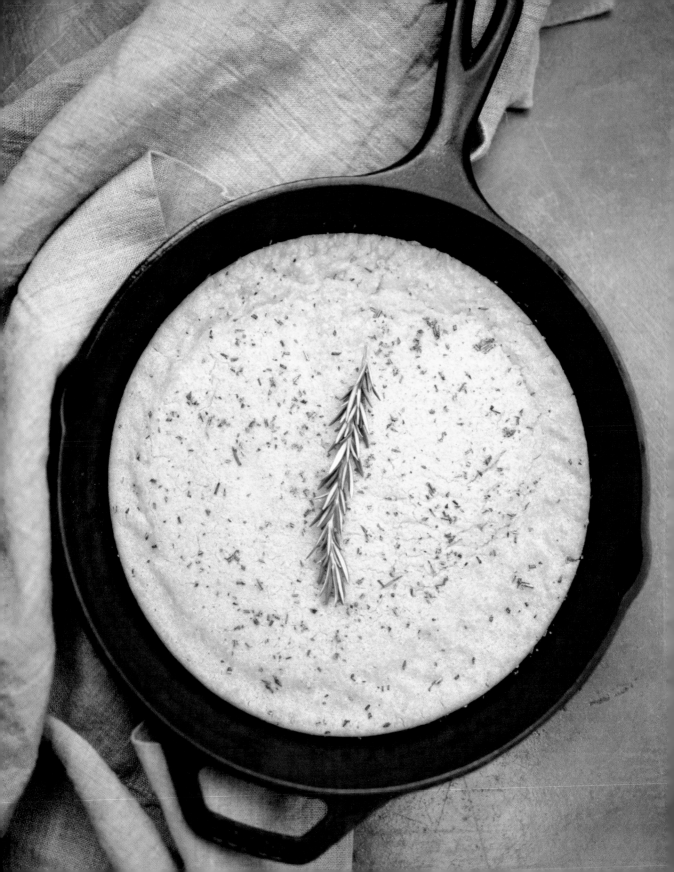

HASHIMOTO'S FOOD PHARMACOLOGY

Nutrition Protocols and Healing Recipes
to Take Charge of Your Thyroid Health

IZABELLA WENTZ

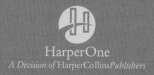

HarperOne
A Division of HarperCollinsPublishers

Also by Izabella Wentz

Hashimoto's Thyroiditis: Lifestyle Interventions for Finding and Treating the Root Cause

Hashimoto's Protocol: A 90-Day Plan for Reversing Thyroid Symptoms and Getting Your Life Back

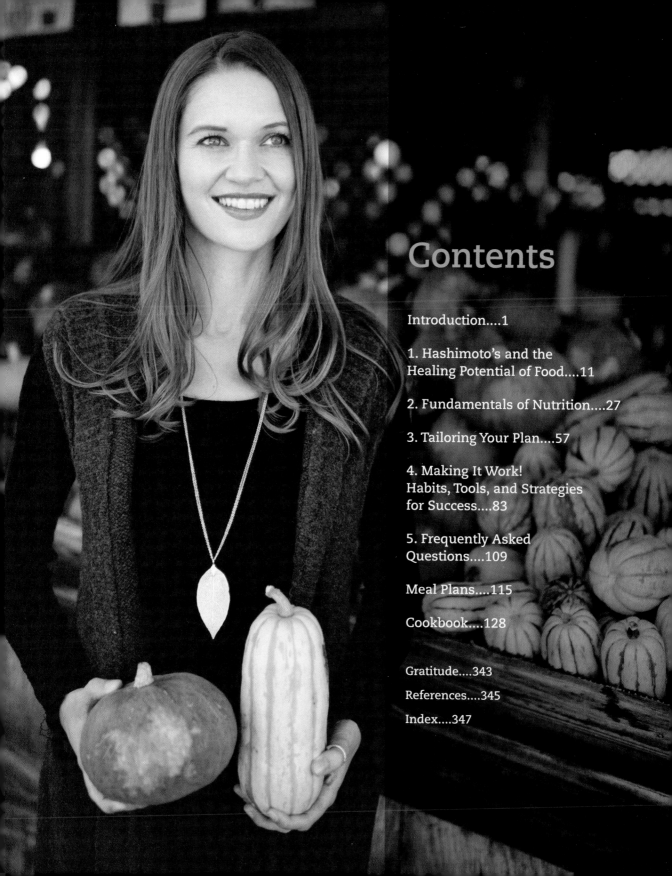

Contents

FIRST EDITION

Designed by Kris Tobiassen of Matchbook Digital
Photographs by Charlotte DuPont
Photograph on page 104 by Kyla Berry; used with permission.

Library of Congress Cataloging-in-Publication Data

Names: Wentz, Izabella, author.
Title: Hashimoto's food pharmacology : nutrition protocols and healing recipes to take charge of your thyroid health / Izabella Wentz.
Description: First edition. | New York, NY : HarperOne, [2018] | Includes bibliographical references and index.
Identifiers: LCCN 2018039829 (print) | LCCN 2018052042 (ebook) | ISBN 9780062571632 (e-book) | ISBN 9780062571595 (hardcover) | ISBN 9780062571625 (pbk.)
Subjects: LCSH: Autoimmune thyroiditis—Popular works. | Autoimmune thyroiditis—Diet therapy—Recipes. | Hypothyroidism—Popular works. | Hypothyroidism—Diet therapy—Recipes.
Classification: LCC RC657.5.T48 (ebook) | LCC RC657.5.T48 W448 2018 (print) | DDC 616.4/44—dc23
LC record available at https://lccn.loc.gov/2018039829

19 20 21 22 23   LSC   10 9 8 7 6 5 4 3 2 1

*To my dear readers—may Food Pharmacology
awaken your inner healing capabilities!*

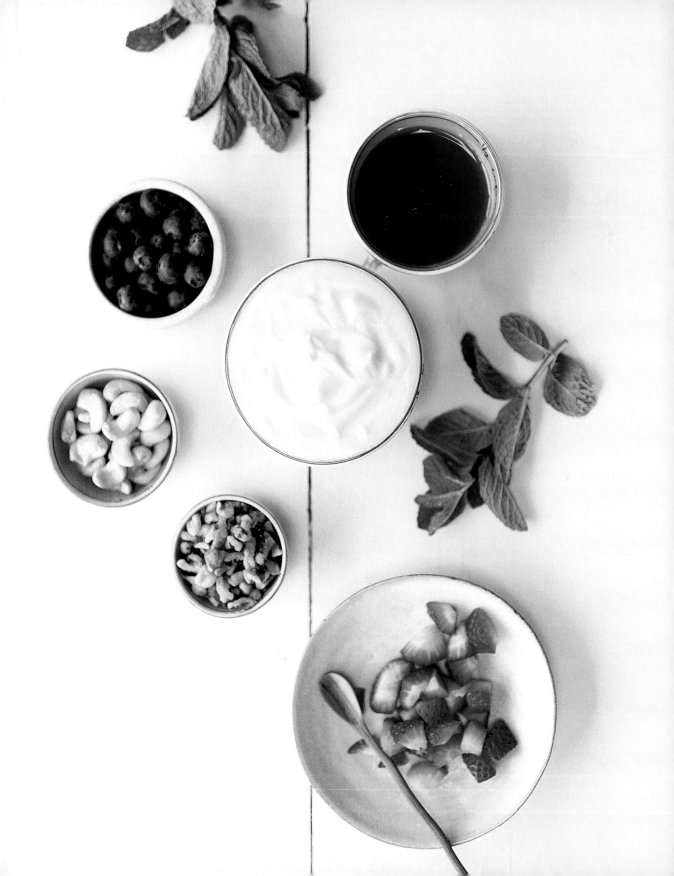

Introduction

If you picked up a copy of this book, there's a good chance you may be asking yourself, "So why is a pharmacist writing a cookbook?" In short, because I know that *all the* substances we put in our bodies can have a profound impact on how we feel.

As a pharmacist, I've spent countless hours learning pharmacology, the study of how various molecules interact with the cells and tissues of our bodies. Traditionally, when we think of pharmacology, we may think only of synthetic substances such as prescription drugs, but pharmacology is really the study of any substance, whether synthetic, naturally occurring, or produced within our body, that can affect our physiology and biology.

I became a pharmacist because I was fascinated by how tiny amounts of certain substances could have such a profound impact on us humans. I was amazed that a teeny 20 milligram dose of lisinopril could drop the blood pressure in the entire body of a 200-pound man and that mere *micrograms* of LSD (a microgram is 1/100th of a milligram) could make the same man hallucinate!

Like the tiny substances found in medications, tiny amounts of substances in foods we eat every day can have a profound effect on the body. Food molecules send thousands of messages to our bodies every day! The right foods can send positive and nourishing messages, giving us plentiful energy, shiny hair, and flawless skin and allowing our bodies to function like the high-performance machines they're meant to be. The wrong foods, on the other hand, can send negative signals, causing inflammation, pain, and countless other symptoms.

In the same way that we use pharmaceuticals to impact our biology, we can use food as our medicine! I call this concept *food pharmacology*. Food can be a powerful ally in your healing journey, and just as you want to be sure that the medications you take are right for your body, you will want to tailor your diet accordingly to get the best results.

What countless hours of research, my own Hashimoto's journey, and my work with thousands of people with Hashimoto's has taught me is that even though each person is unique, there are predictable and repeatable nutrition solutions that will work for most people with Hashimoto's thyroiditis, an autoimmune condition that attacks the thyroid gland and is the leading cause of hypothyroidism in most developed countries, like the United States. Many of these solutions may also work for people with other types of autoimmune disease.

Through my research and work with people with Hashimoto's, I have found that nutrient depletions, food sensitivities, an impaired stress response, an impaired ability to get rid of toxins, intestinal permeability, and infections can trigger Hashimoto's. What do all of these things have in common? According to my Safety Theory of Hashimoto's, all of these factors are evidence that our body has received messages that the world we are living in is not a safe place and that it should go into an energy-conservation mode.

THE SAFETY THEORY

The Safety Theory of Hashimoto's came about through my work with thousands of people with Hashimoto's and the study of biology, medicine, the concept of adaptive physiology, and the leading theories of autoimmune disease, including the bystander effect, molecular mimicry, thyroid-directed autoimmunity, and the three-legged stool of autoimmunity. It was developed as a way to better understand why so many people develop this common condition.

In essence, this is a theory about survival. Research has shown that the thyroid gland works with our immune system to sense our environment and to help us survive. A 2013 study found that the thyroid gland can sense danger and initiate an inflammatory autoimmune response against itself through molecules known as danger-associated molecular patterns (DAMPs).

A concept referred to as adaptive physiology suggests that our bodies develop chronic illness as an adaptation or in response to our environment. In other words, chronic illness serves a protective role. It sounds counterintuitive, but it makes sense when you think of it as a manifestation of our innate drive to survive.

Our bodies have evolved, or were brilliantly designed, to achieve two main goals: to help us survive and to help us reproduce and perpetuate our species. To ensure the best chances for survival (as individuals and as a species), our bodies are constantly sensing our environment and adapting to it.

In addition to predators, infections, and accidents, a main threat to survival for early humans was food scarcity. One very effective way to survive a famine is by reducing our metabolism so we don't have to eat as many calories. The body can do this by slowing down the thyroid gland, which is our master gland of metabolism.

I believe that early humans developed the propensity toward thyroid disorders because they helped us survive in times of famine! Many of these survivors were likely our ancestors, who have passed on this "survival advantage" to those of us with thyroid disease as a predisposition for developing thyroid disorders in times of danger.

We would like to believe that we are modern humans, but the truth is we still live in bodies that respond to danger the same way our ancestors' bodies did. In modern times, although famines are rare in the developed world, we may send the same signal to our body by eating processed foods (things with hardly any nutrients that our ancestors would not have considered food), being on a calorie-restricted diet, eating things that cause inflammation or digestive difficulties, and even eating when stressed. All of these signal the body that food is scarce and that we are in a famine. The food we eat, or don't eat, can send signals to our bodies that our environment is not safe, and we need to go into survival mode.

So if you have thyroid disease, thank your body for having this genius design that has helped keep you safe and helped you survive. And also think about what may be making your body feel as though its going through a time of famine, war, toxic crisis, or illness.

HOW TO TELL YOUR BODY IT'S SAFE

I consider myself to be a problem solver, pattern recognizer, and guinea pig, a person who loves to figure out puzzles through any means necessary. I'm not athletically or artistically inclined, but I do think I have a gift for taking in large amounts of information and seeing patterns. And what I can tell you from studying the patterns and problems related to Hashimoto's is that there are universal things that everyone with Hashimoto's can do to feel better. One way to really outsmart autoimmune thyroid disease is to make your body understand that it's safe!

Wouldn't it be great if we could just send a message to our immune system to stop attacking our thyroid gland and our body, to say that we are actually relatively safe in this unsafe world? I have great news—we can! The key, however, is to *communicate to your body in a language that it will understand*. In simple terms, you must eliminate the things that make your immune system believe that you need to conserve your body's resources and add things that make it believe that it is safe. One of the fastest ways to let your body know that it is safe and that it can thrive is through nourishing your body with food pharmacology!

THE JOURNEY TO TRANSFORMATION

Now, I'm not just a health-care professional sharing this information. I'm also a patient who has been there. My own personal health journey has been the creative driving force behind this Hashimoto's cookbook as well as my other two books, *Hashimoto's Thyroiditis: Lifestyle Interventions for Finding and Treating the Root Cause* and *Hashimoto's Protocol: A 90-Day Plan for Reversing Thyroid*

Symptoms and Getting Your Life Back; my Root-cology supplement line; and a host of other solutions for Hashimoto's.

When I was twenty-seven years old, I was diagnosed with the "incurable" auto-immune condition known as Hashimoto's thyroiditis. My diagnosis came after many years of frustrating, painful, and even debilitating symptoms. Some interfered with my undergraduate studies, some emerged during my doctorate program, and yet others appeared when I began working as a clinical pharmacist. It seemed as though every year I was collecting more and more symptoms. What started off as depression and fatigue eventually progressed into irritable bowel syndrome (IBS), panic attacks, acid reflux, a chronic cough, year-round allergies, brain fog, memory loss, emotional dysregulation, palpitations, hair loss, cold intolerance, dry and dull skin, carpal tunnel syndrome in both arms, and that sudden awful realization, "Wow, even my sweatpants are getting too tight!"

Like many thyroid patients, it took me at least a decade to get the right diagnosis. Let me be clear here: it wasn't for lack of trying. I saw numerous doctors who gave me various unhelpful labels including, "You're just stressed," "You're depressed," "You likely have IBS," and my all-time favorite, "You're just getting older"—which I heard at the ripe old age of twenty-five!

When I received the diagnosis of Hashimoto's and hypothyroidism, a large part of me was relieved and hopeful—finally I had an answer (and maybe a solution) to all of my symptoms! As a pharmacist, I was well versed in thyroid medications and excited at the prospect of taking a pill to replace the hormones my body was no longer making. At the same time, a part of me was devastated; I had an *incurable autoimmune condition*. The condition was progressive and would likely worsen each year; my thyroid gland would incur more damage with each passing day! Additionally, I could potentially end up with a second or third autoimmune condition! According to conventional medicine there was nothing that could be done other than taking replacement thyroid hormones (the hormones do not stop the progression of the condition). And, as I came to learn from personal experience, many people who took medications nonetheless continued to struggle with numerous symptoms.

As a pharmacist and a rational human being, I am a firm believer in cause and effect. I wanted to know if there was anything I could do to improve my condition and if my lifestyle was somehow contributing to making the condition worse.

I was trained in lifestyle as well as medication interventions during pharmacy school. We often recommended lifestyle changes like dietary modification and exercise for people with chronic diseases like diabetes, hypertension, and high cholesterol before we recommended medications. And if people needed medications, we would always still recommend that they focus on lifestyle. Granted the lifestyle changes recommended by conventional medicine are not quite where they should be yet, but hey, at least we were trying, and at least there was some hope that patients' conditions could be improved and even reversed with lifestyle changes.

Yet at the time of my diagnosis, the only type of intervention for Hashimoto's that was being recommended by endocrinologists was a pharmacological one. Don't get me wrong—as a pharmacist, I *loved* using medications (*when appropriate of course!*). In fact, appropriate medication use was my passion and the foundation of my training. I even had postgraduate certifications in medication therapy management and chose a career path as a clinical consultant pharmacist focused on optimizing medication outcomes.

I'm still a firm believer that the right medicine, for the right person, at the right time can be absolutely life changing (and sometimes even lifesaving). But c'mon, asking one tiny substance to shift your body into a positive healing mode when you have thousands of other substances sending negative disease signals is just not realistic. This is the reason many people who take thyroid medications, whether synthetic, compounded, or natural desiccated, continue to struggle with symptoms as I did.

When I started on thyroid hormone medications I was hopeful. And they did help! I was able to sleep eleven hours instead of twelve (I sure was glad to have that extra hour), and I no longer needed to wear two sweaters and a scarf in southern California. But I continued to have carpal tunnel syndrome that made computer work and yoga almost impossible; fatigue that interfered with my goals and social life; diarrhea, stomach pains, and acid reflux that resulted in embarrassing exits from meetings and presentations; hair loss that reduced my lion's mane to a third of its former glory; and a myriad of other symptoms.

My symptoms, along with my high thyroid antibodies (my thyroid peroxidase antibodies were over 2000 IU/mL when I was diagnosed, while my thyroglobulin antibodies were over 600 IU/mL) and a strong desire to get at the root cause of my condition, led me to dig deeper and deeper to see if I could somehow help myself get better.

And thus began my journey to seek out lifestyle interventions for Hashimoto's. My search for information included a review of the latest and greatest scientific literature (yes, I'm a professional nerd), an evaluation of various online patient boards (don't you just love how connected we can be to one another thanks to the internet?), a deep dive into numerous health books, visits to health conferences, consults with healthcare professionals, professional training in integrative and holistic medicine, and most notably turning myself into a human guinea pig to try various interventions that would eventually make me feel like a human again and help me get my condition into remission!

I was personally shocked to learn that my three-year bout of acid reflux and chronic cough and my ten-year struggle with irritable bowel syndrome could be solved within three days—just by getting off two foods I was sensitive to! Other symptoms soon disappeared, and eventually I learned how to properly nourish my body and listen to its subtle (and not so subtle) signals that something was not working for me!

In time, I was able to reduce my thyroid antibodies to the remission range, grow my hair back (very important to a Leo), ditch my carpal tunnel braces, unearth a flat stomach that was hiding under mountains of bloating and stomach pains, and become an overall healthy, happy, and fit person once more (no more panic attacks, mood swings, or bouts of depression).

Perhaps the best part of my own healing is that I was finally able to follow my dreams, to turn them into goals and then into reality. The brain fog, fatigue, and weakness lifted and revealed the strong and powerful person that was hiding underneath all along. I finally got the chance to become the person I hoped I would be when I was a little girl. I went from a fatigued, moody, and self-doubting couch potato who could barely take care of herself to a woman who feels as though she could do anything on most days. My brain is back, and I can't even describe the amount of self-confidence that has instilled in me. I've become an author, a documentary director, and even a new mom, things I never

thought would be possible when I was sick. I'm blown away at the way my life has been transformed through healing my body.

The butterfly is a symbol for transformation, and I sometimes think it's no coincidence that the thyroid gland is a butterfly-shaped gland. If you let go of feeling like a victim of your illness and step into your power, your thyroid condition can be the very thing that transforms you into the person you were always meant to be! I love the saying, "Just when the caterpillar thought its world was going to end, it became a butterfly!"

Ultimately, what I found in my own body and what's been true for most of the thousands of people with Hashimoto's I've worked with is that *Hashimoto's requires a multifaceted approach.* Hashimoto's symptoms often result from a combination of thyroid hormone imbalances, nutrient deficiencies, food sensitivities, an impaired ability to handle stress, an impaired ability to handle toxins, intestinal permeability, and sometimes one or more chronic infections.

All this may seem complicated and like a lot of ground to cover, but the good news is that nutrition is the cornerstone of recovering your health, dietary changes can produce profound improvements in your symptoms, and those changes may in some cases produce a complete remission of your condition. Changing your *output* often starts with changing your *input*, and there's no better way to do this than to start with the fuel you put into your body! Yes, you can feel beautiful, fit, calm, and healthy once more!

BRINGING DIET FRONT AND CENTER

When I discovered how much lifestyle, diet, and functional-medicine changes helped me, I wanted to let the world know. As a healer and empath, I was saddened that millions of people were suffering because they didn't have access to this life-changing information. Although I've always been somewhat of a reserved and private (albeit very friendly) person, I realized that this information was bigger than me and that I needed to share it with the world. I knew that my unique qualifications as a pharmacist (that is, a trained skeptic of all things nonconventional) and a patient who had been in the trenches was the perfect combination to get this message out into the world!

Once I found that I could change my health, I felt powerful and limitless. So I decided to follow a lifelong dream of mine, which was to write a book about my experience and newfound knowledge. Despite the fact that my high-school writing teacher called my writing melodramatic and unrelatable and my attempts at humor corny, I decided to step out of my comfort zone and publish my first book, *Hashimoto's Thyroiditis: Lifestyle Interventions for Finding and Treating the Root Cause. Hashimoto's: The Root Cause,* as readers have been calling it, was published in 2013 and became a surprise *New York Times* bestselling book. My biggest shock was at the number of people who related to the book and told me that they saw themselves in it, that I had captured the same emotions they had encountered. I was amazed to discover how many people with Hashimoto's were looking for ways to take charge of their own health. I was also pleased to receive messages from people who said that the book was so easy to read that they read it in one sitting (and that my corny jokes made the information more digestible).

In the *Root Cause* book, I dedicated a chapter to the topic of different diets that had been reported to reverse Hashimoto's and other autoimmune conditions. My goal at the time was to encourage and empower others to identify their own root causes, that is, the triggers that led to the development of Hashimoto's, and to give them the tools to establish an approach to feeling better. The book was a manual for healing, but in many ways it was a do-it-yourself manual—there was a lot of personal digging required.

While many readers found this approach helpful, others felt overwhelmed by the need to do a lot of their own "detective" work as it related to their health; what they wanted was a specific, streamlined protocol, a "Done-for-You Guide" (as one of my readers, Tereska, called it). So I dove back into emerging science in the growing field of functional medicine and evaluated my personal experiments and experience along with my ongoing work with Hashimoto's patients. Ultimately, I was able to distill all of the information I gathered into three comprehensive and detailed fundamental protocols, which came to represent the core of my second book, *Hashimoto's Protocol*.

Each of these three protocols contained within it a focused dietary approach designed to address vulnerabilities and/or overstressed systems common in people with Hashimoto's. The *Hashimoto's Protocol* also contains Advanced Protocols that focus on additional interventions to take back your health, such as optimizing medications and addressing infections, toxins, and traumatic stress.

The dietary modifications included in *Hashimoto's: The Root Cause* and *Hashimoto's Protocol* are essential to the healing process, but as they are only *part* of that process and a book only has so many pages, readers began asking for more in-depth guidance in food and nutrition. Many people expressed a desire for expanded insight on how to make the diets happen in real life. Could I share more of my favorite recipes? What were my secrets for adding flavor? How do you eat real food without cooking all day? What type of diet was I eating today, so many years after going into remission?

Although I'm not a professional chef, I love to cook and share nutrition tips with my family, friends, clients, and readers, so I decided to turn my focus to a cookbook and nutrition guide. And it's finally here, in your hands! It's been an honor and a pleasure to distill my nerdy nutrition knowledge for you and to share my family's favorite recipes in the pages ahead!

You'll also discover the best strategies for making diet changes an easy part of your life. To make healing approachable and fun, I wanted to create the most helpful, informative, and practical Hashimoto's nutrition book for you. By design, most of the recipes are really easy to make. I chose these recipes with you in mind, as I know what it's like to be fatigued, busy, and overwhelmed.

In sharing this cookbook with you, I am sharing a piece of my heart. Most of the recipes in this cookbook are our family's favorite recipes, ones that my husband and I cook in our day-to-day life. You'll notice that many recipes in this cookbook are traditional Polish recipes—many that have been passed on from my mom, grandmother, and aunts. These traditional recipes have been modified to remove reactive ingredients yet keep their delicious taste. I'm excited to introduce these recipes to you and your family. I hope that you enjoy reading and eating from this book as much as I enjoyed creating it.

As you start using this book in your day-to-day life, I hope it will awaken your inner healing capacities and help you connect with your body's needs. The goal of this book is to provide you with the tools you need to nourish yourself properly, as nourishment is what can send safety signals to your body, allowing and encouraging it to heal. If you have Hashimoto's, your nourishment needs are specific, and both the healing nutrition protocols and recipes I've created have been designed to help you meet these needs.

I also want to provide you with enough information regarding your nourishment needs that you feel empowered to become the undisputed queen or king of your own self-care. This includes understanding how much of each type of macronutrient you will want to consume for optimal healing, what micronutrients and vitamins will be most important to your recovery, and what supplements you can take to support your digestion.

In *Hashimoto's Food Pharmacology*, food and nutrition take center stage and get the full treatment, and what you get as a reader is a deep dive into how to heal yourself with nutrition. This isn't to say that diet can heal everything—there's a reason there are other crucial elements in the protocols I created—but strategic adjustments to what you eat each day can produce profound improvements in how you feel.

This book is written for the nonnutritionist and nonchef. It's written for the men and women who are ready to take charge of their own health and need a friendly guide that can provide the tools and confidence to optimize their nutrition as well as delicious recipes that don't require them to spend all day in a kitchen!!

Are you ready to dive in?

1.

Hashimoto's and the Healing Potential of Food

After my own Hashimoto's diagnosis in 2009, I wanted to figure out what I could do to be the healthiest person with Hashimoto's that I could be. I wanted to know if there was anything I could do to address my symptoms, and if there was anything that could be done to reverse my condition or at least stop its progression. So I set out to find the root cause of my condition and ended up on a health journey that got me out of my comfort zone—which was that of a conventionally trained pharmacist, skeptical of all things natural—and on the way to vibrant health!

Throughout this journey, I've been able to eliminate all of my symptoms and get the condition into remission by using a variety of interventions, most of which have been discussed in my books *Hashimoto's: The Root Cause* and *Hashimoto's Protocol*. The most profound of these strategies were those that centered around food and nutrition, and although there may be many moving pieces to resolving a Hashimoto's

diagnosis, we can always start to heal ourselves using food and nutrition!

As I've gone on to work with thousands of other people with Hashimoto's, either in person or through my programs (as well as hearing feedback about interventions shared in my first two books or my blog), I've found that food always plays an indispensable role in helping people feel better. In this book, I'll show you how to use food for healing. Before we get into the dietary details—and the cooking fun!—I want to offer an overview of Hashimoto's thyroiditis and why it is that diet has such a powerful impact on the condition.

WHAT IS THIS THYROID GLAND YOU SPEAK OF?

Chances are, if you picked up this book, you already know what the thyroid is. Just so that we're on the same page (no pun intended), the thyroid gland is a butterfly-shaped organ located in the neck below the Adam's apple. It produces thyroid hormones, which affect the function of just about every organ system in the human body, including stimulating the metabolism of the foods we eat, extracting vitamins, and producing energy from food. They are also vital to the production of other hormones as well as to the growth and development of our nervous system. The thyroid has been called the "thermostat" of the body, as it maintains our temperature. Indirectly, thyroid function affects every reaction in the human body, since the temperature has to be just right for these reactions to take place properly.

UNDERSTANDING HASHIMOTO'S

Hashimoto's thyroiditis is an autoimmune condition, which means it is a disease characterized by the immune system's attack on our own cells. In Hashimoto's, the cells under attack are located in the thyroid gland; in other autoimmune conditions they are in different parts of the body. When the immune system attacks the thyroid the way it would attack a bacterium, virus, pathogen, or other harmful invader, it causes damage to the thyroid gland, which will likely result in a reduced ability of the thyroid gland to make sufficient thyroid hormones for the whole body. This is known as *hypothyroidism*, or *an underactive thyroid*.

Hashimoto's causes most cases of hypothyroidism in developed countries, including the United States, Canada, Europe, and other countries that add iodine to their salt supply (in developing countries that do not fortify with iodine, iodine deficiency is the primary cause of hypothyroidism). Yet very few of those who are diagnosed with hypothyroidism will ever be tested for Hashimoto's or even informed that they may have an autoimmune condition. Instead, they are usually advised to take synthetic thyroid medication to correct their underactive thyroid, a step that, although necessary and helpful, does not address or correct the underlying destruction of the thyroid gland. This unfortunate oversight can allow the immune system's attack on the thyroid to continue.

In many cases, this oversight is a product of the conventional medical model, which instructs doctors to treat the majority of thyroid disorders, no matter what the cause, with synthetic thyroid medicine. Once on this path, a person's typical treatment plan will entail regular testing of thyroid hormone levels and adjustments of medication as needed, as well as screening for additional autoimmune conditions.

One of the problems with this treatment plan is that pharmacological restoration of normal thyroid-stimulating hormone (TSH) levels doesn't always result in the resolution of symptoms. In other words, on-paper improvement doesn't translate to a state in which the person actually feels better. I've had some clients share with me that this is the "worst part of the condition," because a doctor will end up insisting that their symptoms must be all in their head, since the blood-test results are normal. In this scenario, no one wins. The patient only grows increasingly frustrated, and the doctor, even a well-meaning one, comes across as increasingly dismissive. And still the discussion of Hashimoto's is unlikely to arise.

If you have an autoimmune thyroid condition, there is another factor that can add to the confusion: a fluctuation between or even simultaneous occurrence of hypo-thyroid and hyperthyroid symptoms. As thyroid cells are damaged and destroyed by the immune system, thyroid hormones that are usually stored inside of the cells are released into circulation, leading to an *excess level of thyroid hormones*. This causes what is referred to as transient or temporary *hyperthyroidism*, which can create symptoms such as weight loss, anxiety, and irritability. Then, once the extra thyroid hormones are cleared out of the body, the damaged thyroid gland will have a difficult time making enough thyroid hormones, and symptoms of hypothyroidism will emerge. These symptoms include fatigue, cold intolerance, and joint pain (see the sidebar on page 15 for a more complete list of symptoms).

Beyond the clinical discussion of symptoms, another aspect of Hashimoto's that doesn't get enough attention is what it really feels like to be someone with the condition—what thoughts and feelings can dominate your life and how profoundly the condition can impact your internal world. I know what it's like, and I hope sharing my experience and the experience of others with the condition will reassure you that you're not alone, and you can get better!

WHAT IT FEELS LIKE TO HAVE HASHIMOTO'S

I have a confession: I used to think that thyroid conditions were "boring" in pharmacy school! After all, you either had too much thyroid hormone and needed a pill to lower your levels or not enough and needed a pill to boost your levels! My own personal health journey has taught me that Hashimoto's is anything but boring and that there's much more to it than just thyroid hormone levels. Of course, working with thousands of people with the condition has confirmed this every time! What I've discovered is that the experience of Hashimoto's is one that is filled with not just a wide range of symptoms, but a wide range of emotions too.

In reality, medications don't always resolve thyroid conditions or lead to a disappearance of symptoms. For people with Hashimoto's, this can lead to feeling a loss of control over their physical body and even their mind. When I asked my Facebook community, "What does it feel like to have thyroid disease?" a lot of the responses centered around this sense of loss. One woman described it as feeling "like you don't recognize yourself anymore in many ways."

She said, "You keep trying to find the old 'me,' but she's long gone. I miss the girl I was before Hashimoto's." Another said, "I feel like a completely different person, and I can't seem to get that person back. I hate that. What is worse is, no one gets it, not your friends, family, doctors. Kind of breaks the spirit."

After my thyroid diagnosis, I experienced a feeling of dissociation from myself. I became numb and apathetic toward life, unable to feel any emotion, good or bad. I no longer had a desire for the things that made me human, such as being close to others, making friendships, following my passions, and loving the people in my life.

Although I like to focus primarily on solutions and steps for healing, these feelings can be a very real part of the experience of Hashimoto's, and I want you to feel that your emotions are validated. It's important to take some time to comfort yourself and show yourself kindness for what you are going through. I want you to understand that you're not going crazy, that many of your symptoms may be related to Hashimoto's, and that you can get better!

TESTING FOR HASHIMOTO'S

Because the symptoms shift and can sometimes be nonspecific, it can be tough to get a definitive diagnosis of Hashimoto's. As I mentioned, I personally experienced symptoms for almost a decade before being diagnosed. Sadly, ten years between the appearance of symptoms and the proper diagnosis seems to be the norm among the patients I've talked to. Even when they receive the proper diagnosis, they usually don't get the right treatment. Of course, my goal is to help shorten your path to healing by providing information that lets you become a proactive, empowered patient, one who doesn't need to wait for answers and instead knows what action steps to take. An essential part of this is having an understanding of the most important thyroid tests. Let's take a look at these.

Hashimoto's is usually diagnosed through either blood tests, thyroid ultrasounds, or biopsies of the thyroid gland. Blood tests are typically the most accessible option, and the right ones can often uncover autoimmune thyroid disease.

Most of these tests will be covered by health insurance if ordered by a licensed physician. If your doctor will not order these tests for you, you can get them through direct-to-consumer lab services and pay out of pocket, and in some cases submit the claim for insurance reimbursement.

Blood Tests

TSH (Thyroid-Stimulating Hormone)
TSH is a pituitary hormone that responds to the level of circulating thyroid hormones. The TSH test is used as a screening test for thyroid function and is likely what your doctor would suggest if you reported thyroid symptoms.

THE MANY SYMPTOMS
OF HASHIMOTO'S

Hashimoto's thyroiditis has a unique set of symptoms when compared to nonautoimmune hypothyroidism. If you have Hashimoto's, your symptoms may fluctuate between those of hypothyroidism and those of hyperthyroidism, or you may even experience symptoms of both conditions simultaneously. You may also have symptoms related to autoimmune inflammation. Here are some of the symptoms of each:

HYPOTHYROIDISM	HYPERTHYROIDISM
Cold intolerance	Anxiety
Constipation	Eye protrusion
Depression	Fatigue
Dry skin	Hair loss
Fatigue	Heart palpitations
Forgetfulness	Heat intolerance
Hair loss	Increased appetite
Joint pain	Irritability
Loss of ambition	Menstrual disturbances
Menstrual irregularities	Tremors
Muscle cramps	Weight loss
Stiffness	

Additional symptoms, which can be seen in other autoimmune conditions, include: acid reflux, adrenal fatigue, allergies, balance disorders, bloating, constipation, diarrhea, feelings of disconnection, gum disorders, irritability, irritable bowel syndrome, loss of ambition, mood swings, panic attacks, rashes, vertigo, weakness, and numerous other inflammatory symptoms.

A comprehensive approach is needed to resolve all of your symptoms and to get to the root cause of the condition!

In advanced cases of Hashimoto's and primary hypothyroidism, TSH will be elevated. In advanced cases of Graves' disease and hyperthyroidism, TSH will be low. Unfortunately, the TSH test does not always catch Hashimoto's in earlier stages. During these stages, you can have either high or low TSH or lab work that reveals "normal" readings even while you are experiencing unpleasant thyroid symptoms. I was told that my thyroid was "normal" when I was exhausted, forgetful, losing hair by the handfuls, and sleeping for twelve hours each night under two blankets in southern California.

At the time my TSH was 4.5 mIU/L, and this was considered normal based on the reference range of 0.2–8.0 mIU/L, which most labs still use. The problem is that when this original "normal" range of TSH was created, scientists included elderly patients and others with compromised thyroid function in the calculations, leading to an overly wide reference range. Based on this skewed range, many doctors may miss identifying patients with an elevated TSH (this is one reason why you should always ask your physician for a copy of any lab results).

Thankfully, the accepted TSH reference range is on the path toward change. In recent years, the National Academy of Clinical Biochemists indicated that 95 percent of individuals without thyroid disease have TSH concentrations below 2.5 mIU/L, and a new normal reference range was defined by the American College of Clinical Endocrinologists to be between 0.3 and 3.0 mIU/L. Functional-medicine practitioners have further defined normal reference ranges as being between 1 and 2 mIU/L for a healthy person not taking thyroid medications.

Thyroid Antibodies

The best blood tests for Hashimoto's are those that measure thyroid antibodies, because these will indicate an autoimmune response to the thyroid gland. The two antibodies that are usually elevated in those with Hashimoto's are:

- Thyroid peroxidase antibodies (TPO antibodies)

- Thyroglobulin antibodies (TG antibodies)

If you have Hashimoto's, you may have an elevated level of one or both of these antibodies. In general, the greater the number of antibodies, the more aggressive the attack on the thyroid gland.

Current medical reports state that 80 to 90 percent of people with Hashimoto's will have TPO antibodies. That said, researchers at the University of Wisconsin Thyroid Multidisciplinary Clinic found that only half of the patients who came up positive for Hashimoto's through cytology (when thyroid cells are withdrawn through a thin needle and then evaluated under a microscope; see more on this type of test below) had TPO antibodies. Even if your thyroid antibody test is negative, you could have a less aggressive variant of Hashimoto's known as seronegative, or antibody-negative, Hashimoto's, which does not present with elevated levels of either of the above mentioned antibodies, but may be seen on ultrasound or when running more invasive tests such as the fine needle aspiration.

Free T3 and Free T4

Blood tests can also measure levels of the two most active forms of thyroid hormone, triiodothyronine (T3) and thyroxine (T4). These levels will be low when Hashimoto's progresses to hypothyroidism. These hormone tests are sometimes helpful for diagnosis and can be useful too in determining a correct dosage of thyroid medications. I recommend utilizing the free T3 and free T4 tests instead of the total T3 and T4 tests, as they reveal the thyroid hormone that is unbound, or "free," to interact with thyroid hormone receptors.

Thyroid Ultrasound

Some individuals may have Hashimoto's despite no detectable alterations in their blood work. In these cases, a thyroid ultrasound may need to be used to help determine a diagnosis. Clinicians have found that the changes consistent with Hashimoto's may be visualized on thyroid ultrasounds even when a person does not test positive for antibodies.

Fine-Needle Aspiration Cytology

In a fine-needle aspiration cytology test, cells are extracted from the thyroid gland through a very thin needle and then studied under a microscope for signs of Hashimoto's. Due to its invasive nature, this type of test is usually reserved for determining whether thyroid nodules are benign or cancerous. In some cases, patients will learn they have Hashimoto's when they have suspicious nodules examined this way.

Although I don't recommend this test as the first test for a diagnosis of Hashimoto's, I'm mentioning it here, because this test is more likely to pick up additional cases of Hashimoto's when other advanced tests may miss it. As my friend Dr. Alan Christianson, world-renowned thyroid doctor, always says, "Test results can be negative, and it's really important to listen to the patient. You can't completely rule out Hashimoto's unless you look at every cell inside of the thyroid gland under a

TESTING, TESTING, ONE-TWO-THREE

Most conventionally trained doctors will say that once you test positive for thyroid antibodies, you will never need to test for them again. "You will always test positive, so it doesn't matter," they say. I disagree! Testing thyroid antibodies is helpful to determine a baseline for the aggressiveness of your condition (the higher the number, the more aggressive the condition) as well as to track the progress of your interventions. I generally recommend testing antibodies every one to three months when doing active interventions to improve your thyroid health. You will see the full effect of your interventions within a time span of three months to two years; however, you may be able to see a trend within one month. Reduction in thyroid antibody levels by at least 10 percent should be considered a positive change, an indication that your interventions are helping.

In general, antibody levels over 500 IU/mL are considered aggressive, while levels under 100 IU/mL are considered "in remission" for Hashimoto's. That said, there is no standard definition of remission, and I consider any reduction in antibodies (when correlated with improved symptoms) a positive step on the remission journey! Antibody levels under 35 IU/mL are considered "negative" for Hashimoto's according to some tests, while other tests consider levels under 9 IU/mL to be negative. However, as I already mentioned, a negative antibody test does not rule out Hashimoto's, so I encourage you not to get too hung up on having perfect numbers and focus on feeling better!

microscope." I share this because some people who have thyroid symptoms and will likely benefit from lifestyle interventions for Hashimoto's are often told that they don't have Hashimoto's based on blood tests and even ultrasounds and unfortunately delay taking part in strategies that could help.

Although these tests can reveal to us a diagnosis of Hashimoto's, they don't offer any insight into root causes of the disease, something that can be even more helpful when it comes to understanding solutions. For that, we need to look to the origins of autoimmunity, since all autoimmune disease requires the same factors to be present.

THE ORIGINS OF AUTOIMMUNITY

We know that Hashimoto's is an autoimmune condition. This means that understanding how autoimmunity works can give us important clues about how Hashimoto's happens—and how we might heal from it.

There are at least eighty known autoimmune conditions, including Hashimoto's, type 1 diabetes, rheumatoid arthritis, lupus, and celiac disease (an autoimmune reaction to gluten). Although these are all different conditions, research has shown that all autoimmunity requires the presence of the same factors. Dr. Alessio Fasano, Director of the Center for Celiac Research and Treatment at Massachusetts General Hospital, found that three things must be present for autoimmunity to develop:

- The genetic predisposition

- Triggers that turn on genes

- Intestinal permeability
  (gaps in the intestinal barrier that can let inflammatory pathogens pass into the bloodstream; otherwise known as "leaky gut")

There was a time when it was believed that once these factors had combined to activate the immune system, there was no going back; autoimmunity was thought to be irreversible. Thankfully, we are no longer living in that time.

Researchers have shown that autoimmune expression is much like a "three-legged stool." All three factors need to be present in order for autoimmunity to find expression. Although we can't choose or change our genes, we can impact the expression of both our genes and autoimmunity. We have two potential options to address with autoimmune disease: the triggers—finding and eliminating autoimmune triggers, such as infections or toxins; and intestinal permeability—looking for the root causes of why the gut may be permeable.

The amazing thing is, when we address triggers and/or the health of our gut, we can see significant improvements in autoimmune disease and, in some cases, even get the condition into remission! I've spent the last several years researching Hashimoto's triggers and developing strategies to address and eliminate them. I'd like to take you into

THE FIVE STAGES OF HASHIMOTO'S

Hashimoto's is a progressive autoimmune condition that can lead to the development of other autoimmune conditions if not addressed properly. The five stages are:

In **Stage 1** a person discovers a genetic predisposition to develop Hashimoto's. The thyroid function is normal, and there's no attack on the thyroid. For all intents and purposes, the person does not have thyroid or autoimmune disease at this stage.

In **Stage 2** of Hashimoto's, the attack on the thyroid gland starts, but the thyroid can still make enough thyroid hormone. Although most thyroid tests may be normal at this stage, many people will test positive for thyroid antibodies and may have changes consistent with Hashimoto's on a thyroid ultrasound, but will have normal TSH levels according to the TSH screening test. This is the stage when symptoms begin, yet many people are misdiagnosed with another condition, such as depression, anxiety, or hypochondria, because most doctors don't do the right tests. This stage is also the optimal stage when lifestyle changes and a Root Cause Approach to the condition should be started, because it's much easier to prevent damage than try to fix it later.

In **Stage 3**, the thyroid gland starts to lose its ability to make enough thyroid hormone for the body, and a person will have a slightly elevated TSH with normal T4/T3. More symptoms will be seen at this stage, and there is a higher likelihood of a diagnosis, though some doctors may miss or dismiss the slight TSH elevation and many doctors will recommend a "wait and watch approach." At this stage, in addition to lifestyle changes, a thyroid hormone–supporting medication may also be extremely helpful and in my opinion warranted, though many conventionally trained doctors will refuse to prescribe thyroid hormones until Stage 4.

In **Stage 4** of Hashimoto's the thyroid gland has fully lost its ability to compensate, and the person becomes hypothyroid. Hashimoto's is relatively easy to diagnose at this stage with the current "standard of care tests," which will reveal that the person has elevated TSH and lowered T3/T4. This is the stage in which a person will be even more symptomatic and will finally be offered a thyroid-hormone prescription by most traditionally trained doctors.

Stage 5 is when other types of autoimmune conditions develop. We know that autoimmune conditions can be progressive, and taking thyroid hormones or surgical removal of the thyroid gland will not stop the progression of autoimmunity. People with one autoimmune condition may find themselves diagnosed with other types of conditions such as lupus, psoriasis, or Sjogren's syndrome. The good news is that addressing lifestyle, nutrition, and the root causes of autoimmune conditions can help not just autoimmune thyroid disease, but also the symptoms and progression of other types of autoimmune issues.

what's going on in Hashimoto's to deepen your understanding of my approach.

WHAT'S GOING ON IN HASHIMOTO'S?

In Hashimoto's, in addition to the issue of intestinal permeability there are six potential types of triggers: food sensitivities, nutrient depletions, an impaired ability to handle stress, an impaired ability to handle toxins, digestive issues, and chronic infections. Each person with Hashimoto's will have his or her own combination of triggers, which means that creating a universal approach to healing can be challenging. However, I've found that nearly every person with autoimmune thyroid disease has underlying root-cause commonalities—the same factors and imbalances are present—and many of these imbalances *can* be reliably addressed with proper nutrition.

Although triggers and stressors for the condition can vary from person to person, the body usually responds to them in a very predictable fashion by moving us away from a "thriving state" toward a "surviving state." In just about every person with Hashimoto's, I see the same recurring patterns.

I've called these patterns the "Vicious Cycle of Hashimoto's." This cycle is interrelated and simply adding thyroid supplement to the mix will not result in full recovery for most thyroid patients. But although the triggers of Hashimoto's can break the body down, nutrition can build it back up.

HEALING HASHIMOTO'S PATTERNS WITH NUTRITION

The recognizable patterns in Hashimoto's that lend themselves to nutritional healing include the following.

1. Micronutrient deficiencies. Most people with Hashimoto's have numerous micronutrient deficiencies. These micronutrient deficiencies can occur as a result of eating the Western diet, eating nutrient-poor foods, following a calorie-restricted diet, digestive enzyme deficiencies, inflammation from infections or food sensitivities, medications, or an imbalance of gut bacteria. Lack of sufficient thyroid hormones can also lead to nutrient deficiencies, as it makes nutrient extraction from food more difficult and less efficient.

These nutrient deficiencies contribute to the development of Hashimoto's as well as many of its symptoms. Restoring the nutrients through nutrient-dense foods, supplementation, and optimizing digestion are some of the fastest ways to feel better with Hashimoto's and begin to build the body back up!

2. Macronutrient deficiencies. Oftentimes people with Hashimoto's have diets that are deficient in protein and fat, two essential macronutrients that support the body's growth and repair processes. These deficiencies can develop as a result of our carb-heavy Western diet, fat phobia, and vegetarian/

vegan diets as well as impaired protein or fat digestion.

Impaired protein digestion can also lead to deficiencies in the amino acids L-tyrosine and L-glutamine, both of which may play an important role in healing from Hashimoto's. L-tyrosine is necessary for production of thyroid hormones, while L-glutamine is essential to proper gut lining and immune function. Both amino acids are often depleted in people with Hashimoto's. Improving protein digestion can help restore levels of these important amino acids and promote an anabolic (building up), instead of a catabolic (breaking down) state within the body.

3. Deficiencies in digestive enzymes. Studies have found that people with Hashimoto's and hypothyroidism often have a deficiency in the digestive enzyme hydrochloric acid, resulting in low levels of stomach acid (hypochlorhydria) or a complete absence of it (achlorhydria). Low stomach acid can make it more difficult to digest proteins, which in turn can lead to deficiencies in the amino acids mentioned above.

Additionally, around a third of people with Hashimoto's may also have deficiencies in bile and/or pancreatic enzymes, which can lead to issues with fat absorption. Lastly, up to 80 percent of people with Hashimoto's may have difficulty digesting plant fibers. The digestive process demands a lot of energy, so when it requires more metabolic work than nor-

mal, you may notice yourself feeling tired more often. Utilizing easy-to-digest foods and targeted digestive enzyme supplementation can restore proper digestion and eliminate symptoms like fatigue, virtually overnight.

4. Blood-sugar swings. Many people with Hashimoto's have an impaired tolerance for carbohydrates. If you are one of these people, you are likely to experience blood-sugar swings characterized by a rapid spike in blood sugar after eating carbs followed by an excessive release of insulin. As insulin surges, your blood sugar will crash in a response known as reactive hypoglycemia. Reactive hypoglycemia can lead to unpleasant symptoms such as nervousness, lightheadedness, anxiety, and fatigue, and it can place stress on the adrenals.

When the adrenals become stressed, they are likely to release an excess of cortisol, which can also lead to an increased production of inflammatory proteins that are associated with a heightened immune response. This pattern eventually leads to altered cortisol release, which can in turn lead to numerous symptoms, including chronic fatigue, mood swings, and muscle wasting. Learning how to eat to promote stable blood sugar is an important part of protecting your adrenals from excess stress and in healing from hypothyroidism. Improvements in mood, energy, brain function, and weight are positive side effects of proper blood-sugar balance!

5. A toxic backlog. We are bombarded with toxins every day—they are on and in our foods, in the water we drink, in the personal-care products we put on our bodies, the cleaning products we use in our homes, and so on. Many of these toxins can interfere with hormone production, affect thyroid activity, and perpetuate autoimmunity. For example, fluoride, found in drinking water, bottled beverages, certain teas, and some supplements and medications, may act as a trigger in inducing thyroid cell death and inflammation, leading to the development of thyroiditis or autoimmune thyroiditis. The toxic backlog can lead to numerous symptoms as well! We can take proactive steps to minimize our toxic exposure, freeing ourselves from symptoms in our very own kitchens, by choosing low-toxin tools and foods (see Chapter 4 for more information) and utilizing foods and nutrients that support our detoxification pathways.

6. Food sensitivities. Food sensitivities represent one of the most common patterns I see in those with Hashimoto's. *Food sensitivities* are not the same as *food allergies*. *Food allergies* are reactions to food that are immediate and often life-threatening (think the child who stops breathing after eating nuts), and are readily acknowledged and tested for by conventional medical doctors, especially allergists. These reactions are known as type I hypersensitivity reactions and are governed by the IgE branch of the immune system.

Food sensitivities are known as type IV delayed hypersensitivity reactions governed by the IgG branch of the immune system. As the name implies, they do not occur right away. In fact, it can take up to four days for them to manifest, and this is one of the reasons why it's so hard for most people to correlate food sensitivities with symptoms. For example, you may eat corn on Monday and have a panic attack on Wednesday!

Here's the connection I've made. Hashimoto's is also considered a type IV delayed hypersensitivity reaction and often presents with IgG antibodies to the thyroid gland. In my experience, whenever we eat foods that cause our IgG system to flare up, this also seems to result in a flare-up of thyroid antibodies and thyroid symptoms. More research is needed to reveal exactly why this is the case, but it could be a result of an opening of the flood gates or perhaps inflammatory food proteins cross-reacting with the thyroid gland. What I have seen is that this overlap gives us an incredible opportunity for healing—most people with Hashimoto's (88 percent of my clients and readers) will have a reduction in thyroid symptoms and antibodies after removing the most common reactive foods.

7. Intestinal permeability. According to researchers, every person with an autoimmune disorder has some degree of intestinal permeability, or "leaky gut." A leaky gut has gaps in the gut lining that allow irritating molecules and substances to escape from the digestive system into the bloodstream. This irritation can interrupt the immune system's ability to regulate itself and put the body into a perpetual attack mode that will be counterproductive to healing.

Intestinal permeability can cause such symptoms as bloating, stomach pains, irritable bowel syndrome, and acid reflux. These same symptoms are commonly experienced by people with Hashimoto's, although not everyone with intestinal permeability and/or Hashimoto's will have these symptoms. Both asymptomatic and symptomatic intestinal permeability can lead to a reduced absorption of nutrients required for detoxification and other important functions as well as a reduced output of toxins, which, if not addressed, can interfere with recovery.

There are numerous factors that can initiate or perpetuate damage to the gut lining such as stress, strenuous exercise, surgery/trauma, adrenal hormone imbalances, intestinal infections, toxins, enzyme deficiencies, the use of nonsteroidal anti-inflammatory drugs (NSAIDs), alcohol, nutrient deficiencies, infections (of the gut, sinus, or mouth), and food reactions. We can support the health of the intestines by addressing nutritional factors, such as eliminating reactive foods; addressing nutrient deficiencies; and replenishing enzymes and beneficial bacteria. These three key steps can be life-changing for most people with Hashimoto's.

The Hashimoto's and hypothyroidism lifestyle interventions I have researched and tested aim to dismantle the vicious cycle piece by piece. We repair the broken systems to restore equilibrium, allowing the body to rebuild itself. Nourishing your body will help you shift these patterns and will make you feel so much better! Although the body breaks itself down in Hashimoto's, through nutrition we can build it back up.

HOW NUTRITION CAN HELP YOU REACH YOUR HEALTH GOALS

Through my work with my clients, I have seen hundreds of people recover their health with my Root Cause Approach, and I have now received hundreds of success stories from people who discovered and implemented the approach in my books *Hashimoto's: The Root Cause* and *Hashimoto's Protocol*.

Scientists have said that there is no cure for Hashimoto's, but I believe we have the capacity and knowledge to put the condition into remission for most people. Each autoimmune condition has a different definition of what remission may mean. I like to think of remission as a journey, not necessarily a destination. Remission to me is progress, not perfection. Where you are is an improvement over where you've been. Here are the scenic stopping points on the remission journey: feeling better, eliminating most or all of your symptoms, reducing your thyroid antibodies, regenerating thyroid tissue, and experiencing a functional cure (which here means no symptoms, no antibodies, and no evidence of autoimmune thyroid disease in your body or on your thyroid).

Many people will be able to see a reduction in their thyroid antibodies, and some may no longer test positive for Hashimoto's. A small subset may even be able to regenerate thyroid tissue and discontinue thyroid medications (under a doctor's supervision).

I'll share the full nutritional plans and some success stories from readers just like you who were able to take back their health using the nutrition guidance in Chapter 3 of this book!

WHAT DIET CAN AND CAN'T DO

Optimizing your nutrition can do wonders for your health. This is why following a nutrient-dense diet that is free of reactive foods is one of the first steps I recommend in an approach to healing. A lot of people have had great success by taking this step alone, even going into complete remission from Hashimoto's. But this isn't always the case. Although dietary modifications are powerful, there are limitations to what they can accomplish, and although most will see improvement with nutrition, many may need to dig deeper into the other root causes and interventions to continue improving.

I mentioned that Hashimoto's can be caused by food sensitivities, nutrient depletions, an impaired ability to handle stress, an impaired ability to get rid of toxins, and

intestinal health issues as well as chronic infections. A person may have anywhere from one to all of these root causes! In my work with thousands of Hashimoto's patients, I've found that diet modifications can usually help address and/or heal food sensitivities, nutrient deficiencies, adrenal issues, some gut imbalances, and certain toxic imbalances. In other cases, diet can *sometimes* help with profound nutrient deficiencies, although supportive supplements and/or digestive enzymes may also be needed to fully address deficiencies. In more complicated cases, nutrient deficiencies can result from infections or toxins that require additional treatment.

In certain cases, food sensitivities may be improved by nutrition and elimination of foods; in other cases, food sensitivities can be caused by infections, and the infections can result in the loss of more and more foods and the need for a progressively more restricted diet. Please note, diet can sometimes help manage the symptoms of a gut infection, but no amount of food restriction will heal most gut infections, and many gut infections can produce ongoing food sensitivities and reactions to whatever foods we're eating. Most infections require treatments such as antimicrobial, antiparasitic, antifungal, and/or antiviral herbs or medications.

Severe toxicity may require supplements, medications, and other advanced treatments to clear. Current stress or past traumatic stress can leave our bodies in the

THE STANDARD OF CARE VS.
THE ROOT CAUSE APPROACH TO HASHIMOTO'S

If this is the first time you are hearing about any proactive strategies (or any strategy other than medication) that may help address your Hashimoto's, you might feel overwhelmed, frustrated, and even angry. But I encourage you to feel empowered instead. My Root Cause Approach is different from the current standard of care offered through conventional medicine, which generally overlooks opportunities for healing. Let's review the key differences.

The standard of care approach to Hashimoto's is what I consider to be a lab-number, T4-centric, and reactive model that consists of primary reliance of the TSH test for diagnosis of Hashimoto's and determining the need for more or less thyroid hormone:

Levothyroxine is the thyroid hormone of choice prescribed to most people with Hashimoto's, although it's not the only thyroid hormone that's missing with Hashimoto's.

Often patients are not given appropriate doses of medication, because outdated and cookie-cutter lab reference ranges are used that measure the levels of one thyroid hormone in the pituitary, but not in the rest of the body.

Patients who continue to be symptomatic are referred to other specialists for additional medications, such as dermatologists for hair loss, psychiatrists for depression, and so on.

There are no lifestyle recommendations and no attempt to find triggers for the autoimmune response against the thyroid, and thyroid antibodies are rarely tracked, though patients are offered testing for additional autoimmune conditions.

In contrast, my Root Cause Approach to Hashimoto's is a patient-centered approach that looks at the underlying issues and the person's individuality. The Root Cause Approach to Hashimoto's includes:

Utilizing comprehensive thyroid tests to determine diagnosis and the need for thyroid-hormone therapy.

Using optimal and functional ranges of thyroid hormones instead of outdated reference ranges.

Optimizing thyroid hormones utilizing the T1, T2, T3, and T4 hormones when necessary (all are produced by the thyroid gland, but only T4 is present in levothyroxine, the most commonly prescribed thyroid drug).

Optimizing nutrition through eliminating reactive foods and addressing deficiencies and digestion.

Addressing the stress response.

Addressing the health of the detoxification system.

Addressing the state of the gut.

Identifying the person's unique triggers such as chronic infections, toxins, or traumas.

Tracking thyroid antibodies every three months to see if the interventions are making the condition less aggressive.

Appreciation of the person's experience and always utilizing the person's symptoms as a guide for adjusting treatment.

For a detailed overview of my full approach, check out *Hashimoto's Protocol* and *Hashimoto's: The Root Cause.*

"break it down" mode that no amount of good nutrition can solve, but stress reduction or working with a therapist can help here.

Additionally, when damage to the thyroid gland has occurred and the person can no longer produce adequate amounts of thyroid hormone, supplemental thyroid hormone will be needed. Proper nutrition can prevent damage to the thyroid gland and in some cases thyroid tissue can regenerate, but this is not a quick or even certain process—it's much easier to prevent tissue damage than to grow a thyroid back. No amount of food or special diet will provide thyroid hormone to a damaged thyroid.

I share this information with you about the limitations of diet because I have met plenty of people with Hashimoto's who have locked on to the idea that diet can heal everything. With this belief in place, they continue removing more and more foods from their diet with the expectation that this will lead to healing. My recommendation is that if you've been on a clean diet for three months and you're not seeing results or you are getting stuck, you likely have an undetected infection or other underlying issue that is causing inflammation within your body. I recommend utilizing the full Root Cause Approach shared in my books *Hashimoto's Protocol* and *Hashimoto's: The Root Cause* and working with a functional-medicine practitioner to get on the right path.

THE NOURISHING NEXT STEPS

My goal in writing this book was to create a one-stop, nutrition-centered resource for cooking and nourishing your way to recovery from Hashimoto's. When we begin to see foods for their healing or harmful potential for our bodies, we acknowledge the power of our diet to change our lives. This is food as medicine. To take the reins of this power, we have to dig a little deeper and see the foods that make up our diet for their chemical properties, for it's not just the whole, but the parts of the whole that interact with our internal systems. This more granular understanding of food is what I call food pharmacology.

The only way to see how you will respond to optimizing your nutrition is to take the leap into strategic dietary modifications, which you'll learn more about in the next chapter and will easily be able to implement when you follow the recipes in the Cookbook section.

Now that you have a greater understanding of Hashimoto's, including the tests that can help with diagnosis, the stages of the disease, common triggers and patterns, and how you can use nutrition to promote healing, it's time to take a deeper dive into the specifics. In the next chapter, you'll discover the factors that create an optimal diet for autoimmune thyroid disease!

2.

Fundamentals of Nutrition

A lot of people ask the question: "What is the right diet to heal Hashimoto's?" This question is very complicated, since nutrition is the only science in which multiple answers can be both right and wrong. In other words, there is more than one way to skin a cat, and one person's medicine may be another person's poison. We are all different, and although we may have the same condition, different interventions may be required for each of us to heal.

You may have seen success stories and even perhaps heard what I like to call "diet dogma" from various personalities in the media or online about the best type of diet that *everyone* should follow. Some claim to have "cured" everything with *their* dietary plan; others make the same claim about a completely conflicting diet plan.

I love seeing success stories of people who take back their health and inspire others, but it's important to remember that something that worked for one person may not work for others. What works for most

people may also not work for you as an individual.

As a health-care professional and scientist, I consider myself to be diet-agnostic and I try not to form too many attachments to any dogmas, whether they are about diets, herbs, medications, or other treatment modalities. My goal is to simply try to find the most successful solutions and to show my clients and readers what works!

I personally don't have a preference for any specific diet. In fact, if I were to develop *my* ideal diet, it would largely consist of mojitos, margaritas, croissants, tiramisu, and menthol cigarettes (my diet during spring break in college!). Although you may see some elements of *my* preferred diet in the Cookbook recipes, such as my modified mojito recipe, rather than promoting my own views on diet or adhering to a dietary dogma or the latest food fad, I derived the recommendations for Hashimoto's in my books from clinical data of the diets that are most helpful to most people with Hashimoto's.

In this chapter, I'll introduce to you some of this science—for the science and health nerds (like me!) among you—along with some key diet concepts, including how to optimize macronutrients and micronutrients for Hashimoto's and which healing foods will be vitally important to your recovery.

MY EARLY EXPERIMENTS IN NUTRITION

In 2011, I realized that my own health significantly improved with the use of nutrition, and I had a hunch that I was not the only person who could see improvements in Hashimoto's symptoms with diet, though I wasn't fully convinced that one particular diet was the answer for every single person with the condition. When I began working with clients with Hashimoto's, however, I noticed that most clients got better with a dietary approach that was very similar to my own.

Again, not wanting to jump the gun, in 2015 before I made "official" recommendations, I decided to conduct a survey of Hashimoto's patients. I wanted to know how many people felt better with which dietary protocol, how many people felt worse, and how many people were able to reduce their thyroid antibodies with a dietary protocol. Although I am a big believer in the patient experience and I always recommend trusting your own

body as a guide as to what is working best for you, I decided to include a reduction in antibodies as an objective measure.

Objective measures, such as a reduction in thyroid antibodies, are the types of evidence scientists and doctors prefer to track to determine the severity of a condition and whether the improvements seen by patients are measurable and "real." Generally speaking, the higher the number of thyroid antibodies, the more aggressive the attack on the thyroid gland, so seeing a reduction in thyroid antibodies is a potential indication that the condition is becoming less aggressive.

Over two thousand people answered the survey, and the results were astounding: over 70 percent of respondents reported improvements based on six nutritional modifications. (You can see more on the specific results in the accompanying table.) The big diet winner for most people with Hashimoto's was the gluten-free diet! Eighty-eight percent of people felt better gluten free, and up to 33 percent saw a reduction in thyroid antibodies with the removal of gluten.

Furthermore, 81 percent of people reported feeling better following a grain-free and Paleo diet. Additionally, 79 percent of people felt better off dairy, and another 63 percent felt better off soy. Eating a diet that was blood-sugar balanced helped 76 percent of people feel better. Less than 5 percent of people reported feeling worse with these types of dietary regimens. Furthermore, more than 25 percent of people

2015 SURVEY OF 2,232 PEOPLE WITH HASHIMOTO'S

DIET TYPE	FELT BETTER	FELT WORSE	REDUCED THYROID ANTIBODIES
Based on food-sensitivity test results	62%	4.2%	43%
Autoimmune Paleo Diet	75%	4%	38%
Soy free	63%	1.2%	34%
Gluten free	88%	0.73%	33%
Grain free	81%	0.74%	28%
Paleo	81%	3.2%	27%
Low FODMAP	39%	0%	27%
Vegan	30%	28%	23%
Low Glycemic Index	76%	2.3%	22%
Dairy free	79%	1.5%	20%
Egg free	47%	3%	19%
Nightshade free	48%	2%	14%
Red meat avoidance	40%	14%	8%

reported reducing their thyroid antibodies with a diet based on food-sensitivity tests, the autoimmune Paleo diet, and the soy-free, gluten-free, grain-free, Paleo, and Low FODMAP (fermentable oligo-, di-, and monosaccharides and polyols) approaches.

Although I conducted this survey with a likely biased group (most survey takers were my educated readers), I was pleased that a new research study came out in 2016 that echoed very similar results—and the results were seen in as little as three weeks!

GROWING SCIENTIFIC SUPPORT

In the 2016 study, 180 people with Hashimoto's were randomized to receive either the study diet or a standard low-calorie diet. Ultimately 108 patients followed the study diet, and 72 patients served as the control group. Those in the control group ate a low-calorie diet without any food restrictions or guidelines. Thyroid antibodies (TPO antibodies, TG antibodies, and antimicrosomal antibodies), TSH, free T3, and free T4 as well as body weight, mass, and composition were measured before the start of the study and after the study ended three weeks later in both the study group and the control group.

After just twenty-one days, all the patients in the study group showed a significant decrease in the levels of thyroid antibodies, which are known to indicate how aggressive the attack is on the thyroid gland. This means that their condition was getting better! The antibodies decreased as follows:

- TG antibodies dropped by 40 percent (–40 percent, P<–0.013).

- TPO antibodies dropped by 44 percent (–44 percent, P< 0.029).

- Antimicrosomal antibodies dropped by 57 percent (–57 percent, P< 0.000).

I consider a drop of 10 percent or more in antibodies an improvement, and you can see the numbers above show decreases of 40, 44, and 57 percent—these were amazing results to see!

In contrast, the people following the "normal diet" saw an increase in thyroid antibody markers. This means that their condition was worsening:

- TG antibodies increased by 9 percent (+9 percent, P<0.017).

- TPO antibodies increased by 16 percent (+16 percent, P<0.004).

- Antimicrosomal antibodies increased by 30 percent (+30 percent, P<0.028).

After twenty-one days, those following the study diet also showed a slight decrease in body weight, body mass index, and lost fat mass: "With regard to the body parameters measured in patients who followed this diet, reduction in body weight (–5 percent, P<0.000) and body mass index (–4 percent, P<0.000) were observed."

I'm guessing you probably want to know about the diet, right?! It consisted of 12 to 15 percent carbohydrates, 50 to 60 percent protein, and 25 to 30 percent fat (compare this to the standard Western diet, which contains 50 percent carbohydrates, 15 percent protein, and 35 percent fat). Additional specifics:

Veggie rich: Patients were told to eat vegetables, including large leafy greens (but to exclude goitrogens, foods that can interfere with thyroid function).

Included meats: Patients were told to eat only lean parts of red and white meat and were also allowed to eat fish.

Excluded goitrogens: The goitrogens that patients were told to eliminate were "cruciferous [vegetables] of the (Brassicaceae) family (rapeseed or canola, cabbage, turnip, watercress, arugula, radish, horseradish), milk, soy, spinach, millet, tapioca, and lettuce, including certain food additives (e.g., nitrates used for fish and meat preservation)."

Additional exclusions: Other items excluded were eggs, legumes, dairy products, bread, pasta, fruit, and rice.

I was really excited to see that a diet very similar to what I've been recommending since 2012 now had research to back it up! There were a couple notable differences between this diet and my Root Cause Dietary Approach to Hashimoto's.

In the Root Cause Approach, *not all goitrogens are created equal.* A goitrogen is a name for any substance that has the potential to interfere with thyroid function. The tricky part is that not all of them work in the same way. I like to look at research studies and clinical outcomes before I determine if a food is on the "No" list for Hashimoto's. There are certain goitrogenic mechanisms that make me cautious right off the bat, such as the inhibition of either the thyroid peroxidase enzyme or the thyroid hormone release. I do recommend avoiding certain goitrogens that do this, including milk, soy, and iodine excess.

I also look at the scientific and clinical evidence showing that a substance may be harmful to the thyroid. Research studies have documented that canola (made from rapeseed) and nitrates found in processed foods have direct toxic effects on the thyroid gland. However, the evidence of harm from other goitrogens such as cruciferous vegetables (broccoli, cabbage, turnips, and the like) is lacking.

The goitrogen categorization of crucifers is due to the fact that they contain substances known as glucosinolates. Glucosinolates, when consumed in large quantities, can prevent the absorption of iodine into the thyroid gland. This could be a major issue in someone who has iodine deficiency–induced hypothyroidism (iodine deficiency used to be a top cause of hypothyroidism in the 1950s). However, most people with Hashimoto's today do not have an iodine deficiency, and most cruciferous vegetables do not have enough glucosinolates to induce iodine deficiency.

In my experience, most cruciferous vegetables are well tolerated and offer health benefits for most people with Hashimoto's. They help the body detoxify, especially when cooked, fermented, or lightly steamed. Even in their raw state, I have not seen issues with cruciferous vegetables in most clients, with the exception of those with small intestinal bacterial overgrowth (SIBO) (because crucifers are high in FODMAPs, which aggravate SIBO) and in those with CBS genetic mutation (due to the high sulfur content of crucifers). If I have a client with concerns about iodine deficiency and crucifers, I recommend steaming, cooking, or fermenting the vegetables. This alone will be enough to break down the small amount of glucosinolates contained in them.

In the Root Cause Approach, *there's no set carb/protein/fat ratio.* I don't recommend a set of macronutrient percentages for everyone. Instead, I often have people play around with their ratios of carbs to protein to fat to find what fits them best. Some people (especially if they're more active) benefit from more protein. Others benefit from more fat, such as those with brain fog, pain, and depression. Some may even benefit from ketosis (the use of fat instead of carbs as fuel). The bottom line is that you have to adjust the diet to your needs, and your needs may change!

There were some limitations to the 2016 research study. Based on the way it was conducted, it's difficult to tell whether the carb restriction, goitrogen restriction, avoiding highly reactive foods (gluten, dairy, soy, eggs), or all of the above played a role in improving patient outcomes.

I also wish that the control group was an actual control group (the control group should have kept eating their "normal" diet) and that "low-calorie" was defined. How low are we talking? Some low-calorie diets specify a total of 800 calories, some 1,500. Obviously, there's a big difference between the two!

Last, I would love to see a study that isolated a low-carb diet versus allergen avoidance and goitrogens. This would offer even greater clarity on what spe-

TOO MUCH IODINE?

Scientists have long known that iodine is a crucial nutrient for thyroid health. In fact, iodine deficiency is the primary reason for hypothyroidism worldwide. In an effort to reduce the incidence of hypothyroidism, public-health officials began adding iodine to the salt supplies in many industrialized countries. However, this effort backfired, as iodine turned out to be a narrow therapeutic index nutrient, or a "Goldilocks nutrient." A deficiency of iodine created hypothyroidism due to a lack of building materials for thyroid hormone, but an excess of it also created hypothyroidism, but through a different mechanism. Today, iodine excess is recognized as a risk factor for developing Hashimoto's!

This has to do with the way that iodine is processed in the body. Iodine from foods and supplements is processed by the thyroid gland so that the body can properly use it. During this process, hydrogen peroxide, a free radical, is released. In cases when the body has adequate levels of selenium and it is used properly, the selenium neutralizes the hydrogen peroxide. However, in cases of iodine excess, excess hydrogen peroxide can cause oxidative damage to the thyroid gland.

The use of iodine supplementation in autoimmune thyroid disease is a controversial topic, and in my experience iodine needs to be dosed appropriately to provide benefit and prevent harm. Some research has shown that low-dose daily supplementation when combined with thyroid hormone therapy can improve outcomes and reduce thyroid antibody levels. I've found that for most people with Hashimoto's, low-dose iodine supplements (such as in the range of 150–220 mcg, found in multivitamins and prenatal vitamins) are usually safe and potentially helpful.

However, I have received countless messages from people with Hashimoto's who have

cific modifications were most successful. I would especially like the myth of goitrogen avoidance put to bed, because it's a common misconception in Hashimoto's circles that these are all bad, all the time, and this is simply not true.

There are a handful of other common myths and questions I hear about food, the thyroid, and Hashimoto's that I will be addressing throughout this book, as in many cases misunderstood facts can lead to missed opportunities for healing.

SHOULD YOU BE VEGAN OR VEGETARIAN WITH HASHIMOTO'S?

Another question I hear often is whether I recommend a vegan or vegetarian diet for Hashimoto's. Although research by Seventh-day Adventists suggests that a vegan diet may be protective against thyroid disorders, I have not found the vegan diet to be especially helpful for most of my clients with Hashimoto's. The research was

tried *high-dose* iodine (above 500 mcg per day from supplements, seaweed, kelp, or spirulina). Researchers and my readers have reported that these high doses can lead to adverse reactions such as reduced thyroid hormone levels, increased thyroid antibodies, an exacerbation of thyroid symptoms, and even an accelerated destruction of thyroid tissue! Even those who may initially feel "more energetic" while taking a high-dose iodine supplement are often left feeling much worse after some time—this is because the bump in energy is often a result of the destruction of thyroid tissue, which dumps thyroid hormone into circulation!

Certainly I won't deny that some people with Hashimoto's have been helped by high-dose iodine. However most feel that the risks outweigh the benefits for people with Hashimoto's, and I caution people against the use of high-dose iodine. Out of my Root Cause readers who were surveyed, 356 tried high-dose iodine. Out of that group, 25 percent said that high-dose iodine made them feel better, 28 percent said

that it made them feel worse, and 46 percent saw no difference in how they felt (although this doesn't mean that their thyroid markers weren't affected). The takeaway from this survey is that more people felt worse on high-dose iodine than felt better.

In those who have been exposed to high doses, I may even recommend short-term iodine restriction. Research has shown that a low-iodine diet has been helpful in reducing the autoimmune attack on the thyroid gland and in normalizing thyroid function in people with iodine-induced Hashimoto's. In my survey, iodine restriction made 31.7 percent feel better and 7 percent feel worse. In this case, a person would temporarily restrict iodine to less than 100 mcg per day for a period of one to three months (the thyroid gland needs approximately 52 mcg per day of iodine, which you're likely getting if you take thyroid hormone medications). I'm including iodine in the nutrient analysis of the recipes in this book for those who wish to monitor their iodine intake.

based on a questionnaire that was deployed to 97,000 Seventh-day Adventist Church members asking them about their dietary habits and health conditions. The study reported that people who followed a vegan diet were less likely to develop hypothyroidism compared to those on the Standard American Diet (a diet high in meat, fat, dairy, refined carbohydrates, and salt). In contrast, people who followed a lacto-ovo vegetarian diet were more likely to develop hypothyroidism compared to those on the Standard American Diet. It's possible that the reduction in hypothyroidism seen in the vegan diet was due to excluding dairy and eggs, which are two common reactive foods in people with Hashimoto's.

I've also actively sought out success stories from various places to find Hashimoto's remission stories. Time and time again, I've been led to cases of vegan Hashimoto's remission stories, only to find that, upon deeper investigation, the person continues to struggle with symptoms such as low body temperatures, depression, brittle hair, irritable bowel syndrome, dry, pale skin, and numerous other symptoms correlated with Hashimoto's.

Another study cited by proponents of the vegan diet noted the connection between antibodies formed to the thyroid and antibodies formed to Neu5Gc, a protein found in mammalian meats like lamb, pork, and beef. This study, published in 2014, reported that the majority of people with Hashimoto's present with anti-bodies to Neu5Gc. However, the study did not attempt to demonstrate if exclusion of mammalian meat made any difference in Hashimoto's outcomes. In practice, most of my clinical experience points to the fact that people actually improve with the inclusion of mammalian meat.

In surveying my readers, out of 595 people who tried to avoid red meat, 40 percent reported that avoiding red meat made them feel better, while 14 percent reported that avoiding red meat made them feel worse. Only 8 percent saw a reduction in thyroid antibodies with avoidance of red meat.

Clinically, I had not seen a lot of success in people with Hashimoto's who followed a vegan diet, a vegetarian diet, or a red meat–restricted diet. Additionally, some former vegans have been able to get their Hashimoto's into remission by transitioning to a Paleo-like diet. In surveying my readers, similar results were reported. Although 30 percent of people felt better while following a vegan diet, 28 percent of people with Hashimoto's felt worse with this type of diet! In contrast to the gluten-free diet, which has become my gold standard for Hashimoto's, 88 percent of people with Hashimoto's feel better gluten free, while less than 1 percent feel worse!

Notably, the vegan diet did show a reduction in thyroid antibodies. As I mentioned, my hypothesis is that the antibody reduction resulted from the exclusion of dairy and eggs, two common reactive foods for people with Hashimoto's.

For those with Hashimoto's, vegan and vegetarian diets are problematic for a variety of reasons, especially because they may:

- **Exacerbate blood-sugar issues:** People with Hashimoto's often struggle with blood-sugar issues, which will only be worsened by carbohydrate-heavy vegan and vegetarian diets.

- **Prevent the gut from healing:** Vegetarian protein sources such as legumes (beans), dairy, grains, soy, and some seeds may be incompatible with trying to heal a leaky gut. Pea protein is a vegan alternative that may be easier to digest and is less likely to cause food sensitivities (I developed the Rootcology Organic Pea Protein for people who are looking for a plant-based protein). For vegetarians, eggs, some seeds, and nuts would be the preferred sources of protein, but some people with Hashimoto's may be intolerant of those as well, especially in the early stages of healing.

- **Contribute to nutrient deficiencies that may exacerbate Hashimoto's:** Vegan diets put us at risk for deficiency in many nutrients, including vitamin A, vitamin B_3, vitamin B_9, vitamin B_{12}, vitamin D, calcium, chromium, copper, iodine, iron, magnesium, manganese, zinc, and omega-3s. Vitamin B_{12} and iron deficiencies are extremely common in those with Hashimoto's and contribute to many symptoms.

It's important to point out that the vegan diet is likely to be healthier than the Standard American Diet, but that in cases of Hashimoto's a diet closer to the hunter-gatherer diet seems to work best for most people.

HOW TO TELL IF YOUR DIET IS WORKING FOR YOU

There is a dark side to using food as medicine that I'd like to share with you. In some cases, we may become so attached to a specific diet that we lose our natural ability to

IS MEAT INFLAMMATORY?

Some people are surprised to discover that I recommend a diet that contains meat, since they have heard that eating meat is inflammatory. This is true if you consume meat from conventionally raised animals, which tend to have more inflammatory omega-6 fatty acids than anti-inflammatory omega-3 fatty acids. The reverse is true in naturally raised animals, from which foods higher in beneficial omega-3s and lower in omega-6s are produced. Look for grass-fed, pasture-raised, wild-caught, and free-range options to ensure that you get the quality proteins that will help most with the processes of healing and repair.

determine whether it is beneficial or detrimental to our health. *Orthorexia nervosa* is the newly coined term for this condition, where people become obsessed with clean or healthy eating. A key feature of the condition and what makes it pathogenic, is that the eaters lose perspective and do not realize that their diet is actually making them sicker; they have lost the ability to eat intuitively.

Another feature of orthorexia is an exaggerated faith that inclusion or elimination of particular kinds of foods can prevent or cure a disease or affect daily well-being. They believe that what they're doing is healthy despite all other evidence. So their thyroid antibodies might be going up, they might have more symptoms, and they might be feeling worse or even be malnourished, yet they still think they're doing the right thing. Of course good nutrition is vital, and food is very important in our healing journey, but food is not the "be all and end all."

Although I've never had a history of past eating disorders, I had my own experience with orthorexia in my healing journey. After seeing initial significant improvements with the gluten-free and dairy-free diet but hitting a plateau, I decided to try the GAPS (Gut and Psychology Syndrome) diet (the Specific Carbohydrate Diet is similar), which was touted to be helpful for autoimmune disease. These diets can be helpful for many people, but they did not work for me, yet I continued to follow them despite all evidence of the contrary.

I had gone from slightly overweight to very underweight, to the point that people began asking if I had anorexia. My hair grew thinner and thinner, and I had horrible new cystic breakouts. My skin was dull and gray, and I felt exhausted all of the time. I was losing more and more foods from my diet and thought that if I just kept restricting more foods, I would get better. At one point, I was reduced to eating only a few foods and well-cooked meats and veggies.

I lost the ability to eat in a natural, intuitive manner, and I kept getting sicker. The true healing came when I learned to listen to my body's subtle signals for help, signals that are often communicated as symptoms (you can read more about what your symptoms are trying to tell you in Chapter 3).

Symptoms can mean that you are having a reaction to a food or foods. They could also mean that you have deficiencies in nutrients or digestive enzymes or other root causes like intestinal infections, toxicities, or an impaired ability to handle stress. It's important to remember that these other factors exist. Some people may get stuck on the idea that "diet can heal everything" and that if they just eliminate more foods, they'll be healed—but this isn't always the case. (If you've been on a clean diet for three months and you are not seeing results or getting stuck, you should get tested for gut infections ASAP, so you don't run the risk of losing more foods. The two tests I recommend are: the GI MAP stool test, for parasitic, bacterial, and yeast infections in the gut, and the Bacterial Overgrowth Breath Test, for SIBO.)

The turning point for me came when I began to incorporate nutrients, digestive enzymes, and more healing foods like bone broth, green juices, and green smoothies into my diet. I started to feel and look better and began to tolerate more foods. Continuing to nourish my body, while treating gut infections and toxins, allowed me to incorporate more and more foods back into my diet, and I've now been able to include most foods I was once sensitive to. Today, the way I eat is guided primarily by how I feel, by my body's messages and my intuition.

Although I continue to follow a gluten-free and dairy-free diet, I have incorporated all other foods into my diet, because my body has healed to the point where I can tolerate them. One day I'll research gluten and dairy reintroductions in greater depth, but for now I am too busy and too happy enjoying life to mess with a good thing! You can read more about my day-to-day diet in Chapter 4.

WHAT ALL HEALING DIETS HAVE IN COMMON

When it comes down to it, multiple diets have been reported to reverse Hashimoto's. Most commonly, I see success and remission stories from people who followed diets such as the gluten-free diet, the Paleo diet, the autoimmune Paleo diet, the soy-free diet,

FODMAPS, SIBO, AND HYPOTHYROIDISM

One small study reported that about 50 percent of people with hypothyroidism have SIBO, or small intestinal bacterial overgrowth. SIBO can be a root cause for Hashimoto's and can lead to intestinal permeability and irritable bowel syndrome. Symptoms such as bloating, gas, diarrhea, and constipation are common in SIBO and may be exacerbated by eating foods that contain FODMAPs (fermentable oligo-, di-, monosaccharides and polyols), which are found in foods such as wheat, soy and other legumes, certain fruits and vegetables, dairy, and sweeteners such as fructose and high-fructose corn syrup. The low-FODMAP dietary approach has been shown to be potentially effective in treating symptoms of SIBO-induced IBS; however, it does not get to the *root cause* of the SIBO. About 39 percent of people with Hashimoto's reported feeling better with the low-FODMAP dietary approach, which leads me to believe that the people who benefited from it likely had SIBO.

The recipes in the Cookbook section are not tailored specifically to the low-FODMAP approach, as they contain many foods high in FODMAPS, such as artichokes, leeks, garlic, shallots, onions, peas, cauliflower, mushrooms, apples, cherries, figs, mango, banana, honey, cashews, and black beans. However, many recipes in the book can be modified to low-FODMAP by removing these ingredients (typically just one or two items in any given recipe).

Some low-FODMAP recipes that don't need any modifications include:

Chicken Burgers and Kale Chips (p. 261)
Citrus Salmon (p. 265)
Duck with Date Sauce (p. 217)
Hashi-Mojito Smoothie (p. 170)
Quail with Grapes (p. 270)
Pumpkin Pie (made with pureed dates, p. 331)

In addition to the low-FODMAP diet, you may benefit from peppermint oil and peppermint tea—both have been reported to suppress SIBO (try my recipe for Mint Tea, p. 157). You may also have an adverse reaction to fermented foods and to certain probiotics containing *Lactobacillus* and beneficial *Streptococcus* bacteria, and require additional supplementation with B_{12} and/or iron. Keep in mind that SIBO cannot be overcome through a low-FODMAP diet approach alone and must be addressed with either a pharmacological or herbal approach or a two- to three-week elemental diet (see *Hashimoto's Protocol* for comprehensive treatment protocols for SIBO).

If you'd like low-FODMAP meal plans, please visit thyroidpharmacist.com/food.

the dairy-free diet, the iodine-free diet, or an individualized diet developed with the help of food-sensitivity testing. The connecting thread behind these diverse diets is that they all *remove various reactive ingredients* and are often more *nutrient dense* than the Standard American Diet. Furthermore, most of the diets do include animal protein.

Healing Foods

Besides removing potentially reactive foods from the diet, let's talk about adding delicious, nutrient-dense healing foods! Here are some of the foods I have found to be especially beneficial for people with Hashimoto's.

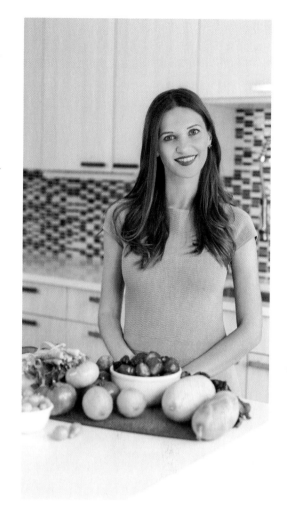

Green smoothies: Sixty-eight percent of people who responded to my survey found green smoothies helpful; 82 percent said that the smoothies gave them more energy, 60 percent claimed improved mood, and 40 percent noticed benefits for normalizing weight. Smoothies are a really great way to increase our intake of nutritious food without the digestive stress. As the ingredients in smoothies are chopped up, the food is easier to digest and the nutrients easier to absorb.

Fermented foods: Few foods are better at promoting healing in the gut than fermented foods. Fermentation is a process of food preservation that produces probi-

---

HOW A GREEN SMOOTHIE CAN HELP YOUR THYROID

I designed the Root Cause Original Smoothie (p. 167) specifically for Hashimoto's healing. Healthy fat from coconut milk, fiber from veggies, and protein from a hypoallergenic powder combine to create a triple boost in thyroid healing as they help to stabilize blood sugar, fight inflammation, and aid in detoxification processes.

Sensitivities to gluten, dairy, soy, and sometimes even eggs take many popular breakfast options off the table for people with Hashimoto's. A green smoothie is a delicious and safe alternative that people have said makes them feel calmer, energized, and free from "hangry" mornings! (Hangry = Hungry + Angry)

otics, or "good bacteria," that can be beneficial in balancing your intestinal flora and help with symptoms of constipation, digestion, and anxiety. Some of my favorite fermented foods include fermented coconut yogurt, fermented coconut water, and fermented cabbage. If you choose to buy fermented foods, be sure to buy the ones that are refrigerated; probiotic bacteria can only survive a couple of weeks at room temperature. In my Hashimoto's survey, 57 percent of responders felt that these foods helped, and the benefits were again seen in energy (64 percent), mood (49 percent), and pain reduction (27 percent).

Bone broth: Bone broth was found helpful by 70 percent of people with Hashimoto's. Specifically, 62 percent saw an increase in energy; 57 percent, an improvement in mood; and 32 percent, an improvement in skin. Bone broth provides healing collagen and nutrients to support our gut lining and skin. You can make your own using my Bone Broth recipe (p. 135) or order it (p. 91).

Gelatin: Gelatin was beneficial for 47 percent of my survey responders; almost half saw improvements in skin, 38 percent saw benefits in hair, and 33 percent saw a reduction in pain and improvement in energy. I love to use gelatin in smoothies and gut-healing desserts. I also have a special traditional Polish treat for you in the Cookbook section, my auntie's Galaretka recipe (p. 189), which is a chicken soup–like gelatin that is especially helpful for healing your gut! Additionally, the Cherry Berry Gelatin Snacks (p. 326) will help with supporting your gut and joints!

Hot lemon water: Lemon juice can help support stomach and liver detoxification pathways and, thanks to its acidity, aid in absorption of certain medications, including thyroid hormone medications. I encourage

THE BENEFITS OF BONE BROTH

Bone broth is an essential part of a nutrient-dense, healing diet for Hashimoto's. Many of its ingredients will directly benefit you and your thyroid:

The gelatin in bone broth helps to seal loose intestinal junctions. It's also easy to digest.

Chondroitin sulfates and glucosamine in bone broth can help increase energy and reduce pain and inflammation.

Amino acids found in bone broth have immune-boosting properties.

Collagen can support the health of your skin, hair, and nails, reduce wrinkles in the skin, restore shine and body in hair, and make nails stronger and longer.

drinking hot lemon water in the morning on an empty stomach and have found that most people who start drinking this in place of caffeinated beverages are surprised by not just how much energy they have, but also how much better they feel overall. You can make your own hot lemon water by squeezing the juice of one-half to one organic lemon into a cup of hot water (cool slightly before drinking).

Beets: Beets are a good source of phytonutrients, which perform anti-inflammatory and antioxidant duties in the body. If you have the MTHFR gene mutation, beets are especially good for you, as they are rich in betaine, a substance that can help break down homocysteine (individuals with the MTHFR gene mutation have trouble processing the amino acid homocysteine, elevated levels of which have been associated with heart disease, difficult pregnancies, birth defects, and possibly an impaired ability to detoxify). I recommend eating one to two servings of beets a week; because they are naturally high in sugar, though, you'll want to combine them with a healthy fat or protein source.

Cruciferous veggies: Glucosinolates, found in cabbage, broccoli, cauliflower, kale, and turnips, help increase detoxification in the liver, which is beneficial for individuals with autoimmune thyroid disease. I recommend buying organic crucifers, especially kale, because kale's hearty green leaves tend to pick up a lot of toxins from the environ-

ment. I've already mentioned the myth that those with Hashimoto's should avoid crucifers; however, if you are concerned about the goitrogen potential of crucifers, you can lightly steam or ferment them, since they mostly only affect the thyroid's absorption of iodine in a raw state.

Cilantro: Fresh cilantro is a natural chelator, which means it will bind to certain toxins and help excrete them from the body. There are other natural chelators, such as chlorella and spirulina, although I do not generally recommend these for people with Hashimoto's due to their high iodine content and their potential to modulate the immune system. You can add cilantro to salads, avocados, green juices, smoothies, and salsas and use it as a fresh condiment topper on chili, stews, and soups.

Fiber: Fiber acts like a sponge as it moves through the digestive system and helps sop up toxins and excess hormones, ultimately supporting their path to excretion. It's best to get fiber from fruits and vegetables rather than from supplements, because supplements have been known to aggravate intestinal permeability and SIBO. I suggest gradually adding fibrous foods into your diet if you don't normally eat a lot of them.

Green juices and chlorophyll: I recommend drinking green juices for a few reasons: first, they are full of healing nutrients; second, they are in liquid form and are therefore easily digestible; and third, they are a wonderful source of chlorophyll. Chlorophyll, a green pigment contained in plants, has been found to have numerous health benefits; it's been shown to help support the process of detoxification in the liver, reduce inflammation and oxidative stress, raise iron levels, and even work as a natural deodorant by neutralizing odors. I have included a recipe for Green Juice (p. 153), but if you create your own combination, be sure that it consists primarily of vegetables with only a small amount of fruit, such as green apples, added for flavor. The best type of juicer to use is a masticating juicer, which "chews" the vegetables instead of cutting them. See Chapter 4 for more info on recommended kitchen tools.

Turmeric: Promoted for its antioxidant and anti-inflammatory effects, turmeric is also antibacterial and antiviral, effective at helping detoxify various metals and toxins and linked to improved mood and memory. These benefits are thanks to a bright yellow chemical called curcumin, the naturally occurring active ingredient found in turmeric. Typically, the effects of curcumin only last about an hour in the body, but I've found that combining curcumin with piperine, an alkaloid found in pepper, will keep it in the body longer.

I recommend turmeric for clients with Hashimoto's because it helps support the gut, liver, and inflammatory pathways. Thanks to its anti-inflammatory effect, it can be especially helpful if you are experiencing pain.

You'll find this ingredient in the Chicken Tandoori (p. 234) and Pork Curry Stew (p. 194).

Berries: Berries are an incredible source of phytonutrients that act as antioxidants in the body. Because they are high in fiber, they also don't cause a spike in your blood sugar as some types of fruit do. I recommend eating a variety of berries, including blackberries, blueberries, raspberries, and strawberries and more exotic types such as boysenberries, currants, and gooseberries. Blueberries are a rich source of myoinositol, a nutrient that has been shown to improve thyroid function and blood sugar. Buy organic fruit as often as you can.

Ideally, you should get one to two servings of berries into your diet daily. It's best to spread these servings out throughout the day, as too much fruit at one time can cause a spike in blood sugar that may lead to tiredness. Even with fruit, you will want to practice moderation, since too much fructose, which is the primary sugar found in fruits, has been linked to insulin resistance and fatty liver disease.

You'll find recipes that feature all of these healing foods—homemade broth, collagen/gelatin, berries, crucifers, fermented foods—plus plenty of recipes for smoothies, healthy proteins, and good fats in the Cookbook section!

In addition to making sure that you're incorporating plenty of healing foods into your diet, I want you to pay attention to your macronutrients and micronutrients. My mentor JJ Virgin, nutrition and fitness expert, always says, "Your body is a chemistry lab, not a bank account!" Most diets focus on counting or restricting calories, but, instead, I want you to ensure you are getting adequate amounts of body-healing proteins, fats, and nutrients.

MINDING YOUR MACROS AND MICROS

I have a little quiz for you:

Which of the following is *not* a required nutrient for humans?

    a. protein
    b. fat
    c. micronutrients
    d. carbohydrates

If you're scratching your head and thinking that there must be a typo in this question, you're likely not alone. This was an actual test question (which I got wrong!!) in my first-year biochemistry course in pharmacy school. The correct answer is D. Carbohydrates are not a required nutrient; protein, fat, and micronutrients are all required. I was shocked to learn carbohydrates were not a required nutrient, whereas fat was required for normal cell function! Based on my previous nutritional knowledge, gathered from store displays and sandwich ads, I thought that carbohydrates were the most important food group!

Not only are carbs not required; they're also the number-one contributor to blood-sugar swings. Blood-sugar swings and blood-sugar imbalances are both common in those with Hashimoto's and can contribute to anxiety, weight gain, hair loss, irritability, weakened adrenals, fatigue, and increased antibodies. Limiting your carbohydrate intake and making sure that you get plenty of good fats and proteins is key to balancing your blood sugar.

Macronutrients Matter More Than Calories

A lot of people look at foods and see either "high calorie" or "low calorie," but I want to steer you away from this commonly used quantitative measurement. My experience has shown that placing too much emphasis on calories inspires a restrictive way of eating that's counterintuitive to eating for health and healing. Although many people can lose weight on a restricted-calorie diet, the weight is typically gained back once the calorie intake is increased again. People who restrict calories, especially those with Hashimoto's, may also continue to struggle with fatigue, anxiety, skin issues, pain, hair loss, and fertility issues. Some of them actually develop these symptoms because of restrictive dieting.

When we think about reduced-calorie diets from an adaptive physiology standpoint, not getting enough calories sends danger signals to our bodies (excessive exercise can do the same). After all, we still live in bodies with the genes of our ancestors', and our ancient bodies interpret an inadequate number of calories to mean we are experiencing a famine. In an effort to help us survive, our bodies will send signals to suppress our metabolism when faced with this "famine." When our metabolism is suppressed, we don't burn as many calories, and therefore we don't need to eat as many calories; that's how a suppressed metabolism can help us survive. As we know, the thyroid gland is the master gland of metabolism; whenever our body receives a signal there's a famine, it will likely try to slow down thyroid function.

Instead of calories, I advise my clients and readers to focus on using food as medicine to balance blood sugar, nourish their bodies with nutrient-dense foods, and reduce inflammation through avoiding personally inflammatory foods. With these guidelines in place, I then encourage eating until they are full and satisfied, thereby increasing the chance that their nourishment needs are being met. The "full" signal sends a safety message to our bodies.

You eat for nutrient density in much the same way; a nutrient-dense diet is one that excludes processed foods (often carbohydrates) and includes nutrient-packed food such as different varieties of meat, all vegetables, all fruit, nuts, seeds, and eggs (some of these may be omitted depending on which diet plan you are following or because of your specific sensitivities). When these are the core foods in your diet, your body can become healthy from the inside out. The "side effects" of nutrient-dense, blood sugar–balancing, anti-inflammatory nutrition include: shiny and full hair; clear and glowing skin; more energy; a calmer, happier mood; reduced pain; balanced hormones; and even effortless weight loss (in addition to improved thyroid markers!).

It's not necessary to pay strict attention to how much of each type of macronutrient you're eating each day, but having a general idea of what to aim for, or even just having the right macronutrient "mind-set" in place, can be helpful. Here are my recommendations for each.

Protein: Proteins are chains of amino acids, which are used within the body to build and repair cells and tissues and to fuel the fight-or-flight response. People with chronic health challenges need more protein in the diet to help support greater repair demands. When you think of protein, I want you to think of your body getting more raw fuel to create thyroid hormones, patch up the leaks in your intestines, and repair neglected parts of your body, such as your joints, skin, hair, and nails.

The average person requires about 1 gram of protein per kilogram of body weight per day (roughly 0.5 gram per pound of body weight). However, people who are over age sixty-five and/or have chronic illness and/or are more active may need up to 1 gram *per pound* of body weight daily. Here's a chart showing how much protein you need.

In addition to getting protein from foods, it may also be helpful to obtain protein from protein powder. As people with Hashimoto's often have deficiencies in digestive enzymes, they may have trouble extracting protein and various nutrients from the foods they're eating. Because it's already broken down into fine form and separated from other ingredients, protein from powder is generally easier to digest than protein from foods. Protein powder is also easy to incorporate into the diets via smoothies!

Even if your digestion is perfect and you eat a 4-ounce serving of steak (31 grams of protein) and a 4-ounce fillet of salmon (25 grams), you will have eaten 56 grams of protein—not enough for most people. In addition to using digestive enzymes (see p. 72 for more info), I also recommend adding hypoallergenic protein powders for most of my clients with Hashimoto's. As an example, one scoop of my Root Cause AI Paleo Protein Powder will give you 26 grams of protein.

Fat: Although we're finally coming out of the decades we spent fearing fat, there's still a lingering mind-set that keeps us from eating enough of this energy-rich macronutrient. My message to you is this: don't fear the fat; it's essential for brain function, healthy skin, shiny hair, and the formation of cell membranes. The key is to eat good fats, which are found in salmon, fish oil, olive oil, coconut oil, and avocados, and stay away from bad fats, primarily trans fats, found in most baked goods, fried foods, margarine, packaged cookies, certain cereals, and some frozen dinners. If you see any type of "hydrogenated oil" on the ingredient list, you should skip it. As a rule of thumb, the more active you are the more protein you'll need. When you eliminate processed foods from your diet, you will essentially have eliminated almost all forms of trans fats.

The other important point to remember regarding fats is that you want to aim to eat more omega-3 fatty acids than omega-6 fatty acids (again, this won't need to be something you pay too much attention to if you've cut out processed foods). You will naturally achieve the right balance of these different types of fatty acids when you eat plenty of good fats and avoid processed oils like sunflower, soybean, corn, and canola oil along with conventionally raised meats.

WHICH PROTEIN POWDER
IS SAFE FOR HASHIMOTO'S?

The problem with most varieties of protein powder on the market is that they are usually based in dairy and/or soy, which are usually highly reactive foods in those with Hashimoto's. Egg white protein is a better option, although unfortunately I've seen people with Hashimoto's develop a reaction to eggs, even when they had not done so before, after using egg white protein. As people in the early stages of their healing Hashimoto's journey have intestinal permeability (which we are aiming to repair!), they are likely to develop food reactions to difficult-to-digest proteins.

The three types of protein powders I've found to be the best tolerated by people with Hashimoto's are hydrolyzed beef protein, pea protein, and hemp protein, respectively. Pea protein and hemp protein are plant-based protein. Although generally well tolerated, they are not complete proteins (don't contain all essential amino acids), and hemp protein may be problematic for some people with estrogen dominance concerns.

Of the three, hydrolyzed beef protein is the best tolerated. Hydrolysis is a process that breaks down the protein into tiny parts to make it easier to digest; therefore it's less likely to be reactive and less likely to cause new reactions, even in people with intestinal permeability. I know that hydrolyzed beef protein powder may not sound that appetizing, but is surprisingly tasty (it has a slight milky flavor).

By popular demand (and because I wanted a hydrolyzed beef protein for my daily smoothies), under my Rootcology brand I created AI Paleo Protein, an unflavored hydrolyzed beef protein that's compliant with even the strictest autoimmune protocol. Rootcology also carries a vanilla-flavored hydrolyzed beef protein, Paleo Protein (appropriate for the Intro and Paleo Diets; see Chapter 4), and an Organic Pea Protein (appropriate for the Intro Diet and, in some circles, the Paleo Diet). You can find them at Rootcology.com, or you can use any other type of hydrolyzed beef or pea protein; just be sure they don't contain soy- or gluten-based fillers. For a free smoothie recipe guide, go to thyroidpharmacist.com/food.

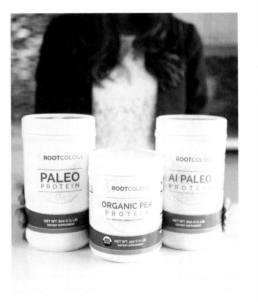

Carbohydrates: As I was shocked to learn in pharmacy school, carbohydrates are not a required element of our diet. Up to 50 percent of people with Hashimoto's may have carbohydrate metabolism issues, and a low-carbohydrate diet has been shown to be beneficial for Hashimoto's.

You will want to limit your carbohydrate intake while healing from Hashimoto's. This will help you balance your blood sugar, and you will likely find that you feel significantly more clearheaded, more energetic, and less anxious with a lower-carbohydrate diet. You should also see your thyroid antibodies trending downward with this kind of dietary plan. Some people with Hashimoto's (though not all) may even benefit from an ultralow-carbohydrate diet such as a ketogenic diet.

I recommend staying away from processed carbohydrates as you set off on your healing path. You can eat natural carbohydrates such as sweet potatoes and berries, but not too much at first! For best results you may want to limit your servings of carbohydrates to one or two a day if you're still in the early stages of your healing journey and struggling with blood-sugar swings. For some of my clients, even too much fruit can throw them off! Generally, having the carbohydrates later in the day seems to be more balancing. You will be able to improve your tolerance for carbohydrates as you heal.

Micronutrients Important to Hashimoto's Recovery

Nutrient depletions are always a factor in Hashimoto's thyroiditis. In fact, I would argue that due to our current farming practices and Western diet, nutrient depletions are a factor for most people! Eating conventionally grown foods, taking medications, and having food sensitivities, gut inflammation, poor digestion, malabsorption, gut infection, an altered flora, and hypothyroidism in itself can lead to nutrient depletions.

Even people who are eating organic, nutrient-dense diets are at risk for nutrient deficiencies, as factors like low stomach acid, fat malabsorption, gut infections, and a deficiency in digestive enzymes will result in an inability to properly break down the nutrients from the foods that they're eating. In addition to addressing digestive challenges, supplementation of important nutrients for Hashimoto's may need to be implemented. Let's take a look at some of the nutrients that you may need to support during your healing journey, starting with those required for thyroid function.

NUTRIENTS REQUIRED FOR THYROID FUNCTION

The thyroid relies on a selection of highly specific nutrients to perform optimally, and each nutrient has its own important job! Various nutrients are required for proper thyroid function, while others are needed for proper immune-system, gut, and adrenal function.

If you develop nutrient deficiencies, your body will send out signals in the form of symptoms. Many of these symptoms may be written off as simply consequences of age or environment, but oftentimes supplementation can eliminate them! On page 49 is a list of common nutrients that can be deficient in those with Hashimoto's as well as some of their respective symptoms.

Any combination of nutrient deficiencies is possible, but among these I've identified seven nutrients that are most likely to be deficient as well as supplements that have proven helpful for a significant number of people with Hashimoto's. Some of these can be taken safely without specific testing, while others require testing to ensure proper use. I have more nutrient solutions strategies for you than I could fit in this book; please visit thyroidpharmacist .com/food to get a free done-for-you guide on these!

Four Safe Supplements

The four thyroid supplements that are safe and helpful for most without lab testing are thiamine, selenium, magnesium, and zinc.

Thiamine (B1)

Thiamine is responsible for converting carbohydrates into energy and also helps with the digestion of proteins and fats. Thiamine is necessary for proper release of hydrochloric acid in the stomach, which is required for proper protein digestion—essential for healing from Hashimoto's. People with Hashimoto's and Crohn's disease have been found deficient in thiamine. Symptoms of deficiency include fatigue, low blood pressure, and adrenal issues, and low levels may contribute to irritability, depression, abdominal discomfort, and trouble digesting carbohydrates.

In 2013, I wrote an article about thiamine, and to this day I still get hugs from readers telling me that they've turned their life around with thiamine. One woman wrote saying that her thyroid fatigue was so severe she had to go on disability, but then supplementing with thiamine allowed her to recover her energy and go back to work. Thiamine also helped me resolve my fatigue along with the low blood pressure I battled for as long as I could remember! My blood pressure has tested normal ever since I started this supplement a few years ago.

Since most of the foods that contain thiamine are restricted throughout two of the three healing diets I will be recommending, supplementation may be necessary to achieve optimum levels. Research studies have shown that a daily 600-mg dose of thiamine for as little as three to five days can produce benefits such as more energy, better brain function, stabilized blood pressure, and improved blood-sugar tolerance. I recommend Benfomax from Pure Encapsulations for thiamine supplementation.

Magnesium

Magnesium has been shown to help improve form and function in damaged thyroid glands; it also supports detoxification pathways in the liver and is essential to the production of hundreds of enzymes utilized by the body. People with Hashimoto's who follow a grain-free diet, thereby omitting cereals that have been fortified with magnesium, or exclude natural dietary sources of magnesium such as nuts, seeds, and legumes may become inadvertently deficient. Deficiency can cause migraines, headaches, insomnia, menstrual cramps, anxiety, joint pain, and a whole host of other symptoms (like intolerance to loud noises).

Magnesium helped me personally resolve horrific menstrual cramps. My clients have also experienced relief from migraines, palpitations, constipation, insomnia, anxiety, and muscle cramps with magnesium supplementation. Studies show that long-term use can also help with normalizing the thyroid gland appearance on ultrasound, and magnesium may also help for thyroid and breast nodules.

pharmaceutical companies are "voluntary" for supplement companies. For this reason, most supplement companies do not take the extra steps to test their products to ensure safety and purity.

Evaluating the safety, efficacy, and cost of various treatments was a large part of my training as a pharmacist. I have put my training to good use in overcoming Hashimoto's, researching the best supplement brands and, now, in the development of my own supplement line, Rootcology. Rootcology is a blend of my two passions and areas of expertise, root causes and pharmacology: *root*—going after the root cause of disease—and *cology* (as in pharmacology)—understanding how tiny amounts of substances affect the human body! Rootcology is dedicated to creating innovative, bioavailable products that are made with the greatest care and with the highest-quality ingredients available. All of the supplement ingredients have been carefully chosen by yours truly to address the needs and sensitivities of people with autoimmune thyroid disease.

All Rootcology supplements are:

- Gluten free
- Dairy free
- Soy free
- Pesticide free
- Toxin free
- Pharmaceutical grade
- Free from potentially harmful fillers

Furthermore, all Rootcology supplements undergo third-party testing to ensure that the ingredients on the label are safe and effective and match what's actually inside the bottle. I created Rootcology to give you a trusted source of supplements that are safe and helpful for people with multiple sensitivities and chronic health conditions.

Throughout this book, you'll find charts that contain the supplements I recommend as well as the specific brands, my own and others', to use. I hope that this information is helpful in your journey!

The usual starting-dose ranges for magnesium are magnesium citrate at 400 mg or magnesium glycinate at 100 mg; you can increase your dosage according to the recommendations of the manufacturer.

I recommend two specific forms of magnesium: magnesium citrate or magnesium glycinate. Choose citrate if you tend to be constipated; glycinate, if your stools tend to be on the looser side. Also, for some people glycinate can worsen anxiety while citrate can reduce anxiety and promote sleep.

Be sure to give yourself four hours between your thyroid medications and magnesium dose. For most clients, I recommend taking magnesium at bedtime, especially if they have trouble sleeping. If you experience diarrhea, this could be an indication that you are getting too much magnesium and that you should lower your dose or perhaps switch to the glycinate version. Please note, for pain relief benefits, magnesium should be taken daily preventatively, and the dose can be increased in times of increased pain or stress.

Zinc

Zinc is an essential element required for detoxification and thyroid function. You also need zinc to form TSH, which is why people with hypothyroidism—those who are constantly producing TSH—are more likely to develop deficiencies. A deficiency can lead to poor wound healing, impaired T4 to T3 conversion, increased intestinal permeability, susceptibility to infections, reduced bacterial detoxification, impaired smell, acne, and low alkaline phosphatase. If you have celiac disease or any other malabsorption syndrome that has caused intestinal damage, you may have an impaired ability to absorb zinc.

You can supplement with zinc to address deficiency, but doses should be no more than 30 mg per day without a doctor's supervision. Doses above 30 mg may cause a depletion in copper levels. I recommend zinc picolinate, because of its improved absorption profile compared to other forms. To ensure optimal absorption, zinc supplements should be taken with food.

Supplements That Require Lab Testing

Other nutrient deficiencies require lab testing prior to supplementation. This is the case with certain minerals and fat-soluble vitamins that may accumulate in the body, leading to excess. Lab results can help determine the specific dosing and duration that are right for you. The three most important nutrient tests I always recommend for people with Hashimoto's: vitamin D, B_{12}, and ferritin. These require testing before supplementing and during supplementing to track progress.

Most doctors will order these tests for you if you ask, and the tests should be covered by your insurance. If you do not have a doctor who is willing to order the tests for you or if you have a high-deductible insurance plan, please visit www.thyroid

pharmacist.com/resources for self-order options.

Please note, the lab interpretation guide I provide below is based on optimal labs. In some cases, doctors may consider your numbers "normal" when you are indeed deficient. Your doctor may not be familiar with research that shows that suboptimal levels can produce numerous symptoms! Make sure to be an educated and empowered patient, and always ask for a copy of your own labs so that you don't miss out on the life-changing effects of these important nutrients!

Vitamin D₃

Vitamin D is an important immune modulator, which could explain why a deficiency of this vitamin is connected to various autoimmune diseases, including Hashimoto's. A vitamin D_3 deficiency may not present any obvious symptoms and will need to be revealed via testing, although people who live in a northern climate; have fat malabsorption, low intake of fatty fish, low exposure to sunlight, and a history of Hashimoto's; or are prone to depression likely need vitamin D.

Vitamin D supplements can improve our mood and can help us reduce thyroid antibodies. Both TPO and TG antibodies were reduced in a Polish trial of 18 women who were supplementing with vitamin D to reach a target of 60 ng/ml. I've personally found that most of my clients who are in remission from Hashimoto's keep their levels of vitamin D between 60 and 80 ng/ml.

A vitamin D_3 deficiency is common among the general population and even more commonly found in people with Hashimoto's—68 percent of my readers with Hashimoto's reported also being diagnosed with vitamin D deficiency—and vitamin D deficiency has been correlated with the presence of thyroid antibodies. Research done in Turkey found that 92 percent of Hashimoto's patients were deficient in vitamin D, and two additional 2017 studies found that low vitamin D levels were associated with higher thyroid antibodies and worse disease prognosis.

I recommend testing for vitamin D deficiency using the Vitamin D, 25-OH and retesting within three months once you start supplementing to make sure that you are getting enough—but not too much. In contrast to most vitamins, which are water soluble and are excreted by the body in excess, vitamin D is fat soluble and can build up.

I recommend spending time in the sunshine to get more vitamin D if you have Hashimoto's. If you don't live in a warm climate, get to one! You have an official prescription for a beach vacation from yours truly! Tanning beds will also do in a bind. (Yes, I said tanning beds.)

Vitamin B₁₂

Vitamin B_{12} helps us with our energy production, and low levels are commonly associated with Hashimoto's and may lead to fatigue, depression, neurological issues, brain fog, tingling extremities, nerve damage, digestive deficiencies, seizures, and anemia. People with Hashimoto's report more energy, improved memory and mood, and much less extremity tingling with adequate supplementation.

Vegans and vegetarians are at greatest risk for deficiency due to the fact that B_{12} is only found in animal foods and cannot be synthesized by the human body. But people with pernicious anemia (a type of autoimmune condition), low levels of stomach acid, and various gut infections common in those with Hashimoto's, including *Helicobacter pylori* and SIBO, can also be susceptible.

Although B_{12} is water soluble and you technically can't overdose on it, I recommend testing for B_{12} deficiency and monitoring your levels to ensure that supplementation is sufficient. B_{12} is readily available in animal proteins, but many people with Hashimoto's may not be able to absorb it properly (especially those with pernicious anemia), and even oral supplements may not be able to restore levels. I recommend either sublingual B_{12} in methylcobalamin form or B_{12} injections to ensure proper absorption.

If you have pernicious anemia, please note that it's often caused by the gut infection *H. pylori*, which can trigger both Hashimoto's and pernicious anemia. Treatment can reverse both conditions!

Ferritin

Ferritin is our iron-storage protein, which has many important roles, including supporting the utilization of T3 and the transport of T3 to cell nuclei. Low levels are a hidden indicator of iron-deficiency anemia and may lead to fatigue, pale skin, cold intolerance, difficulty breathing, tongue abnormalities, big-time hair loss, and ice or carrot cravings (strange, right?).

Women who menstruate or are postpartum may be at increased risk due to blood loss. Additionally, SIBO, *H. pylori*, low stomach acid, a vegan/vegetarian diet, a manganese deficiency, and copper and heavy-metal toxicity can cause low ferritin levels.

Ferritin levels may be low even if all other screening tests for iron and anemia come out within the reference range. You need to request for ferritin to be tested specifically. This is something that can be ordered individually or added to a blood panel.

Food can be an excellent source of iron and ferritin, so if you discover that you are low in ferritin, you can also work on restoring levels by eating cooked liver or beef a few times per week. You might also consider eating a vitamin C–rich food along with an iron-rich food to increase absorption. One option might be to eat a serving of organic steak with a hearty serving of broccoli, a cruciferous vegetable that's surprisingly rich in vitamin C. You can also take a vitamin C tablet and/or betaine with pepsin (more on this in Chapter 3) just after eating iron-rich foods to optimize absorption. Please note,

GUIDE FOR VITAMIN D, VITAMIN B12, AND FERRITIN

NUTRIENT TEST	REFERENCE RANGE	OPTIMAL RANGE	TYPE/DOSE	BRAND
Vitamin B$_{12}$	200–900 pg/mL	700–800 pg/mL	5000 mcg under the tongue daily x 10 days, then 5000 mcg under the tongue once per week x 4 weeks, then 5000 mcg under the tongue monthly for maintenance	B$_{12}$ methylcobalamin, Pure Encapsulations. If you have the COMT V158M gene mutation or mitochondrial issues, the Adenosyl/Hydroxy B$_{12}$ liquid from Pure Encapsulations may work better.
Vitamin D (25, OH)	30–100 ng/mL	60–80 ng/mL	5000–10,000 IU per day	Vitamin D by Rootcology; Vitamin D, Pure Encapsulations
Ferritin (iron storage)	12–150 ng/mL	90–110 ng/mL	Follow package instructions or your practitioner's advice. Iron supplements are the most common supplements indicated in overdose.	Iron Bisglycinate, Thorne; Ferrochel Iron Chelate, Designs for Health; Opti-Ferin C, Pure Encapsulations

even with an iron-rich diet many people may require additional supplementation, and some may even benefit from iron injections.

Ferritin is often something that can be deficient due to numerous root causes, so if supplementing didn't address your levels, you will need to do some more digging.

I have more information in the Advanced Protocols in *Hashimoto's Protocol*.

If you have elevated ferritin levels, you may have iron overload and may benefit from blood donations. Be sure to retest your levels of ferritin, as it can build up in the body and be toxic. Keep this supplement out of reach of children and pets!

BEFORE YOU BEGIN

When I meet with clients, I share with them much of the same information I've shared with you in this chapter. Some people receive this information and are excited, because they finally have a starting point from which to approach feeling better. Others are overwhelmed, especially those who are dealing with debilitating fatigue, because they wonder how they're going to find the energy to incorporate a new diet into their lives. Still others have a reaction that falls somewhere in between these two—they're cautiously optimistic.

What I tell my clients and what I want to tell you is that, no matter what, you have to remember that these dietary plans are not for all of eternity. They are approaches to healing your body from Hashimoto's, but they should be seen as fluid and not fixed; you can try them as they are designed, and then you can let them morph into what works best for your unique body.

It's also important to keep in mind that healing may take longer than we want it to, but there is a reason for this: Hashimoto's doesn't happen overnight, and our healing will take time too. In fact, studies have shown that thyroid antibodies indicative of Hashimoto's can be present for as long as a decade before the person develops impaired thyroid function. Thankfully, symptom improvement and even full recovery often take a great deal less time than this.

What I'm most excited about for you is that you get the opportunity to discover the healing that can occur in your body with the proper nourishment. I hope that the dietary guides and my family-favorite recipes will guide you to getting your health back. You can simply follow the recipes that are marked with the symbol for each diet and know that you are adhering to the specifics of each.

I've designed the recipes in this cookbook specifically with you in mind! You will find that, although abundant in nutrients and tasty, most of the recipes will be incredibly easy to prepare. All of the recipes in my cookbook have been tested by a chef and nutritionist, but you do not need to be a chef or a nutritionist to make the recipes in your own home and benefit from them for healing!

Tailoring Your Plan

All the things that make you unique— your genes, ethnicity, blood type, gender, digestive capability, intestinal environment, food sensitivities, stress levels, and so much more—will make the optimal diet for *you* unique as well. However, what extensive dietary experiments, research, data mining, personal experience with Hashimoto's, and countless client consults have taught me is that, no matter your personal history or present state, there are reliable diet "templates" that can help nourish and strengthen your body to bring it back to a healthy state. Three healing diets have proven the most impactful in my own recovery and in my work with clients. These are the Root Cause Intro Diet, Root Cause Paleo Diet, and the Root Cause Autoimmune Diet. Each of these protocols is distinct, but they also have a lot in common. All three dietary protocols:

1. Limit reactive and processed foods like gluten, dairy, soy, caffeine, and sugar.

2. Are rich in vegetables and recommend aiming for 25 percent meat and 75 percent vegetables per meal, and for 6 cups of veggies/fruit each day.

3. Include fermented foods, which can lead to gut healing and mood improvement.

4. Include green smoothies for five to seven meals per week, which are an excellent source of easy-to-digest nutrients.

5. Are designed to be low on the glycemic index (GI), which is important because blood sugar and adrenal issues are often implicated in those with Hashimoto's. Following a low-GI diet can help with energy and mood swings and reducing the autoimmune attack on the thyroid.

6. Encourage eating a variety of foods and rotating them often. If you have leaky gut, eating the same food over and over again, no matter how healthy it is, can lead to a sensitivity to that food. Rotating foods is an excellent way to prevent new food reactions and to improve nutrient sufficiency.

7. Focus on nutrient density. Each diet recommends that you aim to eat plenty of organic meat and veggies, green smoothies, green juices, bone broth, liver, fermented foods, and gelatins—all foods that are packed with healing and beneficial nutrients.

8. Limit high-iodine foods like iodized salt and seaweed.

9. Are rich in good fats to support hair, skin, and balanced blood sugar.

YOU DECIDE:
STEP UP OR STEP DOWN

I recommend making use of these diets with either a step-up or step-down approach, in which you choose one level and then adjust to another level based on your needs. For example, if you start with the Root Cause Intro but continue to have symptoms after one to three months, you may want to step up to Root Cause Paleo. If you start with Root Cause Autoimmune and find that after one to three months you have reached your health goals, you may want to step down to the Root Cause Paleo and introduce more foods. Each strategy has its pros and cons, and you'll have to decide what's best for you at this time in your journey.

In the *Step-Up Approach*, you start with the least strict diet and work your way up as needed. You will find that it:

- Is easier to handle and implement.
- May prevent unnecessary restrictive dieting.
- May prolong healing time.

In the *Step-Down Approach*, you start with the strictest diet and work your way down. You may find that it:

- Is more difficult to implement.
- May be "overkill."
- May accelerate healing time.

Please note, although the Root Cause Intro and the Root Cause Paleo Diets can be lifelong diets, the Root Cause Autoimmune Diet is not meant to be followed for more than thirty to ninety days. As you heal, you should be able to introduce more and more foods. Becoming sensitive to foods that you were not previously sensitive to is a sign that you are "losing foods," and this is an important signal that you need to dive deeper into other root causes, such as intestinal infections.

No matter where you begin, know that these diets are meant to be a starting point for you and should be tailored to your response. Your needs may also change as time goes on or as you get rid of infections or balance your intestinal flora. Just because one diet worked for someone else does not mean it will work as well for you.

Let's explore each of the diets in greater detail. (If you are already familiar with these, you can skip to Chapter 4 or jump straight to the recipes in the Cookbook section.)

THE ROOT CAUSE INTRO DIET

By following the Root Cause Intro Diet, you will create an internal environment focused on healing and help calm the immune system. Central to this will be the elimination of six commonly reactive substances: gluten, dairy, soy, sugar, caffeine, and alcohol. These dietary irritants, when combined with the toxins we are exposed to in personal-care products, cleaning products, building chemicals, and so on, can overburden your body with toxins. In people with Hashimoto's, who may already have impaired detox abilities due to leaky gut and who have a diminished ability to sweat, this accumulation can overwhelm the liver and lead to a chemical backlog. A buildup of chemicals and toxins can impede the healing you want and need to happen if you are to recover from Hashimoto's.

In *Hashimoto's Protocol*, this diet is part of the Liver Support Protocol, which includes additional strategies for helping heal the liver and improve detox abilities. Starting with foods, however, is the most important step, and the one that can produce the most profound changes. When you eliminate processed foods and transition to a real-food diet, you will automatically remove a significant percentage of your exposure to the trigger foods you want to avoid.

If you've already removed these reactive foods and you are still experiencing symptoms, consider stepping up to the Root Cause Paleo Diet (p. 64).

THE ROOT CAUSE INTRO DIET

EXCLUDED FOODS

Gluten	Sugar
Dairy	Alcohol
Soy	Caffeine

Gluten: Gluten is a protein found in barley, rye, and wheat, which means you will be exposed to it when you eat most types of pasta, cereal, and bread. It's also used in some soups and sauces and in certain types of alcohol. If you have Hashimoto's or any other autoimmune disease, it is highly likely that you have a sensitivity to gluten and may experience symptoms such as abdominal pain, bloating, diarrhea, constipation, headaches, skin rash, and joint pain. It is also possible that you have celiac disease, in which case you could experience a more severe form of these reactions and experience them immediately after eating a gluten-containing food.

In my survey of 2,232 people with Hashimoto's, roughly 88 percent of them reported feeling better after eliminating gluten from their diets. My readers have shared with me some of the benefits they've experienced by going gluten free:

"Going gluten free has helped my hair to start growing back after I lost all my hair—even my eyebrows and eyelashes."

"Going gluten free helped me tremendously. It took eight months to feel the difference, and

now after two years most of my symptoms are gone. Nothing to lose by going gluten free."

"I'm gluten free and have brought my antibodies down to normal range. So thankful!"

"Gluten free and soy free for three months, and I was able to lower my meds and stomach pain, alternating diarrhea and constipation, anxiety, and body aches all gone!!"

If you have celiac disease, gluten elimination can produce a noticeable improvement in how you feel within a matter of days. However, it may take three months to two years for complete healing to take place. If you are gluten sensitive, you may also notice a change in your symptoms in as little as a few days, significant improvement in two to three weeks, and healing in approximately six to eight weeks. (A reminder: if you have other unresolved triggers, those will need to be addressed before you feel completely better.)

Dairy: People with Hashimoto's often have a sensitivity to casein and whey proteins, which are the two proteins found in dairy products such as milk, cheese, yogurt, ice cream, butter, and certain protein powders. Some people have a primary sensitivity to dairy, while others have a secondary sensitivity, meaning that the reaction to dairy proteins is a result of gluten-induced damage to the gut. People in this latter group may be able to tolerate dairy again after intestinal permeability has been repaired or after approximately six months of gluten and dairy avoidance.

WHEN LAB TESTING SAYS YOU'RE NOT GLUTEN SENSITIVE

Lab testing for gluten sensitivity can be very helpful, especially if you get the right kind of test, but unfortunately testing technology is not perfect. More often than not, false negatives can be seen for common reactive foods like gluten, dairy, and soy. The best test for figuring out if you are sensitive to gluten is doing an elimination diet, in which you avoid gluten for two to three weeks and then try it again to see if you react to it.

Getting off gluten helped some people dually diagnosed with celiac disease and Hashimoto's shed their Hashimoto's diagnosis (antibodies went into remission, and thyroid function returned to normal). However, it's not just celiac disease that is caused by sensitivity to gluten. My personal and clinical experience has shown that nonceliac gluten sensitivity is one of the biggest triggers for Hashimoto's. Going gluten free can help alleviate many symptoms associated with Hashimoto's, such as fatigue, hair loss, bloating, constipation, diarrhea, pain, acid reflux, weight gain, and many others as well as reduce the autoimmune attack on the thyroid gland. And this is why it's one of the first things I recommend when you have a thyroid condition, whether it is Hashimoto's, hypothyroidism, or Graves' disease.

Dietary changes can have a big impact on your body. Caffeine, is a well-known addictive substance, and some people may get withdrawal headaches, nausea, irritability, diarrhea, and even vomiting—especially if they quit cold turkey instead of weaning off gradually. #thingsilearnedthehardway

You may also experience withdrawal symptoms if you're reducing your sugar intake. I personally experienced headaches, irritability, unusual vaginal discharge, and lethargy for about two weeks after kicking my sugar habit cold turkey.

Additionally, most people may not realize that gluten and dairy can also be addictive. It has been hypothesized that when gluten is digested, opioid peptides called *gluteomorphins* are released into the gastrointestinal tract and taken up into the bloodstream. These peptides are considered *exorphins*, as they have a morphine-like effect on the brain. In other words, they can have "addictive" properties, so suddenly cutting gluten out of your diet can cause strong withdrawal symptoms.

Similarly, *casomorphins*, which are ingested when milk products are consumed, have been suggested to cause similar withdrawal symptoms when removed from the diet.

Another type of dairy reaction is seen in people who have lactose intolerance. If you are lactose intolerant, you lack the enzyme needed to break down the milk sugar lactose. Although there are similarities in the symptoms caused by lactose intolerance and dairy-protein sensitivity, the difference is that the latter response originates in the immune system.

It's important to point out that all dairy, including raw dairy, should be excluded. Some people claim that pasteurization changes the protein structure of dairy proteins and that this is what makes them more reactive. However, if you've already been sensitized to dairy proteins from drinking conventional milk, you may still have a problem with consuming raw dairy, organic dairy, lactose-free milk, and even goat's milk. Goat's milk and sheep's milk are highly cross-reactive for those with cow's-milk sensitivity, which means there's a good chance it will be a reactive food for you if you are sensitive to dairy. However, camel's milk contains proteins that are different enough not to cross-react and may be well tolerated by people with Hashimoto's.

Soy: "Soy" is short for "soybean" or "soya," which is a type of legume used to make many meat- and dairy-free foods. It's also regularly used in processed foods to bind ingredients together or add texture. A lot of gluten-free products like breads and cookies contain soy, which can be problematic for thyroid patients and worsen the auto-immune attack on the thyroid. This is why I don't recommend simply switching to a "GFJF diet"—a gluten-free junk-food diet—when you eliminate gluten; you may inadvertently end up switching one trigger food for another. I believe that my thyroid condition worsened after eating soy-containing gluten-free products. Once I removed those foods too, my thyroid antibodies dropped from 800 IU/mL to 380 IU/mL (in just one month).

You can eliminate soy from your diet by avoiding edamame beans, soy milk, tofu, tempeh, miso, and soy sauce. You will also want to avoid processed foods and supplements, which often contain soy-based ingredients. This includes vegetarian and vegan products, which can contain soy lecithin, bean curd, hydrolyzed soy protein, and/or hydrolyzed vegetable protein.

Sugar: Eighty-seven percent of my clients and readers reported feeling better on a sugar-free diet. Sugar can exacerbate an imbalanced gut flora that is usually common in those with Hashimoto's and can contribute to blood-sugar swings. To avoid sugar, you will want to eliminate sucrose (table sugar) and high-fructose corn syrup, two ingredients that are commonly used in processed foods. Stevia, xylitol, and trehalose are potential alternative sweeteners, but steer clear of sucralose (Splenda) and saccharine, as they have both been implicated in triggering Hashimoto's.

Caffeine: Caffeine can exacerbate adrenal dysfunction and blood-sugar swings, both of which are common in those with Hashimoto's. Underlying adrenal insufficiency may cause certain symptoms to linger even after you've started taking thyroid medications and shifted to a gluten-free diet. Eliminating caffeine will help reset overworked adrenal glands, but may not be enough to restore them to peak functioning (this may require additional protocols, which you can read about in *Hashimoto's Protocol*).

In addition to wreaking havoc on the adrenal glands and blood sugar, consuming caffeine can prevent us from getting proper sleep, which is vital to healing, and increase gut permeability. For these reasons, an important part of the Intro Diet is avoiding caffeine-containing beverages such as coffee and tea. It's also important to avoid these beverages due to fluoride content (tea) and potential mold or gluten contamination (coffee).

If you regularly consume caffeine, quitting cold turkey can result in unpleasant side effects such as headaches. You may be able to avoid this side effect by weaning yourself off of caffeine instead. To do this, reduce your intake by 50 percent every day. For example, if you usually drink two cups of coffee per day, first drop down to 1 cup, then ½ cup, and ¼ cup, and then none.

In the next section, you'll discover one of my favorite alternatives to caffeine-containing beverages: hot lemon water. I also recommend drinking Mint Tea (p. 157),

SUGAR SUBSTITUTE RECOMMENDATIONS

In my survey of over two thousand people with Hashimoto's, 87 percent felt better after removing sugar from their diet. But transitioning away from it can be difficult at first, which is why most people look for alternative sources of sweetness (I know I did when I initially cut out sugar). When I was considering sugar substitutes, artificial sweeteners were out, since NutraSweet, Equal (aspartame), and Splenda (Sucralose) have been connected to triggering Hashimoto's. Natural sugar substitutes are a better choice, but even they have pros and cons for use.

Stevia is a popular and healthier alternative to sugar. It's derived from the plant *Stevia rebaudiana Bertoni*, or "honey leaf," which contains the sweet-tasting compounds known as steviol glycosides. Stevia can help people lose weight, improve diabetes, lower blood sugar, and lower blood pressure; it has anti-inflammatory and immune-boosting properties, and can even help people with Lyme disease.

Stevia, however, has a strong taste and may not be appropriate for people with adrenal fatigue, low cortisol, low blood sugar, or low blood pressure, due to its effects on blood sugar and blood pressure. One concerned reader reported that stevia had been causing her insomnia and bladder irritation.

Honey and maple syrup are natural and Paleo and Autoimmune friendly, but may contribute to *Candida* and blood-sugar issues, and you'll want to avoid these while you are eliminating sugar.

Xylitol and trehalose are additional sweeteners to consider. Xylitol can reduce cavities, but can cause GI upset and potentially worsen small intestinal bacterial overgrowth (SIBO), a common issue that's present in Hashimoto's. Trehalose can accelerate tissue repair, but like xylitol may exacerbate SIBO and may feed the toxic *Clostridium difficile* (C. diff.) bacteria; thus, if you are struggling with an overgrowth of the C. diff. bacteria, then xylitol may not be appropriate for you.

Myo-inositol, a naturally occurring sugar alcohol with half the sweetness of sugar, may be a better alternative. Myo-inositol, when combined with selenium, has been reported to improve thyroid function, stabilize blood sugar, and help anxiety. However, it may not be appropriate for people with kidney disease or low blood sugar.

Dandy Blend, or Spa Water (p. 168)—purified water with some of your favorite fruit and veggies. Or you might try Maca Latte (p. 158) or Green Juice (p. 153).

Alcohol: Drinking alcohol can lead to leaky gut, blood-sugar imbalances, SIBO, and a backlog in the liver as it works to detoxify ethanol. Even a "healthy" glass of red wine can have these effects, which is why it's advised to avoid all types of alcohol while following the Root Cause Intro Diet. If you miss the taste of alcohol, you can try a few of my favorite substitutes, such as the Hashi-Mojito (p. 154), which will support your liver and gut with probiotics.

THE ROOT CAUSE PALEO DIET

I based the Root Cause Paleo Diet on a traditional Paleo diet, which is the popular approach to eating that is modeled after the way our ancestors ate, and modified it to specifically benefit people with Hashimoto's. The result is a diet that's designed to lower your intake of inflammatory foods and increase your intake of anti-inflammatory foods, including high-quality animal-based proteins, which will help your body repair itself.

The goal of this dietary protocol is to remove stressors that may prevent us from restoring optimal function to the adrenal glands (the majority of my clients with Hashimoto's have presented some degree of adrenal dysfunction). We accomplish this by making dietary choices that reduce inflammation and help balance blood sugar, since both inflammation and

TESTING FOR FOOD SENSITIVITIES

When I was working as a pharmacist, we were always on the lookout for "true IgE-related allergies" to foods and medications (IgE is a class of antibodies). These were the life-threatening reactions that could cause anaphylaxis, shortness of breath, and rashes! I learned about reactions mediated by the other immune branches in immunology during my first year in pharmacy school, but somehow calling the IgE-related reactions "true" led me to believe that the other types of reactions didn't matter. Unfortunately, most conventional medical professionals and insurance companies hold that same misconception, and food sensitivity tests are considered "experimental." This was of course fine with me, because when I "experimented" with removing the foods the tests found to be reactive for me, I felt dramatically better!

The other challenge with food sensitivities is that when we eat the foods that our body is sensitive to on a daily basis, it is very difficult to connect the foods with the symptoms we are having. For example, people who have a dairy sensitivity but continue to eat dairy multiple times a day might be tired, have joint pain, congestion, bloating, and acid reflux daily, but won't be able to pinpoint the foods responsible for the symptoms. I was personally a bread and dairy addict and had no idea that they were causing me issues.

Every time we eat a food we are sensitive to, the body becomes depleted in its ability to protect itself from that food, and the reactions become less specific and more chronic. If the food continues to be eaten, the body will become more and more sensitive. However, once the sensitizing food is eliminated for a few days to a few weeks, we should generally feel better and experience less bloating, less acid reflux, normal bowel movements, more energy, and so on.

When we are exposed to the food again, the body will actually produce a stronger, more specific reaction, allowing us to recognize which particular food is problematic. This is known as an elimination diet and is the gold standard for food-sensitivity testing.

dramatic surges and swings in blood sugar can stress the cells and tissues of the body.

If you began with the Root Cause Intro Diet, you will have already removed alcohol, caffeine, dairy, soy, sugar, and gluten-containing grains. We will add to that list some additional items that can stress the body and possibly interfere with healing.

Grains: When I surveyed my readers, 81 percent of them reported feeling better when they went grain free! If you have pain and symptoms of irritable bowel syndrome such as constipation, diarrhea, nausea, or indigestion and if you are prone to depression, eliminating all grains may help lessen these.

We remove all grains to ensure that any substances that would irritate the intestinal lining are gone and also to help balance blood sugar; even gluten-free products made with grains like rice and corn

The Root Cause dietary protocols are based on the elimination diet, in which we remove the most common sensitizing foods found in those with Hashimoto's; however, some people may benefit from additional trials and testing. There are a multitude of food-sensitivity tests out there, but none of them are perfect. Some may have false negatives; others may have false positives or a combination of both.

The test that I found to be highly accurate for my clients and myself is the Alletess Lab food-sensitivity test. If a food comes up positive on that test, I know that it is a reactive food for that person. However, if the person has been off the food for some time, this test may have false negatives; so if people come up negative for one of the big reactive foods, I recommend going off it anyway and reintroducing it. If you are not quite ready to do an elimination diet or you need to see things in black and white, you may want to look into food-sensitivity testing.

Alletess Lab works primarily through integrative- and functional-medicine physicians, so if you're working with a physician in that category, you can ask your doctor to order the test for you. I'm also really excited to let you know that I've worked with MyMedLab to offer self-order food-sensitivity testing without a doctor's prescription. The test kit comes with a little blood-spot collection paper that can be mailed from just about anywhere in the world!

MyMedLab offers two options to test for the most commonly eaten foods, a 96 and 184 food panel. I started with the 96 food panel, and it was enough to uncover most of my food triggers. I now repeat the 184 food panel on an annual basis to be sure that I'm staying on top of potential triggers, as our sensitivities and reactions to foods can change with time. Please go to www.thyroidpharmacist.com/resources for self-ordering options and special discounts.

If you already had the Alletess food-sensitivity test done (or another credible test), it may reveal that you are sensitive to something that may be included in the Intro, Paleo, or Autoimmune Diet. If this is the case, don't eat it!

THE ROOT CAUSE PALEO DIET

EXCLUDED FOODS	INCLUDED FOODS
Gluten	Meats (all)
Dairy (we also exclude butter and ghee, which are allowed in traditional Paleo)	Fish and shellfish
Soy	Vegetables (except hot peppers)
Sugar	Fruits (all)
Alcohol	Nuts
Caffeine	Seeds
Grains	Eggs
Legumes (except green beans and pea protein)	Oils: avocado, coconut, and olive
Hot peppers	Hydrolyzed beef protein
Iodine-rich foods	Pea protein

can wreak havoc on our blood sugar. Blood-sugar imbalances have been described by many practitioners who focus on reversing Hashimoto's as adding "fuel to the fire" in autoimmune thyroid disease.

Hot peppers: Due to their ability to cause leaky gut, spicy peppers that produce capsaicin, such as cayenne pepper, chili peppers, red pepper flakes, and so on, are omitted from the Root Cause Paleo Diet. Bell peppers, which do not produce capsaicin, are appropriate to eat on the Root Cause Paleo Diet, as is black pepper, which is produced from peppercorns and is "spicy" due to piperine, a different substance.

Legumes (except green beans and pea protein): The most commonly known legumes are beans, including black beans, soybeans, fava beans, garbanzo beans (chickpeas), kidney beans, and lima beans. Lentils and peas, such as black-eyed peas, green peas, snow peas, and snap peas, are also considered legumes, as are peanuts.

Legumes contain phytates that bind various nutrients and can lead to poor zinc absorption, which may interfere with healing. Deficiencies in zinc have been linked to increased intestinal permeability and susceptibility to infections, so we want to take steps to eliminate anything that may prevent zinc absorption.

I've made two exceptions in the legume category, and those are for green beans and pea protein. They are both relatively well tolerated by most people with Hashimoto's.

Iodine-rich foods: Because we know that excessive iodine intake can be a trigger for Hashimoto's in those genetically predisposed to it, I recommend eliminating iodine-rich foods such as iodized salt and all types of seaweed, including nori, kombu, kelp, and wakame, from your diet during the Root Cause Paleo Diet. Other iodine-rich foods like spirulina and chlorella (there are some versions that have lower iodine) should also be avoided. Spirulina and chlorella have immune-stimulating properties that can worsen autoimmunity and even cause new-onset autoimmunity.

THE ROOT CAUSE AUTOIMMUNE DIET

After following the Intro Diet and the Paleo Diet, you will have already excluded gluten, dairy, soy, and grains, the most common reactive foods for those with Hashimoto's. If you are still experiencing symptoms, especially gut-related symptoms, after following these two diets, my recommendation is to step up to the Root Cause Autoimmune Diet. In *Hashimoto's Protocol*, this diet appeared as part of the Gut Balance Protocol, which included the use of enzymes (read about the best enzymes for digestion later in this chapter) and other supplements to help heal the gut. The diet adds to the list of excluded foods eggs, nightshades, nuts, and seeds, which have proven to be reactive foods for some people with Hashimoto's. It is also recommended that you add 1 to 2 cups of homemade Bone Broth (p. 135) to your daily regimen, which will assist in the healing of your gut.

Eggs: Eggs are an excellent source of protein, but can be a reactive food for some people with autoimmune conditions such as Hashimoto's. In my reader survey, 48 percent of people reported that they felt better on an egg-free diet. Eggs contain the enzyme lysozyme, which has the ability to bond with bacteria and proteins as it

---

MY FAVORITE BLOOD SUGAR–STABILIZING SOURCES OF FATS AND PROTEINS

Avocados	Lamb
Chia seeds	Nuts (except peanuts)
Chicken	
Coconut milk	Olives
Coconut, avocado, and olive oils	Pea protein
	Pork
Duck fat	Salmon
Eggs and egg white protein (if not sensitive)	Sardines
	Seeds
	Tallow
Grass-fed beef	Turkey
Hydrolyzed beef protein	Whitefish

THE ROOT CAUSE AUTOIMMUNE DIET

EXCLUDED FOODS	INCLUDED FOODS
Gluten	Meats (all)
Dairy (including butter and ghee, which are allowed in traditional Paleo)	Fish and shellfish
Soy	Vegetables (except nightshades)
Sugar	Oils: avocado, coconut, and olive
Alcohol	Fruits (all, especially coconut)
Caffeine	Hydrolyzed beef protein
Grains	
Legumes	
Hot peppers	
Iodine-rich foods	
Eggs	
Nuts	
Nightshades	
Seeds	
Stevia	

moves through the digestive process, collectively forming what's referred to as a lysozyme complex. A lysozyme complex is sort of like a fireball of potential irritants, which, if you have leaky gut, can pass through intestinal gaps and activate the immune system.

Nightshades: Similar to those eliminating eggs, 47 percent of people who responded to my survey said they felt better eating a nightshade-free diet. Symptoms associated with eating nightshades included joint aches, pain, swelling, tingling, and numb-

ness. Nightshades are a specific family of flowering plants and the fruits and vegetables they produce, including: tomatoes, potatoes, eggplant, bell peppers, tomatillos, spicy peppers (such as Thai peppers and chili peppers and the spices produced from them), goji berries, and cape gooseberries. Nightshades contain alkaloids, which are chemical compounds that can be reactive substances in some people.

Nuts: Nuts are a highly nutritious source of protein and healthy fats, which is why I encourage keeping them in your diet until you reach this level. Despite these nutritious qualities, however, nuts can be tough to digest; they contain oxalates and phytates, both "antinutrients" that can interfere with mineral absorption. Nut allergies are also increasingly common, which suggests that the number of people who are sensitive to them is probably growing too. For people with Hashimoto's, almonds in particular are reported as one of the top reactive foods (it is the fourth most common after gluten, dairy, and soy). This may have something to do with the fact that people are more likely to eat them every day as a snack (the Almond Board has been doing its job!), increasing the risk for a sensitivity to develop. In the Root Cause Autoimmune Diet, almonds and other nuts are excluded, but even if you don't react to them now and you add them back in later, I recommend rotating them with other foods, eating them every three to four days.

Seeds: Although seeds don't to seem to be a reactive food for an overwhelming number of people with Hashimoto's—only 7 percent of those who completed my survey reported a seed sensitivity—they have the potential to aggravate an already irritated gut. Seeds tend to resist digestion and might contribute to symptoms if you have trouble digesting proteins.

The list of included foods on the Root Cause Autoimmune Diet may seem short, but in practice it translates to countless options for delicious eating. Some of my favorite

meals to enjoy while following the Autoimmune Diet include Creamy White Chicken Stew (p. 193), Mango Salsa (p. 296), and Twice-Baked Sweet Potatoes (p. 300). You'll find recipes for these, and several others that you can try while sticking to this diet, in the Cookbook section.

KNOW THAT HEALING IS POSSIBLE: SUCCESS STORIES

In case you're hesitant about trying a radical diet, I wanted to share a few stories from readers just like you from around the world who have implemented the various healing diets mentioned in this chapter. If they did, you can too.

SUE: I did both the food-sensitivity testing and the autoimmune Paleo diet for about a year. My moderate autoimmune psoriasis cleared about 90 percent. Also, I lost weight, which put me into a healthy weight range. I also reduced my Tirosint [hypothyroidism med] from 88 mg to 75 mg.

LANE: Huge difference!! Eliminating gluten-containing grains and dairy completely as well as limiting sugars, alcohol, and processed food changed my life. My thyroid and Crohn's symptoms are not all-consuming anymore. I don't have bloating and stomach discomfort after I eat anymore. I don't constantly pass gas, so I can attend group yoga classes again . . . and not embarrass my teen daughter! I'm not glued to the toilet half the day. I can think again in my engineering job. I can't even imagine how awful my life would be if I didn't make these relatively easy changes. These changes are not big sacrifices—I still eat out just fine—and I have a wonderful future to look forward to! Thank you Izabella Wentz for all you've done to help inspire us to take healing into our own hands!

BONNIE: After reading *Root Cause*, I gradually gave up gluten, then dairy, sugar, alcohol, and coffee. Then I followed Paleo for six months before going completely AIP. About then I started following recommendations from Dr. Wentz's Hashimoto's self-management course and then her book *Hashimoto's Protocol*. I was on my way to remission! After eighteen months on AIP, my thyroid antibodies were in the normal range, and I gradually started reducing my dosage of thyroid hormone. Now I am in the process of gradually reintroducing foods with the eventual goal of staying Paleo 80 percent of the time. I have never felt better!

JOANNA: With the elimination diet, no gluten, no dairy, no sugar, no grains, etc., I reversed Hashimoto's and got best results in ten years!! Hair grown back! Sleep galore! Bloating gone! Puffy face gone!! Miracles!!!

CHRISTINA: Started strict AIP plus good probiotics in October and noticed a difference within a week—the terrible morning joint pain was almost completely gone. Next, my energy started returning and brain fog started lifting. Within a month, joint pain was almost completely gone, energy was so great, brain fog way better, superdry skin improving, hair starting to grow back, and I had lost almost 10 pounds of water weight. I was honestly shocked that just diet and supplements had made such a difference. I've been able to reintroduce a few things, and that's made the diet changes more doable.

SARA: I was diagnosed with Hashimoto's in October, and after reading your books in November I gave up gluten, grains, dairy, refined sugar, and junk. My thyroid gland has dramatically decreased in size. I was getting to the point where I was choking on foods because of my enlarged thyroid. This is so much better. I have a follow-up with ultrasound in March and am excited to see the objective outcome of my diet changes. My brain fog is improved, though there are still days it's there.

My endocrinologist never once mentioned that diet would/could help. She literally told me there was nothing I could do about my new diagnosis. So thank you, Izabella, for your books and your guidance!

NICOLE: Went gluten, dairy, soy, sugar, canola oil, iodized salt, and alcohol free for four months. Added selenium, vitamin E, and vitamin B_{12}, betaine with pepsin, and liver support . . . lost 8 kilograms, had more energy, less bloating, and less inflammation in joints.

CATHARINE: Gluten free, brain fog gone for good in three days after having it for fourteen years.

CAROLINE: I had a huge moment that I would like to share. I was a bestselling author here in the UK and suddenly got sick with Hashimoto's. (Looking back it wasn't sudden—it had been creeping up for years.)

I found myself unable to focus, unable to write even though my thyroid numbers were within range, and I was on Armour. I removed gluten seven months ago, along with adding a few more tweaks here and there as suggested by Izabella Wentz. Along came my "Aha!" moment. My brain is sharper—my ability to write has come back. A few months ago the mere thought of going into a meeting would have terrified me, yet last week I sat in front of a publishing house and landed a book-trilogy deal.

Thank you, Izabella.

WHICH HEALING DIET SHOULD YOU IMPLEMENT NEXT?

You can use the step-up or step-down approach to determine where you want to start with the diets. The chart below can also provide some dietary direction, depending on where you are today.

NOURISHMENT KNOWLEDGE THAT CAN HELP YOU HEAL

"Bad digestion is at the root of all evil," said Hippocrates, the ancient Greek physician who is considered to be the father of medicine. Although he was born in 460 BC, I think he was onto something! Another way

WHERE SHOULD I START?

IF...	THEN...
You are just starting and don't know which one to do	Do the diet that will be the easiest for you to implement. Just take action!
You're losing foods	Consider functional-medicine gut testing ASAP and working with your functional-medicine practitioner to clear infections.
If you're already gluten free but hit a plateau in healing	Move to the Intro Diet (gluten free, dairy free, soy free).
If you're already on the Intro Diet (gluten free, dairy free, soy free) but hit a plateau in healing	Move to Root Cause Paleo Diet.
If you're on the Root Cause Paleo but hit a plateau in healing	Move to Root Cause Autoimmune Diet.
If you're on the Root Cause Autoimmune but hit a plateau in healing	Consider gut testing, food-sensitivity testing, *Hashimoto's Protocol*, the Hashimoto's Self-Management Program, and/or the Root Cause Rotation Diet.*
If you have puzzling symptoms but have not had food-sensitivity testing	Test for food sensitivities.

*Please visit thyroidpharmacist.com/food for more information and resources.

to put this is, "You are what you absorb." People with Hashimoto's usually have a combination of nutrient deficiencies, food sensitivities, impaired ability to handle stress, digestive issues, infections, and an impaired ability to get rid of toxins. Many of these are related to a compromised ability to absorb from our diet the nutrients that the body's systems require for optimal function.

In my personal experience and in my work with clients, I've found that supportive enzymes can help improve digestion and thus may increase nutrient absorption from foods. An enzyme deficiency can, directly and indirectly, contribute to thyroid symptoms and autoimmunity. Using enzymes can help with overcoming symptoms of Hashimoto's including fatigue, hair loss, nutrient deficiencies, infections, and food sensitivities as well as reducing thyroid antibodies.

There are five types of enzymes that may be beneficial on various parts of your healing journey with Hashimoto's:

1. Protein digestive enzymes

2. Systemic enzymes

3. Fat digestive enzymes

4. Vegetable digestive enzymes

5. Gluten/dairy digestive enzymes

Protein Digestive Enzymes

Studies have found that most people with Hashimoto's and hypothyroidism have either low stomach acid or no stomach acid, which contributes to food sensitivities, increased risk of gut infections like *H. pylori*, SIBO, and parasites (potential root causes for Hashimoto's) as well as difficulties in protein digestion. Poor digestion of proteins results in fatigue, because we often become deficient in nutrients derived from protein, such as B$_{12}$, iron, and amino acids, and because the digestive process requires a lot of energy! One of the reasons nutrient supplements, green smoothies, and green juices can boost our energy is that we get a shot of partially or fully digested nutrients without doing the energy-consuming work of digestion.

Betaine hydrochloride (betaine HCL) and pepsin are both naturally occurring components of gastric juice that can help raise levels of stomach acid, making nutrients and amino acids from our protein-containing foods more bioavailable. Betaine and pepsin are often found together in digestive supplements; most brands have around 500 to 750 mg of betaine and around 20 to 50 mg of porcine-derived pepsin per capsule.

Discovering the connection between my deficiency of stomach acid and Hashimoto's was an "Aha" moment for me. After beginning to take betaine with pepsin with my protein-containing meals, my ten-year-long debilitating fatigue was lifted practically overnight! I went from sleeping for eleven or twelve hours per night to eight hours—just because I started digesting my foods better! Finally having enough energy gave me the confidence that I could overcome Hashimoto's and my long list of health struggles. I started writing *Hashimoto's: The Root Cause* the morning after I took the right dose of betaine with pepsin. The restored energy gave me hope that I would be able to devote myself to research and find the root cause of my condition and that I might one day be able to share my knowledge to help others.

Clients and readers have reported similar results as well as a reduction in pain, better mood, and even a more balanced weight. My survey has shown that 59 percent of people found that betaine with pepsin made them feel better; 33 percent said that it made them feel worse; and 7 percent saw no difference in symptoms. Many people have been able to improve their levels of ferritin and B_{12} by improving their stomach-acid levels; 50 to 70 percent of people with Hashimoto's are likely deficient in stomach acid, and deficiency can be determined by a trial of betaine with pepsin.

Here's how to do a trial of betaine with pepsin:

1. Start by taking just one capsule right after you've eaten a protein-containing meal.

2. Monitor for any reactions, such as a slight burning in your throat. If you do feel a burning in your throat, this means that you got too much acid. This is because either you do not need the supplement or the dose of the supplement was too high for your protein intake; that is, you didn't need the supplement for the amount of protein in that meal.

3. If you didn't feel anything, increase your dose to two capsules at the end of your next protein-containing meal and monitor again for any discomfort.

4. Keep increasing the dose by one capsule per meal until you feel a slight burning or discomfort. Once you've reached the burning/discomfort stage, you will know that you've had one dose too many and your target dose will be one less than the "too many" amount. You can drink a cup of water with a teaspoon of baking soda to relieve any continued burning sensation.

Here's a dosing example:

- Meal No. 1: Took one capsule, didn't feel symptoms

- Meal No. 2: Took two capsules, didn't feel symptoms

- Meal No. 3: Took three capsules, didn't feel symptoms

- Meal No. 4: Took four capsules, felt symptoms

- Target dose: three capsules

Most people will require anywhere from 1 to 7 capsules (depending on the brand and their needs) and will often find that they are able to wean off the supplement as time goes on and their digestion improves. Once you find your target dose, you may need to vary your dose based on how much and what type of protein you have. Some people find that they don't need as much with protein powders and vegetarian proteins, but need to increase their dose for a nice big juicy steak.

Please note, this enzyme is not for everyone:

- If you have a history of ulcers or current ulcers or take NSAID medications, aspirin, or steroid medications, do not take betaine with pepsin.

- Acid-suppressing medications can negate the effect of betaine with pepsin, so I don't recommend taking them together.

- If you do have a history of ulcers or use acid-suppressing medications, I recommend testing for gut infections, especially *H. pylori* and SIBO, which could be triggers for gut symptoms and Hashimoto's.

Systemic Enzymes

People with autoimmune disease often have a buildup of circulating immune complexes (CICs). CICs are molecular objects that are produced when an antibody and a reactive antigen, the toxin or foreign substance the antibody is attacking, bind together. CICs can be formed by antibodies mobilized against the thyroid gland as well as antibodies produced by the thyroid and can spell trouble, as they can contribute to liver congestion, autoimmune disease, and many associated symptoms, such as pain, inflammation, and even heart attacks!

Systemic enzymes, also known as proteolytic enzymes, can help bring our immune system into balance by breaking down these immune complexes. Proteolytic enzymes can also break down pathogens such as bacteria and parasites, but it is their role in breaking down the CICs that may reduce the antibodies to foods and to the thyroid.

The body does make some internal systemic enzymes, and we can also boost the break down of CICs by taking systemic enzymes externally. Systemic enzymes have been studied extensively in Europe and have become a popular alternative to pain medications for arthritic disease and many inflammatory conditions.

In one study, forty people with Hashimoto's who were taking levothyroxine were given systemic enzymes for three to six months. The patients reported a reduction of thyroid symptoms, a normalization of thyroid tissue was seen via ultrasound, the number of inflammatory cells in the thyroid was reduced, and significant decreases in thyroid antibodies were seen as well. Many of the study patients were able to reduce their dose of levothyroxine, and some were able to discontinue their medications completely. Patients who had high cholesterol levels before starting the enzymes also presented with improved cholesterol profiles.

In my work with Hashimoto's patients, systemic-enzyme supplementation for one to three months has shown to help significantly reduce both thyroid antibodies and food sensitivities. Clients also report less pain and improved wound healing. I also like to recommend them because they act on the whole immune system, and using them is thought to protect against developing future autoimmune conditions.

Systemic enzymes are a blend of plant- and animal-derived enzymes and may contain a mix of some of the following ingredients:

- Bromelain (from pineapple)

- Chymotrypsin (porcine)

- Pancreatin (porcine)

- Papain (from papaya)

- Rutin or rutoside trihydrate (bioflavonoid)

- Trypsin (porcine)

Systemic enzymes must be taken on an empty stomach at least 45 minutes before a meal or 90 minutes after a meal to work on the immune system. If you take them with food or too soon after you've eaten, they will get used up in the process of digestion instead of making their way to the bloodstream, where they can act on CICs.

The daily maintenance dose of systemic enzymes is typically considered to be 6 capsules. However, it should be noted that the dose of enzymes used in the study mentioned above was two and a half times higher, 5 capsules three times per day (on an empty stomach). This is the dose I recommend to my clients, and it's the one other experienced clinicians use. Each dose of 5 capsules should be taken with a full glass of water (at least 8 ounces). In some cases, even 10 capsules three times per day may be used in the acute phase to modulate the immune system effectively.

Fat Digestive Enzymes

Fat malabsorption is easily overlooked by patients and practitioners alike, but commonly affects 40 to 50 percent of people with Hashimoto's. Some signs and symptoms of fat malabsorption include greasy, smelly, floating, light-colored stools; gas or belching after eating; diarrhea; dry skin; stomach pain; gallbladder pain (which is on the right side, under the ribs), gallstones, or gallbladder removal; nausea; weight loss; hormonal imbalances; and adrenal issues. A low fecal elastase test in functional-medicine stool testing can also indicate fat malabsorption.

If you are not properly digesting and absorbing fats from food, you may start to experience low energy and increased cravings for carbs, since fats are an incredible slow-burning source of energy. If you've had fat malabsorption for some time, you may also find that you will start to develop symptoms of fatty-acid deficiency as well as depletions in the fat-soluble vitamins A, D, E, and K. Deficiencies in these nutrients can lead to numerous symptoms including vision problems, immune-system imbalance, fragile bones, poor wound healing, easy bruising, bleeding gums, nosebleeds, dull hair, depression, skin disorders, eczema, dry itchy/flaky skin or scalp, dandruff, oily scalp, rashes, and many other symptoms.

Another clue to fat malabsorption is when a person has been supplementing with vitamin D, but is still showing a deficiency on labs. Potential reasons why a person may have difficulty with fat absorption include bile deficiency, pancreatic enzyme deficiency, liver backlog, and SIBO.

EXOCRINE PANCREATIC INSUFFICIENCY

Some people with fat malabsorption may also have exocrine pancreatic insufficiency, or a deficiency in pancreatic enzymes. In this case, I've found supplementing with pancreatic enzymes to be very helpful. These enzymes are taken with every fat-containing meal. In about 50 percent of cases, I've seen pancreatic insufficiency resolve simply by using pancreatic enzymes for a few weeks to a few months; in other cases, people may need to take the enzymes long-term and do more detective work to identify why they are deficient in pancreatic enzymes. Pancreatic insufficiency may result from damaged microvilli, celiac disease, SIBO, toxicity, stress, or alcohol use.

The Rootcology supplement Liver and Gallbladder Support can help fat digestion in three different ways: it can support the liver's ability to process fat with milk thistle; give us extra bile through ox bile; and support our bile flow with dandelion, artichoke, and beet. If you have issues with fat malabsorption, this is life-changing support.

Chronic fat malabsorption may result in a deficiency of essential fatty acids. If you have signs of fatty acid deficiency such as pain, inflammation, dry skin, oily hair, acne, or eczema, you may benefit from 1 to 4 grams of fish oil per day.

Vegetable Digestive Enzymes

Many people with Hashimoto's may also have an impaired ability to digest vegetables due to their fiber and starch content. In some cases of hypothyroidism, an indigestible ball of plant fiber material known as a phytobezoar has been found to cause bowel obstruction! In the case of poor fiber absorption, undigested vegetable fibers may be found in the stools, and a high-fiber meal may cause bloating.

When fibrous foods aren't properly digested, we miss out on the valuable micronutrients that don't get extracted fully. One way to compensate for this somewhat is to juice vegetables and fruits, so that the nutrients are better absorbed.

A vegetable digestive enzyme that contains fiber-digesting enzymes like cellulase and/or starch-digesting enzymes like amylases might also help reduce symptoms of nutrient deficiencies and create increased energy.

Gluten/Dairy Digestive Enzymes

Gluten and dairy are two of the most common reactive foods for those with Hashimoto's. When the large protein molecules found in these foods are not fully broken down in the body, they may trigger an immune response from the IgG branch of the immune system. Because this is the same branch of the immune system that makes antibodies to the thyroid, every time one of these reactive foods is consumed, there is a greater production of IgG antibodies—including of the antibodies to the thyroid.

Unfortunately, for some people even small amounts of gluten and dairy can produce significant symptoms and delay progress in healing. This makes many individuals scared to go out to restaurants or visit relatives. Even if the meal they get is made without any gluten or dairy ingredients, there may be potential for cross-contamination if the food is prepared in the same kitchen where gluten/dairy-containing meals are prepared.

The enzyme dipeptidyl peptidase IV (DPP-4) can be helpful in splitting gluten into smaller fragments, so that it is easier to digest. It can be found in combination enzyme products that also contain enzymes that break down casein, beta-lactoglobulin (whey), and sometimes lactose (milk-sugar molecules found in dairy).

RAW VEGETABLES

Raw fruits and vegetables can be difficult to digest if you have leaky gut, which is why in the early stages of intestinal healing you may need to focus on eating well-cooked foods. Cooking and/or pureeing softens fibrous content, making fruits and vegetables easier to digest. Once these are tolerated, you can try to work your way back to raw vegetables with a peel. Start by adding in some raw, peeled pureed vegetables, then progress to raw peeled fruits and vegetables, and eventually try the unpeeled variety. As you begin reintroducing raw fruits and veggies, you may benefit from vegetable-digesting enzymes, which can assist in the breakdown of fibers.

Although enzymes may not be enough to allow a person with celiac disease to eat a whole bowl of pasta, the enzymes can be very helpful for those with a gluten and dairy sensitivity.

I utilize enzymes that aid with the breakdown of gluten and dairy whenever I go out to eat and am concerned about cross-contamination issues. I've used them after accidental consumption of small amounts of gluten or dairy and have found that the enzymes effectively minimize my reaction. I still have a reaction, but instead of suffering for two or three days, I have problems for only a couple of hours. Many of my clients and readers carry a bottle of gluten/

dairy digestive enzymes in their purses and travel bags for dining at restaurants and accidental exposures.

CUSTOMIZED DIETARY MODIFICATIONS FOR SPECIFIC CONCERNS

Although enzymes can provide critical support to digestion and increase nutrient absorption, you may find yourself still experiencing specific symptoms that require a more customized approach. Let's explore some of these symptoms and how you might address them directly.

Certain factors such as your ethnic background, current health status, habits, environment, stress levels, infections, toxin exposure, and symptoms may require more specific dietary modifications in addition to those included in the healing diets. Here are some targeted modifications you can consider based on your symptoms or underlying triggers:

- For food-sensitivity reactions such as breakouts, bloating, fatigue, and/or headaches after meals: do a food-sensitivity test and remove foods based on the results.

- If you are an athlete and are finding that you are lacking in fuel: try increasing your carbohydrate intake through healthy carbs like sweet potatoes and whole fruits.

- For fructose malabsorption or blood-sugar abnormalities: reduce fructose intake to less than 50 grams per day.

- For symptoms of copper toxicity, such as acne/hormonal breakouts, fatigue, emotional lability, or a reddish tint to hair: consider a low-copper diet.

- For symptoms of citrus sensitivity such as fatigue, allergies, headaches, sinus issues, rashes, and upset stomach: remove citrus fruit.

- For impaired detoxification: try a two-week vegan/vegetarian diet.

- For *Candida*: try a yeast-limiting diet like the Body Ecology Diet.

- For neurological issues such as depression, anxiety, brain fog, epilepsy, or migraines: try a ketogenic diet—a low-carb diet where the body breaks down fats for fuel instead of relying on carbohydrates.

- For sulfur toxicity with symptoms such as dry skin, breakouts, and rashes: follow a low-sulfur diet to eliminate symptoms.

- For mercury toxicity: follow a low-seafood diet.

- For severe reactions to dairy with continuing symptoms: experiment with a trial beef avoidance (may be especially helpful with pain).

DIGESTIVE ENZYME SUPPLEMENTATION

ENZYME TYPE	PURPOSE	HOW TO TAKE	RECOMMENDED BRAND
Betaine with pepsin	To support protein digestion, low stomach acid	Dose determined by trial, usually 1–7 capsules per day with protein-containing meals	Betaine with Pepsin by Rootcology or Pure Encapsulations
Fat digestive enzymes	To support fat digestion	With meals, follow package instructions	Rootcology Liver & Gallbladder Support; Digestion GB, Pure Encapsulations
Pancreatic enzymes	To support digestion of fats, carbohydrates, and proteins	With meals of protein, fat, and/or carbohydrates, in case of pancreatic enzyme deficiency	Rootcology Pancreatic Enzymes Plus; Pure Encapsulations Pancreatic Enzymes
Systemic (or proteolytic) enzymes	To break down CICs, reduce antibodies against food and the thyroid	5–10 capsules/tablets on an empty stomach, 3 times daily, apart from food	Wobenzym; Pure Encapsulations Systemic Enzymes
Vegetable digestive enzymes	To break down fiber and starch in vegetables	Take with starchy and/or fibrous foods such as raw fruit and veggies	Rootcology Veggie Enzymes; Digestive Enzymes Ultra, Pure Encapsulations
Gluten/dairy digestive enzymes	To minimize reactions from accidental exposures to gluten and/or dairy	Take with meals when eating out, eating foods that may be cross-contaminated with gluten/dairy, or after accidental exposures	Gluten/Dairy Digest, Pure Encapsulations

- For inflammatory issues not resolved by other diets or interventions such as pain, vulvodynia, fibromyalgia, urinary burning, kidney stones, or irritable bladder: follow a low-oxalate diet.

- For cases of malabsorption: consider reducing raw foods and try pureeing foods.

- For improving detoxification: increase your intake of raw foods.

- For mold toxicity: you may benefit from avoiding high-mold foods and beverages such as peanuts, raisins, dried fruit, nuts, coffee, beer, and wine or eating a low-mold diet like the Bulletproof Diet.

If you do remove or eliminate a certain food or foods as recommended in some of these steps, you can test it to see if it is in fact what's causing your symptoms. To do this, remove all sources of the food for three weeks, observing your symptoms throughout, and then reintroduce the food by eating it during three consecutive days. Observe your symptoms over these three days to determine if the food is indeed reactive.

If you didn't see your symptom listed above, see if you can spot it on the chart on page 81—and if you do, give the suggested strategy in the "Also Try" column a go.

I've written about resolving many of these symptoms in great detail on my website. If you'd like more details on any of these symptoms as well as more symptom solutions, please visit thyroidpharmacist .com/food to get my free Thyroid Symptom Solutions eBook.

BRINGING IT ALL TOGETHER: USING NUTRITION KNOWLEDGE WITH THE RECIPES

When you get to the recipes, you'll see a nutritional analysis at the bottom of each one that shares the B_{12}, iron, iodine, magnesium, and selenium content. These key nutrients are included because they are involved in and often deficient in thyroid conditions. It should be noted that in the case of iron, there are two forms: heme and nonheme. Animal proteins contain both heme and nonheme, while plant foods contain just nonheme. Since nonheme is not as easily absorbed, it's best to consume plant foods high in iron with vitamin C–rich foods. My Truffled Veggies (p. 279) is a perfect example of an iron-rich plant-based dish!

The nutritional analysis also includes macronutrient details, which can help you determine your need for specific supporting digestive enzymes. For example, meals that are richer in protein will require more betaine with pepsin compared to foods that have low amounts of protein. If a dish doesn't contain protein, you will not need the betaine with pepsin.

Each recipe is analyzed for one serving, but of course some individuals will consume more than one serving—you can simply double (or triple) the serving figures

WHAT ARE YOUR SYMPTOMS TRYING TO TELL YOU?

SYMPTOMS	COMMON NUTRITIONAL CAUSES	ALSO TRY
Acne	Gluten, dairy, eggs, nuts, toxins	Tanning, organic skin care, sweating, zinc, fish oil, low-copper diet
Anxiety	Caffeine, tea, coffee, chocolate, sugar, blood-sugar imbalances, gluten, dairy, nuts	Selenium, balancing blood sugar, probiotics, fermented foods, magnesium, low-copper diet
Asthma	Dairy, gluten, eggs, nuts	NAC, indoor air purifier, salt therapy, SIBO treatment, address mold/yeast
Depression	Gluten, dairy, grains, soy, nuts/seeds	Blue light during the day, probiotics, fermented foods, fish oil
Fatigue	Poor digestion, gluten, dairy, nutrient deficiencies	Betaine with pepsin, lemon water, thiamine, green smoothies; test for B_{12}, ferritin, and vitamin D levels
Gallbladder issues	Egg, pork, onion, poultry, milk, coffee, orange, corn, nuts, tomatoes	Liver & Gallbladder Support by Rootcology; Digestion GB by Pure Encapsulations
GERD	Gluten, dairy, eggs, nuts	*H. pylori* treatment, digestive enzymes, magnesium
Hair loss	Low ferritin, blood-sugar swings	T3 containing thyroid meds, optimize TSH, biotin, zinc, gelatin, collagen, omega-3s
IBS	Gluten, dairy, grains, raw vegetables	High-dose probiotics, digestive enzymes, parasite cleanse, SIBO testing
Migraines	Gluten, dairy, eggs, yeast, corn, sugar, citrus, coffee, tea, chocolate, beef	Magnesium supplement, Epsom salt baths, *H. pylori* testing
Pain	Gluten, dairy, grains, nightshades	Low-level laser therapy, Epsom salt baths, acupuncture, chiropractic, magnesium
Trouble gaining weight	Not eating enough calories	Support adrenals, gut testing, the Root Cause Building Smoothie (p. 171), track calories (use a calorie-counting app), reduce stress
Trouble losing weight	Carbohydrates, gluten, dairy, processed foods, low-calorie diet	Rest more, test adrenals, probiotics, less exercise, more calories (real food), multivitamins, check medication side effects, test for nutrient deficiencies, check digestion and nutrient absorption

depending on how much you are eating for your meal. Additionally, I've included sodium and potassium for each recipe, for those who wish to track their levels.

I specifically did not include calories, because I feel that we should be focusing on nutrient density for healing rather than counting calories. If you follow my meal plans, you will be consuming appropriate amounts of nutrients with a whole-food approach and therefore your calories will fall into place. You will find that soon enough you will feel and look healthier and begin to shed unwanted symptoms.

4.

Making It Work! Habits, Tools, and Strategies for Success

Changing the way you've been eating, just like changing any habit, can be challenging at first, since it requires paying more attention than we normally do to what we put in our bodies. But it is so worth it! Your body will repay you, and you will soon see that your symptoms will vanish before your eyes. Furthermore, as time goes on, you will get in the habit of eating nutritious foods, and this way of eating will become second nature.

One way to prepare for the challenge is to make sure you are in the right frame of mind. This is the one that sees the attention you are paying to yourself and your nourishment needs as an essential act of self-care, one that will hopefully continue on indefinitely. As I tell my clients, *the practice of compassionate self-care is a long-term strategy for your best health.*

Of course, there are also tangible ways to prepare for and even minimize any stress you may feel about making dietary changes. You may have heard the phrase, "If you fail to plan, you're planning to fail."

After reading up on the theory and guidelines, you may be interested in the practical applications of your new lifestyle. If you're anything like me and my clients, you likely have lots of questions, and I know that sometimes just one of these questions may be a roadblock for getting started or continuing on the road to success.

In this chapter I share some of my best success strategies for making the new lifestyle work for you, including:

- Optimizing your kitchen for your new lifestyle

- Getting the right tools to make life easier

- Choosing the most healing ingredients

- Making healthy replacements for common staples

- Shopping for quality and specialty foods without breaking the bank

- Keeping the new diet exciting

- Making real food in real life when you're busy

- Making the lifestyle work with the whole family

- Dealing with unsupportive people

- Eating out

Let's dive in!

LET'S LOOK AT YOUR KITCHEN

I've found that having a reliable plan of action for making over your diet starts with making over your kitchen! I have two suggestions to do so. I recommend, first, "greening your kitchen" by removing the low-hanging, everyday toxins that are present in your kitchen and may be seeping into your foods, and, second, investing in tools that will help make life easier, either by speeding up or simplifying a cooking process.

Greening Your Kitchen

You may not realize it, but toxic substances are likely lurking throughout your kitchen cupboards and drawers; they exist in cookware, food-storage containers, utensils, and more. Here are seven simple ways you can minimize your in-home exposure:

1. Use glass baking dishes, ceramic-coated pots and pans, and cast-iron skillets instead of Teflon-coated or stainless-steel pots and pans.

2. Use wood utensils instead of plastic or metal-coated ones.

3. Use glass containers, such as wide-mouth Mason jars, instead of plastic containers for food storage.

4. Invest in BPA-free storage bags.

5. Never heat or cook foods in plastic, as this can release toxins.

6. Swap out aluminum foil for chlorine-free parchment paper when baking, grilling, and steaming.

7. Invest in a reverse osmosis filter to remove fluoride, a thyroid toxin, from the water supply you use for cooking and drinking.

Transitioning your kitchen into a space that contains fewer toxins will likely take time. However, you shouldn't feel the need to postpone trying any recipes or removing reactive foods from your diet until you've greened up your cooking space. In fact, the sooner you get started on your healthy diet, the sooner you will likely start to feel better. Make the adjustments in your kitchen as time and money allow, and make cooking healing foods for yourself the number-one priority.

Kitchen Tools That Simplify Your Life

Many of these tools may seem like a luxury but they are a worthwhile investment because they can make your life much easier as you adjust to a real-food lifestyle and increase your likelihood of success! Here is a list of must-have tools:

Slow cooker: A slow cooker is an electric pot that cooks your food slowly over a longer period of time at low temperatures. You throw in raw ingredients, turn the pot on, and can go to work or take a nap while the pot does all of the work! It has become such an essential part of my cooking that I'm not sure how I functioned before I got one. I use it to make Bone Broth (p. 135), Winter Oxtail Stew (p. 191), Cuban Ropa Vieja (p. 181), Hubby's Carnitas (p. 228), and many other favorite dishes. One of my favorite things is to wake up or come home to fragrant food that's waiting for me!

High-powered blender: A high-powered blender is a workhorse that can be used to make green smoothies, cauliflower mashed potatoes, soups, nut butters, and even your own mayonnaise and coconut yogurt. If I could have only one appliance in my kitchen, this would be it!

Masticating juicer: A masticating juicer "chews" fruits and vegetables instead of cutting and spinning them, allowing more nutrients to infuse the juice. Drinking the juice lets you get more nutrients into your body!

Electric pressure cooker: An electric pressure cooker is a fantastic cooking appliance that allows you create hearty, nourishing meals in a relatively short amount of time. When you add your ingredients, along with water or cooking broth, securely fasten the lid, and set the controls to heat the vessel, the contents are under pressure, water reaches a higher temperature than its normal boiling point, and the resulting cooking process is sped up.

Glass baking dishes: Glass baking dishes are an incredibly versatile must-have in your kitchen. I use them for quiches (Mexican Quiche, p. 245; Broccoli and Chicken Quiche, p. 246), Baked Ginger-Lemon Chicken Thighs (p. 259), Bacon and Chive Scalloped Potatoes (p. 282), Almond and Date Snack Bars (p. 310), and so much more. I recommend getting a variety of sizes. Some also come with tops, so you can use them to store leftovers.

Mason jars: I love my Mason jars. They can be used for serving beverages, food storage, and meal preparation for the whole week when you make Jar Salad (p. 196) and smoothies.

Fermenting crock pot: If you want to get fancy, traditional Polish or German fermentation pots can be used to make fermented vegetables, which help to repopulate the gut with good bacteria.

Some optional but fun tools include:

Spiralizer: This awesome tool makes all kinds of veggies into noodles and thin slices that cook much faster. The veggie noodles made at home are much healthier than gluten-free noodles, which are full of processed grains! I love making noodles from zucchini, beets, and sweet potatoes!

Waffle iron: Every now and then you may miss certain textures or comfort foods. Dedicating a waffle iron to gluten-free creations for those slow weekend mornings might be just the thing that hits the spot (speaking from personal experience here!).

Roasting pan: I love using a roasting pan for quick one-pot weekday meals. You can place a whole chicken or duck on top of veggies in a roasting pan, add some fat, such as coconut oil or duck fat, cover, and let them bake! Keeping the moisture in results in juicy meats and yummy veggies.

Cast-iron skillet: Cast-iron skillets are fantastic for making quick stir-frys, hashes, and one-pot stovetop meals. As an added bonus, they can help with supporting your iron and ferritin levels!

CHOOSING QUALITY INGREDIENTS

Over the years, I've learned how to shop efficiently for the highest-quality ingredients. I want to share some tips on how you can do the same.

When it comes to proteins, it's important to remember to choose organic varieties over conventional when possible. Organic practices require livestock to be raised outside at least part of the year and that a percentage of their diet be met through foraging for food (this is where the terms "pasture-raised" and "grass-fed" come from). This more natural lifestyle leads to proteins that are higher in beneficial omega-3s and lower in omega-6s. Omega-3 fatty acids are linked to better immune function, and organic meats have been shown to contain about 50 percent more than conventional meats.

Fish should be wild caught and low in mercury. Some excellent choices are salmon and sardines, while tuna and shark should be limited due to high mercury content.

If you can find a local farmer who raises chickens, ask if you can buy their eggs; chances are they will be from happily roaming chickens. Inquire about the feed—some people who previously thought they were egg intolerant have found that they tolerate eggs from chickens fed a non-GMO and soy-free diet.

Studies have also shown that organic fruits and vegetables have higher levels of antioxidants, which have anti-inflammatory benefits. Organic farmers rotate crops, use compost as fertilizer, and rely on natural alternatives to pesticides—strategies that lead to more nutrient-rich soil (this means more nutrients for the produce), slower growth (more time for nutrients to develop),

MERCURY LEVELS IN FISH

HIGHEST MERCURY: AVOID EATING

Mackerel (king)

Marlin

Orange roughy

Shark

Swordfish

Tilefish

Tuna (bigeye, ahi)

HIGH MERCURY: EAT NO MORE THAN THREE 6-OZ. SERVINGS A MONTH

Bluefish

Grouper

Mackerel (Spanish, Gulf)

Sea bass (Chilean)

Tuna (canned, white albacore)

Tuna (yellowfin)

LOW MERCURY: EAT NO MORE THAN SIX 6-OZ. SERVINGS A MONTH

Bass (striped, black)

Carp

Cod (Alaskan)

Croaker (White Pacific)

Halibut (Pacific and Atlantic)

Jacksmelt (silverside)

Lobster

Mahi-mahi

Monkfish

Perch (freshwater)

Sablefish

Skate

Snapper

Sea trout (weakfish)

Tuna (canned, chunk light)

Tuna (skipjack)

LOWEST MERCURY: ENJOY TWO 6-OZ. SERVINGS A WEEK

Anchovies

Butterfish

Catfish

Clams

Crab (domestic)

Crawfish/crayfish

Croaker

Flounder

Haddock

Hake

Herring

Mackerel (North Atlantic, chub)

Mullet

Oysters

Perch (ocean)

Plaice

Salmon

Sardines

Scallops

Shad (American)

Shrimp

Sole

Squid (calamari)

Tilapia

Trout (freshwater)

Whitefish

Whiting

Adapted from American Pregnancy Association, "Mercury Levels in Fish," http://americanpregnancy.org/app/uploads/2013/03/mercurylevelsinfish.pdf.

and crops that have to fend for themselves (this results in an increase in protective compounds that can benefit us).

Nonorganic produce has varying degrees of pesticide residue; some varieties are safer to buy than others. I rely on the Environmental Workgroup (EWG), a nonprofit consumer-protection agency, to help determine my must-buy organic fruits and vegetables. Every year, they produce the "EWG's Shopper's Guide to Pesticides in Produce," which includes two lists: the Dirty Dozen Plus and the Clean Fifteen. The Dirty Dozen Plus reveals the produce with the highest loads of pesticide residue, and the Clean Fifteen lists the produce with the least. We can use these lists to help make choices that lower your pesticide exposure (and save money when possible).

Organic and nonorganic produce is usually clearly marked when you shop at a grocery store. You can also go to a farmers' market or a local farm to pick up quality ingredients! To help you decide if you want to purchase from a farm:

EWG'S 2018 SHOPPER'S GUIDE TO PESTICIDES IN PRODUCE

THE DIRTY DOZEN PLUS: CONTAIN THE MOST PESTICIDE RESIDUE	THE CLEAN FIFTEEN: CONTAIN THE LEAST PESTICIDE RESIDUE
1. Strawberries	1. Avocados
2. Spinach	2. Sweet corn*
3. Nectarines	3. Pineapples
4. Apples	4. Cabbage
5. Grapes	5. Onions
6. Peaches	6. Sweet peas frozen
7. Cherries	7. Papayas*
8. Pears	8. Asparagus
9. Tomatoes	9. Mangoes
10. Celery	10. Eggplant
11. Potatoes	11. Honeydew melons
12. Sweet bell peppers and hot peppers	12. Kiwis
	13. Cantaloupes
	14. Cauliflower
	15. Broccoli

* A small amount of sweet corn, papaya, and summer squash sold in the United States is produced from genetically modified seeds. Buy organic varieties of these crops if you want to avoid genetically modified produce.

- Ask if the farm is certified organic or if it has any other certifications that would imply safer farming practices.

- Ask if GMO seeds are used or if seeds are heirloom and/or certified organic.

- Ask to take a farm tour. (If you see nets, this is a good sign—they are sometimes used in place of sprays for pest control.)

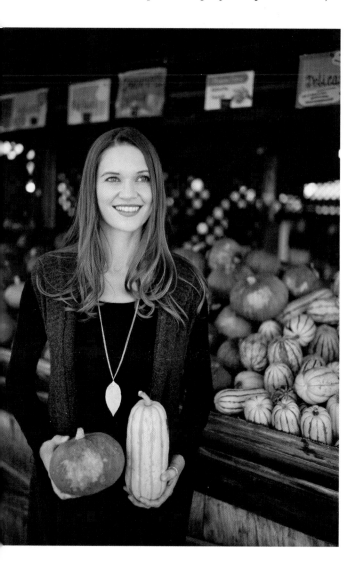

Additional Tips for Choosing Quality Ingredients

- Read the labels—the label will disclose so much about what is in the food. Try to focus on foods that do not carry labels: fresh fruits and vegetables, fresh meats. Canned foods that are organic generally have only water and salt in addition to the food item.

- Shop the perimeter of the grocery store. The outside of the store generally focuses on fresh fruits, vegetables, and protein.

- Food additives and preservatives can cause a host of problems including behavioral issues, headaches, confusion, and gastrointestinal issues, to name a few. Avoid foods that have additives such as:

  Artificial sweeteners

  BHA/BHT

  Carrageenan

  Casein (and anything with the word "casein" in the description)

  Food dyes

  Lactose (and anything with the word "lactose" in the description)

  Monosodium glutamate (MSG)

  Sodium benzoate

  Soy

  Sugar alcohols

  Thickeners

SUBSTITUTIONS FOR TRADITIONAL INGREDIENTS

INGREDIENT TYPE	TRADITIONAL INGREDIENTS TO AVOID	APPROVED INGREDIENTS FOR AUTOIMMUNE, PALEO, AND INTRO DIETS
Cooking oils	vegetable oil, canola oil, corn oil, peanut oil, seed oils, nut oils	AI: cold-pressed oils, coconut oil, avocado oil, olive oil, grass-fed animal lard Paleo: ghee, AI oils (see above) Intro: all of the foods approved for AI and Paleo (see above)
Gluten-containing products	whole-grain flour, couscous, pasta, breadcrumbs, oats not labeled gluten free	AI: cassava, tapioca, arrowroot and coconut flours; spiralized vegetable noodles (zucchini, sweet potato, butternut squash); spaghetti squash Paleo: almond flour, AI flours (see above) Intro: chickpea flour, quinoa, rice, gluten-free pasta, gluten-free breadcrumbs, gluten-free oats, AI and Paleo gluten-free products (see above)
Dairy products	products derived from the milk of cows, sheep, goats, camels (although some may be able to tolerate camel's milk): milk, yogurt, ice cream, cheese, butter, protein powders (whey); sneaky ingredients such as casein, whey, lactose, lactic acid (look for variations of these names in ingredient lists)	AI: coconut milk, coconut yogurt, coconut ice cream, frozen banana/fruit ice cream, coconut butter, hydrolyzed beef protein, nutritional yeast*, coconut oil, vegetable shortening from palm oil for baking, duck fat in place of butter for roasting Paleo: nut milks, almond yogurt, almond ice cream, pea protein, egg white protein,* cashew cream cheese, AI nondairy products (see above) Intro: vegan cheese (such as Daiya), camel's milk*, AI and Paleo nondairy products (see above)
Sweeteners	sugar (cane sugar, dextrose, corn syrup, fructose, brown sugar, raw sugar, Sucanat, turbinado, agave, nectar); artificial sweeteners (aspartame, sucralose, saccharin, acesulfame)	AI: honey, maple syrup, molasses, fruit juice (fresh squeezed), dates Paleo: coconut sugar, stevia, monk fruit, coconut palm sugar, xylitol, trehalose, AI-approved sweeteners (see above) Intro: all of the foods approved for AI and Paleo (see above)
Thickeners	thickeners: cornstarch, potato starch, gums	AI: arrowroot powder, tapioca powder, gelatin Paleo: chia seeds, AI thickeners (see above) Intro: all of the foods approved for AI and Paleo (see above)
Eggs	whole eggs, egg white protein, dried egg	AI: hydrolyzed beef protein (not a binder), gelatin, apple cider vinegar, applesauce (for baking) Paleo: flaxseed, chia seed, pea protein, AI egg replacers (see above) Intro: all of the foods approved for AI and Paleo (see above)

*Denotes that a sensitivity to the food item is more likely to occur.

Stocking Up on Safe Ingredients

As you're getting ready to transition to one of the dietary templates, you may be wondering how you'll ever replace everyday traditional ingredients, like cheese, butter, vegetable oils, protein powders, flours, and other potentially inflammatory ingredients, with ingredients that are safe for people with Hashimoto's. Thankfully, there are plenty of great-tasting substitutes that you can have on hand when you need them. The table on page 90 offers some of the best alternate choices.

Where to Shop for Quality Ingredients

I also recommend developing a reliable list of the places you can get the ingredients you'll be using most. If you are dealing with Hashimoto's-related fatigue or any other energy-draining symptoms, you don't want to spend your entire day searching for the healthy ingredients you need.

Local health-food stores, farmers' markets, and farms: One of the reasons I decided to move to Boulder, Colorado, is because of the abundance of farmers' markets, health-foods stores, and farms that carry high-quality foods. Within a fifteen-minute drive from my home, I can pick up organic, free-range duck eggs from a local farm, gluten-free snacks from the local health-food store, and seasonal organic fruit from the farmers' market! If you haven't been to one of these, I highly recommend you get into the habit of checking them out!

Local Community Supported Agriculture (CSA) delivery: If you want to get deliveries of fresh and seasonal produce from local farms, you may want to consider signing up for a CSA box. Check www.localharvest.org to see what farms in your area may deliver. You can usually customize your order for the size box you would like (for the number people you will be feeding) and how often you would like a delivery.

Online resources: Luckily for us, we are living in a time when a lot of what we need can be found online and shipped straight to us wherever we are. Here are some of the places I like to shop for high-quality ingredients online:

Rootcology.com. The Rootcology website carries the least reactive protein powders I can formulate for people with Hashimoto's, including two hydrolyzed beef proteins (AI Paleo and Paleo Protein), as well as Organic Pea Protein.

Flavor Chef Bone Broth. This excellent brand of flavorful, entirely organically sourced, slow-simmered bone broth in chicken and beef is a go-to base for so many dishes. (Receive 10 percent off by using code Thyroid10.)

US Wellness Meats. This company produces the finest grass-fed and organic meat with no antibiotics or growth hormones that are rich in nutrients and higher in essential vitamins and minerals. You can buy a variety of organic meats and poultry, including beef, bison, lamb, pork, rabbit, chicken, and duck. It also has a selection of wild-caught seafood.

Vital Choice Seafood and Organics. A trusted source for fast home delivery of the world's finest wild seafood and organic fare, harvested from healthy, well-managed wild fisheries and farms, Vital Choice is a leading source of pure, healthful, sustainable foods and omega-3 supplements.

Butcher Box. Butcher Box provides the highest-quality organically sourced, fresh-frozen bone broths on the market. (Get free bacon and $10 off using code THYROID.)

Paleovalley Snacks. Paleovalley provides delicious snacks that are free from additives.

Dry Farm Wines. Dry Farm Wines is a source of natural and organic family-farmed wines that are low in alcohol, sugar, carbs, and sulfites, and additive free.

Thrive Market. A membership community that uses the power of direct buying to deliver the world's best healthy food and natural products at wholesale prices, Thrive Market provides products that adhere to various dietary preferences such as dairy free, vegetarian, organic, Paleo, and gluten-free.

Amazon.com. Amazon carries numerous pantry staples and specialty items such as duck fat, coconut wraps, creamed coconut, maca, chia seeds, and various gluten-free flours.

Desert Farms Camel Milk. Camel's milk is the safest animal milk for people with cow's milk sensitivity; it also has potential gut-healing properties.

For a comprehensive list of resources and special discounts, please visit thyroidpharmacist.com/resources.

Tips and Strategies for Saving Money on Real Foods

Eating real food is an investment in your health and will be more costly than eating processed foods. But you are so worth it! Here are some tips to save money!

SNACKS

Sometimes you need a snack to carry you over between meals! Here are some snack ideas:

Intro: Hummus, Chilly Day Chili (p. 178), all of the options below

Paleo: Almond and Date Snack Bars (p. 310), Red Pepper Turkey Dip (p. 309), nuts, seeds, Paleovalley snack bars, hard-boiled eggs, Epic bars, Tanka bars, Lärabars, Hemp Heart bars, all of the options below

Autoimmune: Cilantro-Lime Guacamole (p. 287), Coconut Yogurt (p. 131), Beef Jerky (p. 307), Lemon–Banana Cream Ice Pops (p. 341), smoothies, sardines, fruit leathers, fruit, veggies

- Purchase canned coconut milk in bulk. I like to buy a dozen cans when they are on sale. It's so versatile and can be used in many recipes, plus it has a long shelf life.

- Get cheaper cuts of organic or grass-fed meats, such as chicken thighs and legs, skirt steak, and organ meats, which are generally more nutrient dense with a smaller price tag. Many times these meats are tougher cuts and need to be slow-cooked.

- Purchase produce that is in season or join a food-share box program through which you receive seasonal fresh produce weekly. Shopping at farmers' markets is one way to ensure that your fruits and vegetables are local and in season, and you can inquire about what is used on the produce for pest control. If you do your shopping close to the end of the market, you may get some "must go" deals.

- Watch for sales on frozen organic fruits and vegetables, and when they arrive, stock up your freezer with produce for later use. Fruits and vegetables that are frozen are picked at their prime.

KEYS TO KEEPING YOUR DIET EXCITING

Of course, knowing where to get your ingredients is great, but knowing what to do with them once they're in your kitchen is equally important, if not even more so. In each of

the recipes in the Cookbook section, you will find specific instructions for preparation, but I also want to share with you some strategies related to general food preparation and variety that I think will be helpful as you start to modify your meals.

As you know by now, the recipes featured in this book are based on diets designed to help you heal from Hashimoto's. You also know that these diets focus on the removal of reactive foods, which will by default exclude most processed foods. What you may not know is that, depending on your dietary habits beforehand, the dietary changes you are going to introduce may produce some cravings and perhaps even elicit a mini-revolt by your palate. Some of the foods you try may taste bland or boring to you at first, but this is to be expected, and I want to reassure you that this won't last.

If you've been eating a lot of processed foods, especially if this includes fast foods, your palate has likely been exposed to a lot of engineered flavors that have been created to trick your taste buds into wanting more, and more, and then some more. When you shift to a diet focused on real foods, you will ultimately crave these healthier-for-you foods too, but it may take a little time for the adjustment to take place. What's critical is that you remain connected to the fact that you are eating with a purpose: to help your body heal.

I've found a few strategies that have made it easier for me and my clients to stick to a nutrient-dense, healing diet. Using a variety of spices and trying different cooking methods to create a mixture of textures and flavors have both proven effective at making the transition easier and at helping prevent diet boredom.

Spice Up Your Life!

Spices add flavor and medicinal properties to our foods. I call this a win-win from a food pharmacology perspective!

Here are some of my favorite spices as well as just a few of the many benefits of each spice:

- Pumpkin pie spice helps to balance blood sugar and promotes tissue regeneration.

- Sea salt may help with adrenals and contains beneficial minerals. (Truffled sea salt has the same benefits as sea salt, with an extra punch of flavor!)

- Basil supports digestion and blood-sugar balance.

- Oregano has antifungal and antiviral properties.

- Turmeric has detoxifying and anti-inflammatory properties.

- Garlic powder has antimicrobial properties.

- Cardamom has antimicrobial properties, especially for the mouth.

- Ginger is an antioxidant and anti-inflammatory and helps with nausea.

- Cilantro helps detoxify the liver and chelates heavy metals.

TIME TO RETHINK YOUR SALT SELECTION

Processed salt consumption has been linked to autoimmune disease, and the fortification of salt with iodine is partially responsible for the Hashimoto's epidemic. In fact, studies have found that iodine fortification has led to an *increased* incidence of Hashimoto's!! So should you avoid salt? No, but you will want to make sure you're using the right kind.

Avoid salt that is processed and/or fortified with iodine; instead, use sea salt with naturally occurring minerals! You can add generous amounts of sea salt in your food to address cravings you might be experiencing (underlying adrenal dysfunction can cause subclinical electrolyte imbalances that can increase cravings for salt). If you're still using processed iodized salt, I suggest tossing it and picking up gray or pink sea salt for cooking and eating.

If you regularly feel light-headed and faint after getting up, you might also consider adding a teaspoon of sea salt to a glass of warm water and drinking it each day to see if this helps.

Please note, salt is not bad for us—it actually helps balance our electrolytes. However, you want to select the right kind of salt!

Autoimmune-Unfriendly Spices

Additionally I want to make you aware that some spices are not allowed on the auto-immune dietary protocol. Thus we avoid nutmeg, cumin, and paprika during the autoimmune diet entirely, but you can make autoimmune-friendly versions your-self. Luckily, you can make your own spice blends! Just add the spices to a bowl and mix thoroughly. Throughout the recipe sec-tion, when you see the comment "(if toler-ated)" next to an ingredient, you will know to make your own blend when necessary.

Additionally, although black pepper, allspice, and cardamom are generally safe on autoimmune diets, they can be reactive for some people. You may want to use them with caution.

Varied Cooking Methods

Varied cooking methods are key to keeping your palate happy, even when you can only tolerate a limited number of ingredients. Oftentimes we miss certain textures more than the foods themselves. We can create and replicate various textures by mixing up our cooking methods. Let's use the humble carrot to demonstrate how many different options we can create with just one ingre-dient. Here are nine ways to enjoy carrots (and some recipes to try!):

1. **Roasted carrots:** Drizzle with olive oil and roast at 350°F for 30 minutes (or make Carrot Fries, p. 312)

SPICE RECIPES

AI Curry Powder

1 tablespoon ground turmeric
1 teaspoon ground ginger
1 teaspoon onion powder
½ teaspoon garlic powder
¼ teaspoon dried dill weed (not seed)
⅛ teaspoon ground cinnamon
⅛ teaspoon ground cloves

Curry powder has a host of ingredients that are not AI compliant, including coriander seeds, cumin, hot peppers, and cardamom. You may wonder why I've included dill in my recipe for curry powder—it adds a bit of tang to the flavor, but surprisingly is minimally detectable!

AI Pumpkin Pie Spice

3 tablespoons ground cinnamon
2 teaspoons ground mace
1 teaspoon ground ginger
¼ teaspoon ground cloves

Nutmeg and allspice are not compliant for AI followers. Simply make your own AI Pumpkin Pie Spice! Replacing these two spices with mace will yield a flavor very similar to traditional pumpkin pie spice.

AI Herbes de Provence

1 tablespoon marjoram
1 teaspoon basil
1 teaspoon savory
1 teaspoon rosemary
1 teaspoon lavender
1 teaspoon oregano
½ teaspoon thyme

You may be able to find an herbes de Provence blend on the market that does not contain fennel, but if not, just try this combination of dried herbs.

2. **Steamed carrots:** Cut into ¼-inch pieces and steam for about 10 minutes or until fork tender

3. **Shredded raw carrots with apple:** Apple-Carrot Salad (p. 293)

4. **Juiced carrots:** Green Juice (p. 153)

5. **Pureed carrot soup:** Carrot-Ginger-Pear Soup (p. 186)

6. **Mashed carrots:** Parsnip-Carrot Mash (p. 304)

7. **Carrot noodles:** Use a spiralizer to create carrot noodles you can use as a side dish for meatballs (Citrus Bison Meatballs, p. 222; Squashghetti and Meatballs, p. 253)

8. **Raw carrots:** Slice into ¼-inch-wide sticks and use with dip

9. **Stewed carrots:** Chop into ½-inch pieces and stew in a slow cooker 6 to 8 hours (as in Beef Stew, p. 174)

In each of these, you will find a different textural or even taste experience. Roasted carrots may caramelize and turn richly sweet; raw carrots provide a fantastically dense and satisfying crunch; pureed carrots enjoyed in a soup taste soothing and nourishing; shredded carrots with a bit of apple are reminiscent of summer picnic fun. I encourage you to try as many of these preparations as possible when cooking for yourself. In the recipes, you'll see that I've used all of the cooking methods mentioned above, but I also love stir-frying, blending, and slow-cooking.

SAVING TIME

One of the biggest challenges of eating a real-food diet is that many meals require cooking from scratch. This can be a big feat when you have a full life and are fatigued, brain-fogged, and overwhelmed by dietary changes. I've created the recipes in this cookbook with this in mind. The majority of the recipes are simple weekday recipes (with some fancy weekend recipes thrown in just for fun!). You'll notice that I try to minimize time-consuming food preparation techniques such as chopping, peeling, or dicing vegetables and instead opt for using whole, unpeeled vegetables whenever possible. This method doesn't just save time but also provides more nutrients. Additionally, many of the recipes work really well with a busy schedule by utilizing freezing, slow-cooking, and batch cooking. Batch cooking is a method I personally use each week to ensure that, no matter how busy I get, I continue to nourish my body.

The Fine Art of Batch Cooking

When I first started cooking all my meals from scratch for myself, there were times when I felt overwhelmed by the effort it took to meet my nourishment needs. This feeling lessened as I got better at food preparation and cooking, and especially when I started batch cooking, which became a life-changing habit for me. I've since encouraged batch cooking as a food-prep strategy to my clients, and everyone who's tried it has come back telling me how much it's helped them.

The idea behind batch cooking is really just that you want to maximize the amount of food prepared for the week and minimize the mess you make. Most people already practice a form of this by doubling a dish and then eating leftovers or freezing food for later use. With a little more strategy, you can cook a week's worth of food in a relatively short amount of time.

You can make batch cooking work even if you have a small kitchen. When I lived in an apartment that had four stovetop surfaces, a medium-size oven, and moderate amounts of counter space, I found a way to do it. I didn't have too many kitchen tools at the time, but I did have a Vitamix blender, a slow cooker, and two roasting/baking dishes (a small one and a large one).

The first thing I recommend is picking part of one day to do some cooking; I like to dedicate my Sunday afternoon to this task. Here's an example of how a batch cooking session might work:

1. Look around your kitchen. What types of surfaces and kitchen tools do you have? Make a plan of your kitchen and pick recipes that will help you maximize your space and time. For example, you may have a counter to chop veggies, a blender to prep smoothies or soups, a stovetop for making a stir-fry, an oven for roasting, and a slow cooker for brewing up some bone broth.

2. Pick five to ten recipes that will spread the activity out over your work surfaces and cooking areas. Get your recipes together and create a shopping list. Shop for all of the food you need (you can also get the groceries delivered), and once you have everything, prep your space before you get started cooking. I also like to have a timer ready to use to keep track of each recipe's time.

3. Review your recipes to determine how to make the best use of your time. Which recipe will take the longest? Which requires the most prep? What can you do while one recipe is in the oven?

4. Look for any "repeat" ingredients that appear in more than one recipe. Include in this tally any fresh ingredients that you may be able to prep for smoothies and salads throughout the week. Figure out the amounts you'll need and write down the totals on a piece of paper. For example, if one recipe calls for 2 cups of chopped carrots and another ½ cup, you'll want to chop 2½ cups of carrots. The goal is to be efficient and not have to go back to repeat a step with an ingredient you've already worked with or even put away.

5. Prep ingredients starting with vegetables first, followed by meats, and then dry or liquid goods.

6. Next, you'll start cooking. I typically start with the recipes that call for roasting, as this often takes the longest (next to slow-cooker dishes). If I can fit different types of ingredients on one sheet pan, I will do that—it's faster and I like when flavors blend together. After that, I like to get my slow-cooker dish going. Then, start steaming, boiling, and sautéing other dishes.

7. Set a timer for each dish so that you know when anything needs to be stirred, turned, removed, and so on.

8. Once everything is up and running, you can set up jar salads and smoothies for the week.

Busy Day Meals

In addition to batch cooking, I also like to keep eight to ten meals in the freezer for days when I know I'm going to be busy. Some great dishes for batch cooking and freezing include:

- Soups, such as Barszcz (p. 176), Chicken Soup (p. 175); Polish Pea Soup (p. 180); Cream of Broccoli Soup (p. 183); and Carrot-Ginger-Pear Soup (p. 186)
- Coconut-Fig Energy Balls (p. 323)
- Cuban Ropa Vieja (p. 181)
- Hashi Hash Hash (p. 231)
- Hubby's Carnitas (p. 228)
- Chicken Tandoori (p. 234)

GET STARTED WITH 10-PLUS BATCH-COOKED MEALS

Here are the kitchen spaces and tools to use for ten-plus meals you can make in a few hours:

Slow cooker: Add all ingredients for Bigos (p. 218) or Bone Broth (p. 135) and turn the slow cooker on low.

Oven and three baking dishes: Preheat the oven to 350°F and put in Root Veggie Bake (p. 303), Hubby's Carnitas (p. 228), and Maple Meatloaf Muffins (p. 233). Note down the time when each will be done baking.

Stovetop: one steamer, one stockpot, two pans: Steam veggies in the steamer, make Cream of Broccoli Soup in stockpot (p. 183), and make Truffled Veggies (p. 279) and Hashi Hash Hash (p. 231) in the pans.

Counter space and Mason jars: Use to make Jar Salads (p. 196) and prep smoothies (Orange Cream Smoothie, p. 162; Root Cause Original Smoothie, p. 167; Hashi-Mojito Smoothie, p. 170; or Root Cause Building Smoothie, p. 171) for five days!

High-powered blender: Make smoothies, soups, and purees in minutes! I like to use it to make Goddess of Detox Dressing (p. 149).

HEALTH FOR THE WHOLE FAMILY: INSPIRING THOSE AROUND YOU

After switching to a nutrient-dense diet, I was pleasantly surprised at how tasty these foods could be. I began sneaking them into potlucks with friends and coworkers as well as dinner parties with family members. I didn't make a big deal out of them or my dietary theories, but people soon took notice of how much better I looked and realized that healthy foods were not as horrible as they thought! Soon enough, one by one, people around me began to ask for recipes and dietary advice. Now countless friends and family members, including my hubby, mom, brother, and sister-in law as well as our dog, Boomer, are on nutrient-dense diets free of inflammatory foods, and so many health miracles have occurred! Here are some examples.

By using my dietary and functional-medicine protocols, my beautiful mom was able to eliminate three thyroid nodules, has been able to see a significant improvement in her asthma symptoms, and has even been weaned off her medications under her doctor's supervision. She was 100 percent symptom free, but had a flare-up after accidentally consuming a bar that contained whey protein!

My husband, Michael, a lifelong athlete, was generally in great shape. Utilizing nutrition, functional-medicine protocols, and food-sensitivity testing results combined with his meditation and exercise routine, Michael has been able to shed the 15 stubborn pounds he wanted to lose, gained more muscle, and resolved his anxiety.

Last but not least, our ten-year-old Pomeranian, Boomer, was previously eating grain-free kibble and is now eating home-prepared, nutrient-dense foods free of inflammatory and reactive foods! His main improvements include better energy, shinier coat, weight loss, and no more needing to go potty every two hours! Each week, we use a pressure cooker and food processor to prepare his feast of stewed lamb and vegetables!

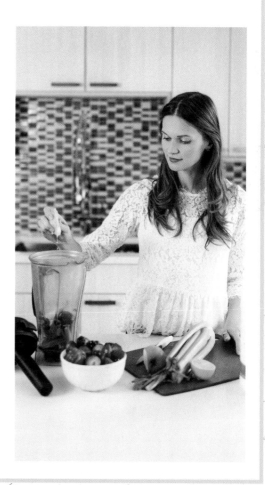

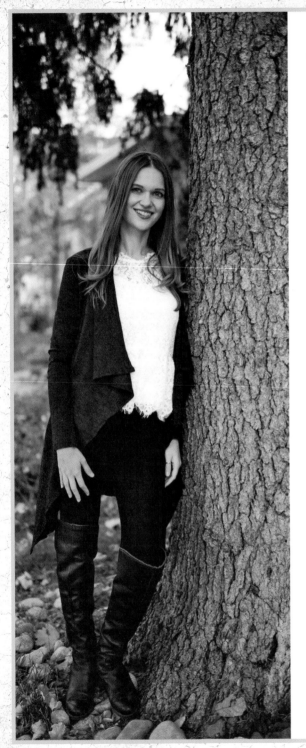

WHAT I EAT

My readers often ask, "What do you eat on a daily basis? How do you stay balanced?"

My diet has changed so much since my Hashimoto's diagnosis. Prior to my diagnosis most of my diet consisted of wheat, dairy, sugar, and processed foods. I hated salads and avoided red meat and pork like the plague, and I suffered dearly from blood-sugar swings, joint pains, mood swings, panic attacks, and a plethora of other symptoms.

At first, stuck in a state of paralysis by analysis, I researched the gluten-free diet for over a year before trying it! Unfortunately, my condition progressed during that time, and I developed even more symptoms!

Finally in January 2011, I decided to fully commit to trying whatever I could to improve my health—and I'm so glad that I did. It actually took doing a food-sensitivity test to get me to change my diet. Hey! I was a skeptical scientist—I needed to see the evidence on paper that foods could be a problem!

After eliminating gluten and dairy and the other reactive foods, I started to feel better in three days. It was quite funny, because I actually didn't think the diet would work. I was shocked when I didn't need to reach for my bottle of acid-reflux medication on the third day of the diet! The rest, my friends, is history. Through optimizing my hormone levels, nutrition, and digestion and addressing my stress response, detox pathways, and infections, I was able to recover my health!

Currently, I avoid gluten and dairy. I have an IgA reaction to dairy, which is a celiac-like reaction. Though I used to have horrific symptoms after exposure to both of these, recent accidental exposures resulted in only mild symptoms like arm tingling and bloating. For a while, I also avoided nuts because they caused me to have skin breakouts and emotional swings. (I would tell people that nuts made me nuts!)

I've changed my diet over the last few years and have an intuitive connection with what I eat. My diet changes with the seasons, with where I'm living, and with what I'm doing.

When I was working on tight deadlines for the *Hashimoto's Protocol* book and the *Thyroid Secret* documentary, my body craved a lot of fat! My Duck Salad (p. 208) was one of the recipes that came out of that time period!

Once the book and documentary had come out and I was no longer on tour for the book, I became more active outdoors and craved more fruit and veggies and fewer heavy foods. I drank lots of green juices, ate lots of salads and salsas like the Mango Salsa (p. 296) and Katy's Greek Salad (p. 200), and incorporated fruit into my smoothies (like the Orange Cream Smoothie, p. 162).

I was writing this very book when I was pregnant with my son, Dimitry, and he too inspired changes in my diet! I ate a lot of methylation-supporting beets (and the recipes for Heirloom Tomato and Beet Salad, p. 199; Barszcz, p. 176; and Sloppy Joes in a HeartBeet, p. 260, were my favorites), and a *lot* of iron-boosting grass-fed burgers with pickles (it later turned out that, like many pregnant women, I was iron-deficient, or as my husband called it, "burger-deficient"). Dimitry also inspired me to make more sweets than I would normally eat! You can thank him for the Lemon–Banana Cream Ice Pops (p. 341) and the AI Very Berry Pie (p. 339)!

The amazing thing I've noticed since switching to a nutrient-dense diet and away from foods that were inflammatory for me is that my body often guides me in choosing the best foods for me! Once you rebalance, your cravings can actually dictate your dietary needs!

I still love starting my day with a Root Cause Original Smoothie. I generally add ingredients based on how I'm feeling that day. I developed the Rootcology AI Paleo Protein for myself, which is a daily staple. The smoothies were especially wonderful after I had my son!

For lunch, I will have a soup, salad, bowl, or a burger, depending on the weather and how I feel. These foods are usually batch-cooked or prepared on Mondays and Thursdays, so I don't have to make them from scratch each day. Some of my favorites are the Maple Meatloaf Muffins (p. 233), Creamy White Chicken Stew (p. 193), Taco the Town Salad (p. 211), and the Bibimbap Bowl (p. 202).

Dinners are a family affair, and I love to have a side salad (like the Chopped BLT Salad, p. 214) with a high-quality meat dish. For snacks I have Coconut Yogurt (p. 131) with berries and seeds, Beef Jerky (p. 307), Cilantro-Lime Guacamole (p. 287), or a smoothie.

On the weekends, I love to make Waffles (p. 336) or Plantain Crepes (p. 329) with bacon and eggs and a nice side of avocados, Coconut Yogurt (p. 131) with fruit and seeds, or Fermented Vegetables (p. 132).

I love cooking, but when I'm busy juggling book deadlines and a newborn, I ask for help from my hubby, my mom, or another angel, order food from local restaurants that offer gluten-free, dairy-free, and health-conscious options, or use delivery services that offer Paleo-friendly meals. I also keep eight to ten freezer meals that can be thawed and cooked or easily thrown into a slow cooker for emergencies!

You can freece these in Mason jars or BPA-free plastic freezer bags and then reheat them on your stove for serving. Side dishes, such as Root Veggie Bake (p. 303) and Parsnip-Carrot Mash (p. 304), can be frozen in glass baking dishes and then reheated in the oven once thawed.

I also love my slow cooker. When I'm prepping, I often put together the raw ingredients for a slow-cooker meal and freeze them. Then on a busy day, all I have to do is thaw them and pop them into the slow-cooker before I leave in the morning. The following recipes are fantastic for busy-day slow-cooker meals:

- Bigos (p. 218)
- Bone Broth (p. 135)
- Chicken Tandoori (p. 234)
- Chilly Day Chili (p. 178)
- Cuban Ropa Vieja (p. 181)
- Pulled Cherry Pork (p. 269)
- Winter Oxtail Stew (p. 191)

MASON JAR HACK FOR SALADS AND SMOOTHIES

Mason jars are lifesavers when it comes to food prep. I use them to create supereasy salads and smoothies that I can enjoy during the week.

To make salads: Set out five 32-ounce wide-mouth Mason jars, one for each week day. Put your dressing in the bottom—Everyday Dressing (p. 138) is my easy go-to. Take the veggies and fruits you've prepped and get ready to stack. Stack the firm vegetables, like cut cucumber, bell peppers, baby carrots, at the bottom of the jar, followed by softer veggies and fruit, like olives, cherry tomatoes, or blueberries. Top off with nuts or seeds, some greens, and coconut shavings or fresh herbs. Seal and refrigerate. In the morning, grab a jar along with some protein or fat (chopped chicken or boiled eggs are some ideas for protein; avocados are a great fat) and take it with you for your lunchtime meal.

To make smoothies: Set out five 32-ounce wide-mouth Mason jars. Add any precut veggies and store in the fridge. In the morning, grab one of the jars and pour the veggies into your blender. Add other ingredients such as coconut milk, avocado, and protein powder and blend. Enjoy before you head out the door to start your day.

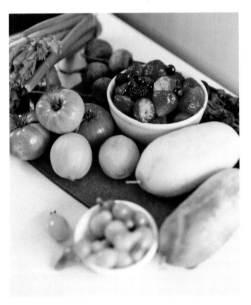

As someone with a growing family, it was really important that I include recipes in this cookbook that could satisfy everyone, kids included. Here are some of my top family-friendly picks:

- Apple-Carrot Salad (p. 293)
- Baked Coconut Bananas (p. 333)
- Baked Ginger-Lemon Chicken Thighs (p. 259)
- Beef Stew (p. 174)
- Broccoli and Chicken Quiche (p. 246)
- Carrot Fries (p. 312)
- Chunky Applesauce (p. 146)
- Citrus Bison Meatballs (p. 222)
- Citrus Salmon (p. 265)
- Cream of Broccoli Soup (p. 183)
- Creamy White Chicken Stew (p. 193)
- Golden Raisin Chicken Salad (p. 195)
- Grilled Fish and Pineapple Salsa Packets with Green Beans (p. 262)
- Hashi Hash Hash (p. 231)
- Hubby's Carnitas (p. 228)
- Lemon–Banana Cream Ice Pops (p. 341)
- Maple Meatloaf Muffins (p. 233)
- Paleo Banana-Almond Muffins (p. 324)
- Shepherd's Pie (p. 241)
- Sweet and Sour Chicken Skewers with Broccoli Salad (p. 221)
- Tropical Grilled Chicken Skewers (p. 236)

DEALING WITH UNSUPPORTIVE PEOPLE

Unfortunately many people who get diagnosed with Hashimoto's will find that the people in their lives are not as supportive as they would like them to be. Hashimoto's is an invisible illness—people can't see what we feel on the inside. Hashimoto's is also a spectrum—one person may have no symptoms, while another may have debilitating symptoms. Additionally, conventional medicine doesn't support the use of nutrition or other advanced interventions at this time. All of these factors may lead friends and family members to disregard our symptoms, dismiss us as hypochondriacs, or disagree with the lifestyle changes we are attempting in order to make ourselves feel better.

There's another factor to consider, however. Although it may sound strange, many times people treat us the way that they do because *we allow them to*, and it's up to us to assert our needs and boundaries. In most cases, relationships can be saved and people can learn how to support us better once we begin to gently demand their care.

At first, my husband didn't understand why I needed to be 100 percent gluten and dairy free. He was supportive of my eating a healthier diet and less sugar, but he was a fan of moderation and thought my new diet had become an unhealthy obsession. He does not have a medical background and did not understand that even tiny amounts of gluten can make a sensitive person sick. He was embarrassed about the fuss I made at restaurants when I refused to eat meals that possibly contained contaminated foods. It didn't help that I didn't seem to be getting better as I tried various interventions.

Of course I was upset that my knight in shining armor wasn't coming to my rescue, but once I calmed down and allowed logic to take over, I said, "Gluten and dairy make my thyroid numbers get out of range and cause me to have acid reflux and stomach cramping. Even tiny amounts can do this. I deserve to eat the things that make me feel good, just like anyone else in the world. It would really mean a lot to me if you were supportive of my diet."

Having this talk with him was enough for him to understand that food was affect-

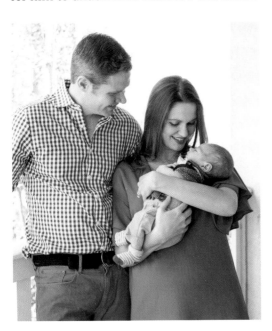

ing my health, and he became very supportive. He even tried a thirty-day Paleo challenge with me later that year and found that he actually felt much better on this type of diet, which has now become our diet.

I hope that you can gently remind and encourage the people in your life to be supportive, but keep in mind that some people just aren't going to be sympathetic. In fact, they may even be toxic, and you might have to let them go. Toxic people get their energy, confidence, and encouragement from the pain and suffering of other people, whether that's through subtle mean comments, manipulation, or causing physical harm.

A woman in a Hashimoto's support group I follow shared the story of a "friend" who invited her over for lunch, assuring her that the meal would be gluten, dairy, soy free. Shortly after the woman with Hashimoto's started eating the meal, she became ill. Her "friend" admitted that she was just testing her to see if she was faking; she had purposely made a meal that hid the very ingredients she promised would be avoided, so that she could "test" her. With friends like that, we don't need enemies.

As a general rule, I recommend that you seek people who will lift you up, not drag you down. Don't be afraid to cut ties with abusive, unsupportive friends and family members and seek out companionship from supportive and loving people.

There are a lot more good people in this world than bad, and letting go of relationships that no longer serve you is often what opens the door to find ones that do.

I've found that removing inflammatory foods from your life can create profound improvements in your health and well-being. I've also found that removing "inflammatory people" from your life can have *even more* profound effects!

SUGGESTIONS FOR EATING OUT

Eating out on a restricted diet can be quite intimidating, especially for those of us who don't like to draw a lot of attention to ourselves or tend to avoid confrontation. I've spoken with women who have celiac disease who were too afraid to speak up at restaurants and fell ill, often for weeks at a time, after dinners out with friends and family members. Some of my readers and clients have also reported feeling bad about speaking up or starting a conversation with a server with negatives like, "I can't have …"

You may think you're a bother or that you're making a big deal out of things. Society has taught us that being "high maintenance" is a very negative thing for a woman, while a "high maintenance" car generally implies that the car is worth more attention and care because of its value.

Let me let you in on a little secret. You too are worthy and deserve proper care and attention, and you deserve to have your needs met.

Here are some tips for keeping on your plan while eating out and enjoying a social life:

1. Review the restaurant's menu online before you go to see if the restaurant offers gluten-free options and accommodates people with food sensitivities (many do!), or call ahead to speak to a manager. I like to use the website OpenTable to make reservations ahead of time and review the menus. Some of my clients love using phone apps like Find Me Gluten Free to find restaurants that offer gluten-free options.

2. Don't be afraid to recommend a restaurant you know to be food sensitivity friendly when dining with friends or work colleagues. When I lived in Chicago, I often asked colleagues to meet me at Francesca's, an Italian chain that offers gluten-free options. Everyone was able to find something they enjoyed, and I didn't have to worry.

3. The chefs and wait staff at most restaurants want to help you and want you to have a great experience. I usually start the conversation with a statement like, "Hey, can you help me out? I'm on a new diet that restricts X, Y, and Z, and I'd love to know if there's anything on the menu that would suit my needs." Most servers are more than happy to go out of their way to help find something that works or to talk to the chef.

I've often had fun and creative meals made for me by excited chefs who enjoy the challenge of creating something out of the ordinary for their guests. An experience that used to be intimidating and anxiety provoking can be turned into a VIP experience with a bit of patience, kindness, and gratitude! Of course, I'm always happy to tip a little extra for the special service! Often when I eat out with friends, they look at my food and comment that it looks better than theirs. I'm happy to have food that truly nourishes me, instead of worrying about eating like everyone else and then being sorry I did!

4. You might also consider ordering what are generally reliable "safe" orders. A Cobb salad (greens, tomato, bacon, grilled chicken, boiled egg, onions, avocado, cheese) or a Greek salad (some variation of grilled chicken, olives, greens, tomatoes, bell peppers, onions, cucumbers, and feta cheese) are good options. Ask for grilled chicken and have them hold the cheese and dressing (many salad dressings contain soy and high-fructose corn syrup), and order olive oil and lemon juice to use as your dressing.

Other go-to meals include any grilled meat served with steamed or grilled veggies (ask for a double serving in place of any grain or cheesy potato side). If you're concerned about cross-contamination from breaded foods, share this with your server and ask if any efforts can be taken to prevent gluten exposure—sometimes a chef will cook food in foil or keep foods separate from certain appliances or utensils.

5. Carry a gluten/dairy digestive enzyme with you when you eat out. The digestive enzymes won't eliminate the reaction, but they can minimize it if you are exposed to gluten or dairy.

6. When in doubt, pack your own food or eat a meal at home before you head out. If you are going to a baseball game where the food options will be limited to beer and hot dogs, bring your own food or eat before you go!

TIPS FOR AN EASY TRANSITION TO A CLEAN DIET

You are about to embark on a journey that may seem scary. I assure you that you can do this, as have many others. You can succeed. Your health can get better, if you invest in yourself. Remember that you are worth it!

- Use a food and symptom journal to help track foods and symptoms associated with foods. This will help you to identify patterns and foods that may or may not be benefiting you.

- Eat simple! Many of my recipes, such as my Carrot-Ginger-Pear Soup (p. 186) and the SAM Salad (p. 213) are simple yet nutritiously satisfying.

- Cook in bulk and freeze for future meals, especially if you find that one day you are in a bind and do not have time to cook for yourself. Freezer meals are quick and convenient. See p. 98 for a list of my favorite freezer-meal recipes.

- Batch cooking is also a great way to help you stay on track. On p. 97 I explain in detail the way I like to batch cook for the week. Setting a few hours aside on a single day can really make a difference!

- If you find it difficult to go "cold turkey," you can slowly transition yourself into the diet that I recommend throughout the book. Pick one type of food each week and slowly use my guide above to switch your foods. An example would be pasta. Instead of eating pasta with my Tomato Sauce (p. 150), start by introducing gluten-free noodles or substitute some spiralized vegetable noodles to boost your vegetable intake!

- I've made some meal plans for you to follow as well. Choose a plan that you would like to begin with, such as Paleo, and start cooking! If it's too much all at once for you, start with my Root Cause Original Smoothie (p. 167) in the morning. When you are comfortable with making smoothies daily, you can incorporate dinners from the book and use the leftovers for your lunch the next day.

- Take things one day at a time, and celebrate small wins and successes! Forgive yourself for "falling off the wagon" and setbacks. Take some time to reflect and be kind to yourself. Remember that you can do this!

Keep in mind that all the tips shared here are just suggestions. You might already have some strategies in place that work for you. If this is the case, hopefully I've shared some ideas that you can add to your success toolbox! If you're new to cooking and to cooking for healing specifically, I hope the suggestions help build your confidence as you get started with self-nourishment.

5

Frequently Asked Questions

1. What are some strategies for avoiding hidden gluten?

Any packaged, prepared, and/or otherwise processed foods may contain gluten, even if you normally wouldn't expect them to. If you don't see "gluten-free" on a food's packaging, you should presume that gluten may be present. Many varieties of wheat contain gluten, including semolina, graham, farro, durum, farina, and spelt (this is why eliminating all grains can be helpful when you're avoiding gluten). Possible hidden sources include sauces and gravies, tortillas, beer, soups, salad dressings and marinades, malt vinegar, certain chips and candy, processed meats, fried foods (the batter may contain wheat flour), bulk foods, Asian rice paper, and some frozen foods. Gluten may also be present in the wax used on fruits and vegetables to make them shiny, and there is likely some residue in and on toasters, cutting boards, and utensils.

Nonfood items that may contain gluten include over-the-counter meds, prescription drugs, and supplements. Depending on how sensitive you are, you may also want to pay attention to personal-care products such as shampoo, conditioner, body wash, and lipstick or lip balm—you can inadvertently ingest any of these, especially the products applied to your lips. Also, powdered rubber gloves and art supplies such as modeling clay, and paint may contain gluten. It's safe to assume that you won't put these items in your mouth, but if you don't wash your hands after use, you could accidentally ingest traces of gluten.

2. How do I reintroduce foods?

You can consider reintroducing a food once you have been off of it for at least three weeks. Once this time has passed, and you feel you are ready to test your reaction to a food, you can reintroduce it—but be sure that you add only one food at a time, waiting at least four days before introducing a second food. Exceptions are gluten, dairy, and soy, which may need to be gone from your diet for good.

3. I'm overwhelmed by the idea of modifying my diet—where do I start?

Give yourself a hug. I'm serious! Wrap your arms around yourself right now and squeeze; take a nice deep breath and know that you can do this. Next, clear out any reactive foods from your fridge and pantry (push them to the side if you have others in your home who aren't making modifications). Then create a shopping list for the recipes you want to make first and go shopping; get home and get cooking. One of my favorite strategies to help if you're feeling overwhelmed is batch cooking. Read about this on p. 97.

Making Bone Broth (p. 135) is also a great getting-started step; it offers a wonderful way to begin your day, plus it is a healthy base for many dishes. Additionally, I recommend that you scan through the Cookbook section and find recipes that appeal to you. There are quite a few simple, tasty recipes that can be made. A few to consider: Slow-Cooked Chicken (p. 274), Moroccan Lamb Stew (p. 184), and Hashi Hash Hash (p. 231).

4. Will I still be able to eat my favorite comfort foods while following the diets?

Most traditional comfort foods like bread, mac and cheese, biscuits and gravy, desserts, and so on contain the reactive ingredients that may be causing and perpetuating your symptoms. Instead of focusing on how you will ever survive without those foods in your life, I encourage you to focus on how much better you might feel if you eliminate them.

If you find yourself craving comfort food, give these recipes a try: Creamy White Chicken Stew (p. 193); Lemon–Banana Cream Ice Pops (p. 341); Maple Meatloaf Muffins (p. 233); Tropical Grilled Chicken Skewers (p. 236); and Taco the Town Salad (p. 211).

5. I have to travel for work and I want to travel for fun—how can I eat for healing while on the go?

When you have a health condition, traveling can be a challenge, especially if your condition requires you to stick to a special diet, and your health and recovery are on the line. But you can protect your health and go out into the world by doing one thing: planning ahead.

If you are flying, I suggest getting TSA Pre Check; this will allow you to skip the security scanners that expose you to radiation (even low-level radiation can exacerbate Hashimoto's) and lead to less travel stress overall. Specific food planning strategies will also make your travel easier:

- If meals will be served, call the airline ahead of time to request a gluten-free meal.

- Look up local restaurants where you're headed and check the menus for gluten-free dishes.

- Pack foods into your carry-on bag; some of my favorite packable foods include meatballs and diced roasted vegetables.

- Bring a stash of snack bars, such as Paleovalley snack bars, fruit-leather bars, Epic bars, Lärabars, Hemp Heart bars, and Wilde bars. (Check specific ingredients to see which ones fit with your diet plan.)

- If you are traveling to a foreign country, get some food-sensitivity cards. These contain printed messages regarding your sensitivity or allergy that have been translated into the local language. Hand these to servers or staff to make sure your dietary needs are clear.

- Take a gluten/dairy digestive enzyme, which can minimize adverse reactions should you be exposed to these reactive foods.

6. Can I ever cheat and include dairy or gluten in my diet, even if it's just once a year?

I recommend that most people with auto-immune thyroid disease consider lifelong removal of gluten, dairy, and soy. However, once your leaky gut has healed and you feel resilient and strong, you will likely be able to tolerate some foods and/or drinks that previously elicited symptoms. In my case, I'll have grains occasionally, but I'm 100 percent gluten free all the time. I will drink wine or a mojito or margarita every now and then or indulge in a gluten-free dessert if it's good. Most of the time, I'm able to tolerate these "treats" without a problem, but if I overdid it for several days or weeks in a row, however, I'm sure my body would rebel. Through trial and error, you will be able to determine your personal tolerance for various foods. Make an effort to get a lot of sleep and try to keep your stress level as low as possible. Whenever we don't get enough sleep and we're stressed out, that's when we become less resilient and our system may not be as tolerant of occasional indulgences.

7. Is there any easy way to make some of your recipes for one person?

Many of the recipes featured in the book are freezer friendly. This means that you can make one recipe and freeze extra portions for other days when you don't have time or energy to cook a meal.

Or consider dividing the recipe by the number of portions specified and make that portion. Some recipes lend themselves to a combination. If a recipe has a protein and a sauce, you can make the full amount of sauce, but cook just one portion of protein. Then enjoy your protein with one serving of sauce and either refrigerate or freeze the remainder for later use.

8. I'm having major cravings for sweets and salty foods—what should I do?

When you modify your diet, you may notice an increase in cravings for sugary or salty foods. This is normal. Eating to balance your blood sugar can help, as can taking an L-glutamine supplement. If you find that your cravings don't subside after a few weeks, you may want to get specific tests done. For sweet cravings, you need to get tested for yeast, which can be done through a gut test, and for salt cravings, get your adrenals tested.

9. What can I eat in place of cheese that will satisfy my craving for it and provide a good source of calcium?

Good dietary sources of calcium include canned salmon and sardines, broccoli, kale, and, when not eliminating legumes, black-eyed peas and white beans. To help satisfy your cheese craving, I recommend trying my recipe for Cashew Cream Cheese (p. 144). You might also snack on something nutritious and salty like olives or something rich and nourishing like avocado slices sprinkled with sea salt.

10. What should I do if I have histamine reactions?

Histamine is a chemical that is released from our cells when an allergic substance enters the body. If you have a healthy gut lining, cells within the lining will produce an enzyme called diamine oxidase (DAO) to break down histamines. If your gut lining is impaired, as it is in those with intestinal permeability, you may not be able to produce sufficient DAO. Histamines can accumulate and in some people create reactions such as headache, stuffy nose, dizziness, itchy/watery eyes, heart palpitations, and hives.

If you have histamine intolerance, your body isn't reacting to the histamine within the food, but rather the bacteria harbored on or within the food that reacts with our histamine receptors (mast cells). This is why if you are histamine intolerant, you may react to foods higher in even good bacteria, such as fermented foods and drinks and cured meats.

Since a leaky gut is often a root cause of histamine intolerance, my recommendation is to first try the healing diets featured in this book, which will help repair your gut. This intestinal repair might also restore your ability to produce enough DAO needed to eliminate histamines properly. If your symptoms persist, however, look into trying a low-histamine diet.

11. I never know what to make for breakfast—what are some of your favorite recipes?

During the week smoothies are my favorite breakfast food. I really enjoy the Root Cause Original Smoothie (p. 167) in the morning; it gives me a ton of energy and is filling without making me feel too full. On weekends I love to make myself a breakfast hash with some grass-fed ground beef and veggies. Other specific recipes you can try for breakfast include:

- Hashi Hash Hash (p. 231)

- Plantain Crepes (p. 329) with Cashew Cream Cheese (p. 144) and mixed berries

- Salmon-Parsnip Cakes (p. 239)

- SAM Salad (p. 213)

- Turkey and Pepper Avocado Boats (p. 226)

- Sweet and Salty "Granola" (p. 289) with Coconut Yogurt (p. 131) and berries

- Broccoli and Chicken Quiche (p. 246)

- Beef Stew (p. 174)

- Frittata with Ham and White Sweet Potato (p. 216)

12. Is intermittent fasting healthy for people with Hashimoto's?

Any type of fasting can have cleansing and healing effects. However, because even intermittent fasts can be stressful on the adrenal glands, I don't recommend them in the early stages of healing. I have found that most people with Hashimoto's (many of whom have underlying adrenal issues) often feel worse when they try fasting too soon after the introduction of dietary modifications.

13. I don't like the taste of coconut or coconut oil—are there alternatives I can use?

Alternatives for coconut oil include avocado oil, animal fats (tallow, lard from grass-fed or pastured animals), palm shortening, red palm oil (sustainable), and olive oil. If you need a replacement for coconut flour for baking, you can try arrowroot flour, cassava flour, tapioca flour/starch, and sweet potato flour/starch.

14. Are there any foods I should avoid or eat more of if I have *H. pylori*?

Helicobacter pylori, commonly known as *H. pylori*, is a bacterial infection that can trigger leaky gut, making it a potential trigger for Hashimoto's and other autoimmune diseases. *H. pylori* can contribute to low stomach acid, which in turn may lead to poorly digested foods and resulting nutrient deficiencies. Symptoms may include nausea, frequent burping, loss of appetite, and unintentional weight loss. A specific protocol needs to be followed to eradicate *H. pylori* (see Hashimoto's protocol). You can try drinking cabbage juice as a supportive dietary strategy; consume 4 ounces daily for twenty-eight days. Black cumin seed oil (*Nigella sativa*) can also be consumed to address an *H. pylori* infection.

15. Is the keto diet safe for people with Hashimoto's?

The purpose of the keto diet is to get into ketosis, which is when your body begins to use ketones from fats as fuel instead of sugars from carbohydrates. Some people with Hashimoto's may benefit from ketosis, such as those with chronic pain and brain fog.

Some people reported feeling more tired on the ketogenic diet. It's important to note that low energy levels could be due to low stomach acid and not a reduced intake of carbohydrates. Low stomach acid can lead to inefficient protein digestion and in turn low energy. I recommend trying betaine with pepsin (p. 72) before determining if low carb is a good choice for you.

Some keto-friendly recipes included in the book include:

- Chocolate Avocado Pudding (p. 320)
- Bone Broth (p. 135)
- Beef Jerky (p. 307)
- Broccoli and Chicken Quiche (p. 246)
- Chicken Burgers and Kale Chips (p. 261)
- Chopped BLT Salad (p. 214)
- Cilantro-Lime Guacamole (p. 287)
- Everyday Dressing (p. 138)
- Italian Meatza Pie (p. 263)
- Mexican Quiche (p. 245)

16. What are the signs of soy sensitivity?

If you are sensitive to soy, you may experience reactions such as anxiety, palpitations, gut issues, and/or increased thyroid antibodies.

Meal Plans

Intro Week 1 Meal Plan

RECIPE NAMES	MEAL TYPE	FOOD TYPE	PROTEIN (G)	FAT (G)	CARBS (G)	MEAL
DAY 1						
Root Cause Original Smoothie	AI	Main	12.79	26.38	15.98	Breakfast
Chicken Burger and Kale Chips	AI	Main	22.65	13.21	5.93	Lunch
Beef Fried Rice	Intro	Main	19.46	28.08	18.62	Diner
Cilantro-Lime Guacamole	AI	Side	1.66	10.38	7.81	Snack
Beef Jerky	AI	Side	20.86	12.64	3.78	Snack
	Total Nutrient Analysis		**77.42**	**90.69**	**52.12**	
DAY 2						
Root Cause Original Smoothie	AI	Main	12.79	26.38	15.98	Breakfast
Chopped BLT Salad	Paleo	Main	7.65	29.35	5.82	Lunch
Kotlety (Polish Chicken Cutlets)	Paleo	Main	32.83	40.93	10.43	Dinner
Katy's Greek Salad	Paleo	Main	3.05	12.55	14.5	Dinner
Cherry Berry Gelatin Snacks	AI	Snack	5.52	0.71	1.84	Snack
	Total Nutrient Analysis		**61.84**	**109.92**	**48.57**	
DAY 3						
Root Cause Original Smoothie	AI	Main	12.79	26.38	15.98	Breakfast
Creamy White Chicken Stew	AI	Main	27.02	53.93	24.31	Lunch
Bibimbap Bowl	Intro	Main	17.01	11.95	25.84	Dinner
Sweet and Salty "Granola"	Paleo	Snack	5.22	13.04	22.03	Snack
Coconut Yogurt	AI	Snack	3.23	23.26	8.65	Snack
	Total Nutrient Analysis		**65.27**	**128.56**	**96.81**	

RECIPE NAMES	MEAL TYPE	FOOD TYPE	PROTEIN (G)	FAT (G)	CARBS (G)	MEAL
DAY 4						
Root Cause Original Smoothie	AI	Main	12.79	26.38	15.98	Breakfast
Chicken Spring Rolls with Almond Dipping Sauce	Intro	Main	6.45	14.44	24.9	Lunch
Squashghetti and Meatballs	Paleo	Main	24.64	30.29	9.34	Dinner
Hashi-Mojito Smoothie	AI	Snack	28.54	1.16	17.21	Snack
	Total Nutrient Analysis		**72.42**	**72.27**	**67.43**	
DAY 5						
Root Cause Original Smoothie	AI	Main	12.79	26.38	15.98	Breakfast
Hubby's Carnitas	Paleo	Main	49.73	35.13	2.16	Lunch
Biscuits	AI	Side	1.34	11.3	28.15	Dinner
Chilly Day Chili	Intro	Main	19.43	6.29	30.36	Dinner
Sweet and Salty "Granola"	Paleo	Snack	5.22	13.04	22.03	Snack
Coconut Yogurt	AI	Snack	3.23	23.26	8.65	Snack
	Total Nutrient Analysis		**91.74**	**115.4**	**107.33**	
DAY 6						
Broccoli and Chicken Quiche	Paleo	Main	21.64	11.97	7.65	Breakfast
Cowboy Caviar	Intro	Side	5.63	4.93	16.19	Lunch
Tropical Grilled Chicken Skewers	AI	Main	16.56	5.48	22.15	Lunch
Paleo Meatloaf	Paleo	Main	20.02	24.26	3.75	Dinner
Parsnip-Carrot Mash	AI	Side	1.64	7.22	19.29	Dinner
Chocolate Avocado Pudding	Paleo	Snack	7.88	23.66	6.05	Snack
	Total Nutrient Analysis		**73.37**	**77.52**	**75.08**	
DAY 7						
Chicken Burger and Kale Chips	AI	Main	22.65	13.21	5.93	Breakfast
Paleo Meatloaf (LO)*	Paleo	Main	20.02	24.26	3.75	Lunch
Parsnip-Carrot Mash (LO)*	AI	Side	1.64	7.22	19.29	Lunch
Gnocchi with Peas and Pancetta	Intro	Main	8.61	13.87	47.17	Dinner
Green Juice	AI	Snack	7.72	11.77	38.82	Snack
	Total Nutrient Analysis		**60.64**	**70.33**	**114.96**	

* LO = leftovers.

Intro Week 2 Meal Plan

RECIPE NAMES	MEAL TYPE	FOOD TYPE	PROTEIN (G)	FAT (G)	CARBS (G)	MEAL
DAY 1						
Root Cause Original Smoothie	AI	Main	12.79	26.38	15.98	Breakfast
Kotlety (Polish Chicken Cutlets)	Paleo	Main	32.83	40.93	10.43	Lunch
Sautéed Rapini	AI	Side	1.09	4.66	1.39	Lunch
Lentil Shepherd's Pie	Intro	Main	8	4.87	35.74	Dinner
Maca Latte	Paleo	Snack	2.75	28.61	14.11	Snack
	Total Nutrient Analysis		**57.46**	**105.45**	**77.65**	
DAY 2						
Root Cause Original Smoothie	AI	Main	12.79	26.38	15.98	Breakfast
Eggplant Lasagna Stacks	Paleo	Main	10.95	21.46	30.14	Lunch
Golden Raisin Chicken Salad	Paleo	Main	19.26	10.94	14.83	Lunch
Pork Chop with Balsamic Glazed Onions	AI	Main	27.45	37.89	8.38	Dinner
Twiced-Baked Sweet Potatoes	AI	Side	3.94	11.75	15.62	Dinner
Chocolate Avocado Pudding	Paleo	Snack	7.88	23.66	6.05	Snack
	Total Nutrient Analysis		**82.27**	**132.08**	**91**	
DAY 3						
Root Cause Original Smoothie	AI	Main	12.79	26.38	15.98	Breakfast
Polish Pea Soup	Intro	Main	11.96	8.19	21.88	Lunch
Beef Jerky	AI	Side	20.86	12.64	3.78	Lunch
Paella	Intro	Main	21.7	7.79	7.88	Dinner
Hot Chocolate	Paleo	Snack	18.18	43.91	23.14	Snack
	Total Nutrient Analysis		**85.49**	**98.91**	**72.66**	

RECIPE NAMES	MEAL TYPE	FOOD TYPE	PROTEIN (G)	FAT (G)	CARBS (G)	MEAL
DAY 4						
Root Cause Original Smoothie	AI	Main	12.79	26.38	15.98	Breakfast
Paella (LO)*	Intro	Main	21.7	7.79	7.88	Lunch
Gołąbki (Polish Stuffed Cabbage Rolls)	Intro	Main	43.1	25.49	39.74	Dinner
Truffled Veggie Blend	AI	Side	13.99	15.83	28.55	Dinner
Turkey and Pepper Avocado Boats	Paleo	Snack	17.46	15.31	10.96	Snack
	Total Nutrient Analysis		109.04	90.8	103.11	
DAY 5						
Root Cause Original Smoothie	AI	Main	12.79	26.38	15.98	Breakfast
Duck Salad	Paleo	Main	13.39	20.02	9.22	Lunch
Bigos (Polish Hunter's Stew)	Paleo	Main	32.38	17.8	8.43	Dinner
Chopped BLT Salad	Paleo	Main	7.65	29.35	5.82	Dinner
Maca Latte	Paleo	Snack	2.75	28.61	14.11	Snack
	Total Nutrient Analysis		68.96	122.16	53.56	
DAY 6						
Mexican Quiche	Paleo	Main	21.97	32.24	5.74	Breakfast
Cream of Broccoli Soup	AI	Main	9.49	30.17	14.34	Lunch
Quail with Grapes	AI	Main	26.68	11.7	12.98	Dinner
Cucumber-Fig Salad	AI	Side	35.59	14.37	5.85	Dinner
Pumpkin Maca Latte	Paleo	Snack	3.28	29.13	15.95	Snack
	Total Nutrient Analysis		97.01	117.71	54.86	
DAY 7						
Waffles	Intro	Main	44.5	30.49	0.11	Breakfast
Cashew Cream Cheese	Paleo	Side	5.84	14	10.57	Breakfast
Mixed Berries	AI	Side	0	0	0	Breakfast
Stuffed Portobello Mushrooms	Paleo	Main	14.01	24.61	25	Lunch
Heirloom Tomato and Beet Salad	Paleo	Side	1.36	4.72	8.03	Lunch
Taco the Town Salad	Intro	Main	31.76	19.97	22.51	Dinner
Pumpkin Pie	AI	Sweet	3.94	11.32	24.7	Dinner
Red Pepper Turkey Dip	Paleo	Snack	16.82	5.18	6.55	Snack
	Total Nutrient Analysis		120.47	110.29	97.47	

* LO = leftovers.

Paleo Week 1 Meal Plan

RECIPE NAMES	MEAL TYPE	FOOD TYPE	PROTEIN (G)	FAT (G)	CARBS (G)	MEAL
DAY 1						
Root Cause Original Smoothie	AI	Main	12.79	26.38	15.98	Breakfast
Chopped BLT Salad	Paleo	Main	7.65	29.35	5.82	Lunch
Bigos (Polish Hunter's Stew)	Paleo	Main	32.38	17.8	8.43	Dinner
Biscuits	AI	Side	1.34	11.3	28.15	Dinner
Coconut Yogurt	AI	Snack	3.23	23.26	8.65	Snack
Sweet and Salty "Granola"	Paleo	Snack	5.22	13.04	22.03	Snack
	Total Nutrient Analysis		**62.61**	**121.13**	**89.06**	
DAY 2						
Root Cause Original Smoothie	AI	Main	12.79	26.38	15.98	Breakfast
Bigos (Polish Hunter's Stew) (LO)*	Paleo	Main	32.38	17.8	8.43	Lunch
Eggplant Lasagna Stacks	Paleo	Main	10.95	21.46	30.14	Dinner
Heirloom Tomato and Beet Salad	Paleo	Side	1.36	4.72	8.03	Dinner
Almond and Date Snack Bars	Paleo	Snack	8.72	15.95	23.46	Snack
	Total Nutrient Analysis		**66.2**	**86.31**	**86.04**	
DAY 3						
Root Cause Original Smoothie	AI	Main	12.79	26.38	15.98	Breakfast
Golden Raisin Chicken Salad	Paleo	Main	19.26	10.94	14.83	Lunch
Duck with Date Sauce	AI	Main	13.96	48.53	34.26	Dinner
Turkey and Pepper Avocado Boats	Paleo	Snack	17.46	15.31	10.96	Snack
	Total Nutrient Analysis		**63.47**	**101.16**	**76.03**	

* LO = leftovers.

RECIPE NAMES	MEAL TYPE	FOOD TYPE	PROTEIN (G)	FAT (G)	CARBS (G)	MEAL
DAY 4						
Root Cause Original Smoothie	AI	Main	12.79	26.38	15.98	Breakfast
Hubby's Carnitas	Paleo	Main	49.73	35.13	2.16	Lunch
Truffled Veggies	AI	Side	13.99	15.83	28.55	Lunch
Winter Oxtail Stew	Paleo	Main	35.9	24.77	12.92	Dinner
Maca Latte	Paleo	Snack	2.75	28.61	14.11	Snack
	Total Nutrient Analysis		**115.16**	**130.72**	**73.72**	
DAY 5						
Root Cause Original Smoothie	AI	Main	12.79	26.38	15.98	Breakfast
Frittata with Ham and White Sweet Potato	Paleo	Main	20.07	15.38	11.69	Lunch
Paleo Meatloaf	Paleo	Main	20.02	24.26	3.75	Dinner
Twiced-Baked Sweet Potatoes	AI	Side	3.94	11.75	15.62	Dinner
Red Pepper Turkey Dip	Paleo	Snack	16.82	5.18	6.55	Snack
	Total Nutrient Analysis		**73.64**	**82.95**	**53.59**	
DAY 6						
Broccoli and Chicken Quiche	Paleo	Main	21.64	11.97	7.65	Breakfast
Paleo Meatloaf (LO)*	Paleo	Main	20.02	24.26	3.75	Lunch
Twiced-Baked Sweet Potatoes (LO)*	AI	Side	3.94	11.75	15.62	Lunch
Pork Curry Stew	Paleo	Main	29.41	10.34	7.94	Dinner
Mizeria (Polish Cucumber Salad)	AI	Side	4.26	3	27.21	Dinner
Almond and Date Snack Bars	Paleo	Snack	8.72	15.95	23.46	Snack
	Total Nutrient Analysis		**87.99**	**77.27**	**85.63**	
DAY 7						
Frittata with Ham and White Sweet Potato (LO)*	Paleo	Main	20.07	15.38	11.69	Breakfast
Duck Salad	Paleo	Main	13.39	20.02	9.22	Lunch
Stuffed Portobello Mushrooms	Paleo	Main	14.01	24.61	25	Dinner
Cucumber-Fig Salad	AI	Side	35.59	14.37	5.85	Dinner
Red Pepper Turkey Dip (LO)*	Paleo	Snack	16.82	5.18	6.55	Snack
	Total Nutrient Analysis		**99.88**	**79.56**	**58.31**	

* LO = leftovers.

Paleo Week 2 Meal Plan

RECIPE NAMES	MEAL TYPE	FOOD TYPE	PROTEIN (G)	FAT (G)	CARBS (G)	MEAL
DAY 1						
Root Cause Original Smoothie	AI	Main	12.79	26.38	15.98	Breakfast
Salmon-Parsnip Cakes	Paleo	Main	36.83	27.11	11.95	Lunch
Apple Carrot Salad	AI	Side	1.13	0.31	26.99	Lunch
Kotlety (Polish Chicken Cutlets)	Paleo	Main	32.83	40.93	10.43	Dinner
Root Veggie Bake	AI	Side	1.4	9.2	14.06	Dinner
Paleo Banana-Almond Muffins	Paleo	Snack	3.47	5.84	10.27	Snack
	Total Nutrient Analysis		**88.45**	**109.77**	**89.68**	
DAY 2						
Root Cause Original Smoothie	AI	Main	12.79	26.38	15.98	Breakfast
Sloppy Joes in a HeartBeet	AI	Main	17.35	18.77	16.51	Lunch
Chicken Burger and Kale Chips	AI	Main	22.65	13.21	5.93	Dinner
Pumpkin Maca Latte	Paleo	Snack	3.28	29.13	15.95	Snack
	Total Nutrient Analysis		**56.07**	**87.49**	**54.37**	
DAY 3						
Root Cause Original Smoothie	AI	Main	12.79	26.38	15.98	Breakfast
Chicken Tandoori	Paleo	Main	33.8	35.61	2.39	Lunch
Cuban Ropa Vieja	Paleo	Main	19.7	9.83	3.68	Dinner
Cucumber-Fig Salad	AI	Side	35.59	14.37	5.85	Dinner
Beef Jerky (Thai variation)	Paleo	Side	14.65	12.16	6.52	Snack
	Total Nutrient Analysis		**116.53**	**98.35**	**34.42**	

RECIPE NAMES	MEAL TYPE	FOOD TYPE	PROTEIN (G)	FAT (G)	CARBS (G)	MEAL
DAY 4						
Root Cause Original Smoothie	AI	Main	12.79	26.38	15.98	Breakfast
Cuban Ropa Vieja (LO)*	Paleo	Main	19.7	9.83	3.68	Lunch
Mizeria (Polish Cucumber Salad)	AI	Side	4.26	3	27.21	Lunch
Shepherd's Pie	Paleo	Main	18.36	20.82	25.56	Dinner
Cilantro-Lime Guacamole	AI	Side	1.66	10.38	7.81	Snack
Cucumber rounds						Snack
	Total Nutrient Analysis		56.77	70.41	80.24	
DAY 5						
Root Cause Original Smoothie	AI	Main	12.79	26.38	15.98	Breakfast
Peaches and Steak	AI	Main	30.89	36.45	23.82	Lunch
Paleo Pizza	Paleo	Main	9.06	30.19	10.82	Dinner
Apple-Blueberry Crumble	Paleo	Snack	6.4	25.12	16.81	Snack
	Total Nutrient Analysis		59.14	118.14	67.43	
DAY 6						
Golden Raisin Chicken Salad	Paleo	Main	19.26	10.94	14.83	Breakfast
Pulled Cherry Pork	AI	Main	45.73	31.83	19.87	Lunch
Biscuits (LO)*	AI	Side	1.34	11.3	28.15	Lunch
Moroccan Lamb Stew	AI	Main	47.48	33	23.31	Dinner
Galaretka	AI	Main	12.3	4.71	7.93	Snack
	Total Nutrient Analysis		126.11	91.78	94.09	
DAY 7						
Mexican Quiche	Paleo	Main	21.97	32.24	5.74	Breakfast
Moroccan Lamb Stew (LO)*	AI	Main	47.48	33	23.31	Lunch
Baked Ginger-Lemon Chicken Thighs	AI	Main	14.17	45.47	11.38	Dinner
Katy's Greek Salad	Paleo	Side	3.05	12.55	14.5	Dinner
Orange Cream Smoothie	AI	Main	14.32	5.11	20.61	Snack
	Total Nutrient Analysis		100.99	128.37	75.54	

* LO = leftovers.

AI Week 1 Meal Plan

RECIPE NAMES	MEAL TYPE	FOOD TYPE	PROTEIN (G)	FAT (G)	CARBS (G)	MEAL
DAY 1						
Root Cause Original Smoothie	AI	Main	12.79	26.38	15.98	Breakfast
Creamy White Chicken Stew	AI	Main	27.02	53.93	24.31	Lunch
Ginger-Peach Pork Tenderloin	AI	Main	32.44	8.4	9.39	Dinner
Apple-Carrot Salad	AI	Side	1.13	0.31	26.99	Dinner
Cilantro-Citrus Cooler	AI	Snack	31.42	11.78	25.49	Snack
	Total Nutrient Analysis		**104.8**	**100.8**	**102.16**	
DAY 2						
Root Cause Original Smoothie	AI	Main	12.79	26.38	15.98	Breakfast
Ginger-Peach Pork Tenderloin (LO)*	AI	Main	32.44	8.4	9.39	Lunch
Katy's Greek Salad	Paleo	Main	3.05	12.55	14.5	Lunch
Italian Meatza Pie	AI	Main	6.18	12.25	4.91	Dinner
Cream of Broccoli Soup	AI	Main	9.49	30.17	14.34	Dinner
Coconut-Fig Energy Balls	AI	Snack	1.62	12.95	2.48	Snack
	Total Nutrient Analysis		**65.57**	**102.7**	**61.6**	
DAY 3						
Root Cause Original Smoothie	AI	Main	12.79	26.38	15.98	Breakfast
Biscuits	AI	Side	1.34	11.3	28.15	Lunch
Sloppy Joes in a HeartBeet	AI	Main	17.53	18.75	18.96	Lunch
Grilled Fish and Pineapple Salsa Packets with Green Beans	Paleo	Main	28.51	0.69	16.14	Dinner
Bacon and Chive Scalloped Potatoes	AI	Side	9.86	43.68	19.28	Dinner
Liver Pâté	Paleo	Snack	11.88	4.35	4.71	Snack
Raw Carrot Sticks	AI	Snack	0	0	0	Snack
	Total Nutrient Analysis		**81.91**	**105.15**	**103.22**	

* LO = leftovers.

RECIPE NAMES	MEAL TYPE	FOOD TYPE	PROTEIN (G)	FAT (G)	CARBS (G)	MEAL
DAY 4						
Root Cause Original Smoothie	AI	Main	12.79	26.38	15.98	Breakfast
Poached Trout with Beets	AI	Main	43.12	14.68	11.55	Lunch
Baked Ginger-Lemon Chicken Thighs	AI	Main	14.17	45.47	11.38	Dinner
Steamed Green Beans	AI	Side	0	0	0	Dinner
Cilantro-Lime Guacamole	AI	Side	1.66	10.38	7.81	Snack
Jicima Chips (raw sliced jicima)	AI	Snack	0	0	0	Snack
	Total Nutrient Analysis		**71.74**	**96.91**	**46.72**	
DAY 5						
Root Cause Original Smoothie	AI	Main	12.79	26.38	15.98	Breakfast
Baked Ginger-Lemon Chicken Thighs (LO)*	AI	Main	14.17	45.47	11.38	Lunch
Katy's Greek Salad (LO)*	Paleo	Main	3.05	12.55	14.5	Lunch
Chicken Burger and Kale Chips	AI	Main	22.65	13.21	5.93	Dinner
Root Veggie Bake	AI	Side	1.4	9.2	14.06	Dinner
Coconut-Fig Energy Balls	AI	Snack	1.62	12.95	2.48	Snack
	Total Nutrient Analysis		**55.68**	**119.76**	**64.33**	
DAY 6						
Galaretka	AI	Main	12.3	4.71	7.93	Breakfast
Chicken Burger and Kale Chips (LO)*	AI	Main	22.65	13.21	5.93	Lunch
Root Veggie Bake (LO)*	AI	Side	1.4	9.2	14.06	Lunch
Beef Stew	AI	Main	29.42	9.18	11.67	Dinner
Cucumber-Fig Salad	AI	Side	35.59	14.37	5.85	Dinner
Coconut Yogurt	AI	Snack	3.23	23.26	8.65	Snack
Mixed Berries	AI	Snack				Snack
	Total Nutrient Analysis		**104.59**	**73.93**	**54.09**	
DAY 7						
Twiced-Baked Sweet Potatoes	AI	Side	3.94	11.75	15.62	Breakfast
Beef Stew (LO)*	AI	Main	29.42	9.18	11.67	Lunch
Quail with Grapes	AI	Main	26.68	11.7	12.98	Dinner
Carrot Fries	AI	Side	1.23	3.7	12.14	Dinner
Hashi-Mojito Smoothie	AI	Snack	28.54	1.16	17.21	Snack
	Total Nutrient Analysis		**89.81**	**37.49**	**69.62**	

* LO = leftovers.

AI Week 2 Meal Plan

RECIPE NAMES	MEAL TYPE	FOOD TYPE	PROTEIN (G)	FAT (G)	CARBS (G)	MEAL
DAY 1						
Root Cause Original Smoothie	AI	Main	12.79	26.38	15.98	Breakfast
Sloppy Joes in a HeartBeet	AI	Main	17.53	18.75	18.96	Lunch
Pork Chop with Balsamic Glazed Onions	AI	Main	27.45	37.89	8.38	Dinner
Parsnip-Carrot Mash	AI	Side	1.64	7.22	19.29	Dinner
Root Cause Original Smoothie	AI	Main	12.79	26.38	15.98	Snack
	Total Nutrient Analysis		**72.2**	**116.62**	**78.59**	
DAY 2						
Root Cause Original Smoothie	AI	Main	12.79	26.38	15.98	Breakfast
Pork Chop with Balsamic Glazed Onions (LO)*	AI	Main	27.45	37.89	8.38	Lunch
Parsnip-Carrot Mash (LO)*	AI	Side	1.64	7.22	19.29	Lunch
Sweet and Sour Chicken Skewers with Broccoli Salad	AI	Main	26.9	4.83	23.5	Dinner
Spaghetti Squash Sauté	AI	Side	0.68	7.34	7.14	Dinner
Chocolate Avocado Pudding	Paleo	Snack	7.88	23.66	6.05	Snack
	Total Nutrient Analysis		**77.34**	**107.32**	**80.34**	
DAY 3						
Root Cause Original Smoothie	AI	Main	12.79	26.38	15.98	Breakfast
Sweet and Sour Chicken Skewers with Broccoli Salad (LO)*	AI	Main	26.9	4.83	23.5	Lunch
Spaghetti Squash Sauté (LO)*	AI	Side	0.68	7.34	7.14	Lunch
Maple Meatloaf Muffins	AI	Main	15.25	20.34	9.24	Dinner
Crunchy Arugula Salad	AI	Main	2.91	7.5	13.47	Dinner
Galaretka	AI	Main	12.3	4.71	7.93	Snack
	Total Nutrient Analysis		**70.83**	**71.1**	**77.26**	

* LO = leftovers.

RECIPE NAMES	MEAL TYPE	FOOD TYPE	PROTEIN (G)	FAT (G)	CARBS (G)	MEAL
DAY 4						
Root Cause Original Smoothie	AI	Main	12.79	26.38	15.98	Breakfast
Maple Meatloaf Muffins (LO)*	AI	Main	15.25	20.34	9.24	Lunch
Carrot Fries	AI	Side	1.23	3.7	12.14	Lunch
Slow-Cooked Chicken	AI	Main	52.01	8.65	0.42	Dinner
Bacon and Chive Scalloped Potatoes	AI	Side	6.57	29.12	12.85	Dinner
Lemon–Banana Cream Ice Pops	AI	Snack	4.63	9.77	6.76	Snack
	Total Nutrient Analysis		**92.48**	**97.96**	**57.39**	
DAY 5						
Root Cause Original Smoothie	AI	Main	12.79	26.38	15.98	Breakfast
Chicken Soup	AI	Main	19.57	3.64	6.37	Lunch
Cucumber-Fig Salad	AI	Side	35.59	14.37	5.85	Dinner
Moroccan Lamb Stew	AI	Main	47.48	33	23.31	Dinner
Galaretka (LO)*	AI	Main	12.3	4.71	7.93	Snack
	Total Nutrient Analysis		**127.73**	**82.1**	**59.44**	
DAY 6						
Chicken Plantain "Nachos"	AI	Main	7.12	8.32	28.3	Breakfast
SAM Salad	AI	Main	19.18	25.62	22.89	Lunch
Cream of Broccoli Soup	AI	Main	9.49	30.17	14.34	Dinner
Beef Jerky	AI	Side	20.86	12.64	3.78	Dinner
Orange Cream Smoothie	AI	Main	14.32	5.11	20.61	Snack
	Total Nutrient Analysis		**70.97**	**81.86**	**89.92**	
DAY 7						
Hashi Hash Hash	AI	Main	24.58	8.82	16.48	Breakfast
Moroccan Lamb Stew (LO)*	AI	Main	47.48	33	23.31	Lunch
Pulled Cherry Pork	AI	Main	45.73	31.83	19.87	Dinner
Biscuits	AI	Side	1.34	11.3	28.15	Dinner
Steamed Green Beans	AI	Side	0	0	0	Dinner
Sweet Potato Pistachio Pudding	Paleo	Snack	8.6	10.2	30.28	Snack
	Total Nutrient Analysis		**127.73**	**95.15**	**118.09**	

* LO = leftovers.

Cookbook

SAVORY MAINS

SIDES AND SNACKS

SWEETS

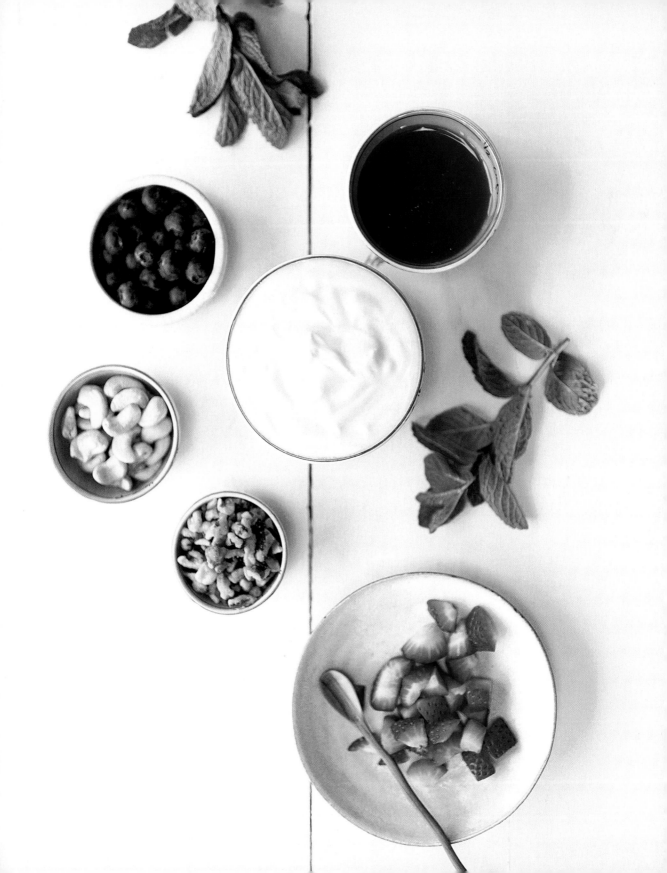

Coconut Yogurt

Ⓐ AUTOIMMUNE

Prep time: 30 minutes

Cook time: 8 to 24 hours in yogurt maker

Serves: 4

14 ounces creamed coconut

½ cup water

2 teaspoons gelatin

1 tablespoon maple syrup

Dairy-free yogurt starter, high-quality probiotic capsules, ¼ cup yogurt starter, or ¼ cup yogurt from previous batch

Coconut yogurt is a delicious way to restore balance to your gut. This creamy homemade Coconut Yogurt provides all of the gut-healing benefits without the extra sugar and other additives that can complicate your health journey. I love using this in salad dressings and smoothies or enjoying it topped with shaved coconut, pumpkin seeds, nuts, berries, or a splash of maple syrup.

1. Blend the creamed coconut with water in a high-powered blender. Heat the coconut milk to 180°F, then cool to 105°F.

2. Add the gelatin and maple syrup.

3. Place the mixture in a yogurt maker or tightly sealed Mason jar at room temperature for 8 to 24 hours.

4. If using yogurt maker, remove and put into sealed containers, such as glass Mason jars.

5. Store in the fridge for up to 2 weeks.

Nutritional Analysis per Serving: Protein (g) 3.23; Fat (g) 23.26; Carbs (g) 8.65; B_{12} (mcg) 0; Iron (mg) 1.67; Iodine (mcg) 0; Magnesium (mg) 37.35; Potassium (mg) 267.52; Selenium (mcg) 6.54; Sodium (mg) 17.35

Fermented Vegetables

Ⓐ AUTOIMMUNE

Prep time: 20 minutes

Cook time: 7 to 10 days fermenting

Serves: 8

2 pounds cabbage, core removed, finely chopped

4 teaspoons sea salt or pink Himalayan sea salt

Water

1 large cabbage leaf per jar to cover and push down the vegetables

Fermenting veggies increases the nutrient content and creates beneficial bacteria that can help with digestion and repopulating the gut. This supersimple recipe is made with cabbage, but you can substitute almost any vegetable, such as carrots, broccoli, chard, beets, spinach, kale, or cucumber to create gut-healing foods you will love!

Fermented vegetables are a staple of Polish culture—my grandmother would make these every fall and would store them in her cellar all winter long. My brother Robert has taken over the tradition and makes a fermentation crock's worth of fermented cabbage each winter for our whole family to enjoy.

1. In a large bowl, gradually salt the cabbage and squeeze until juice forms, about 10 to 15 minutes.

2. Add chopped vegetables to glass jars and compress.

3. Close the lid and store in a cool dark place like a pantry, allowing it to ferment for 7 to 10 days.

4. Store in the fridge until ready to use.

Nutritional Analysis per Serving: Protein (g) 1.45; Fat (g) 0.11; Carbs (g) 6.58; B_{12} (mcg) 0; Iron (mg) 0.53; Iodine (mcg) 0; Magnesium (mg) 13.61; Potassium (mg) 192.78; Selenium (mcg) 0.34; Sodium (mg) 800.41

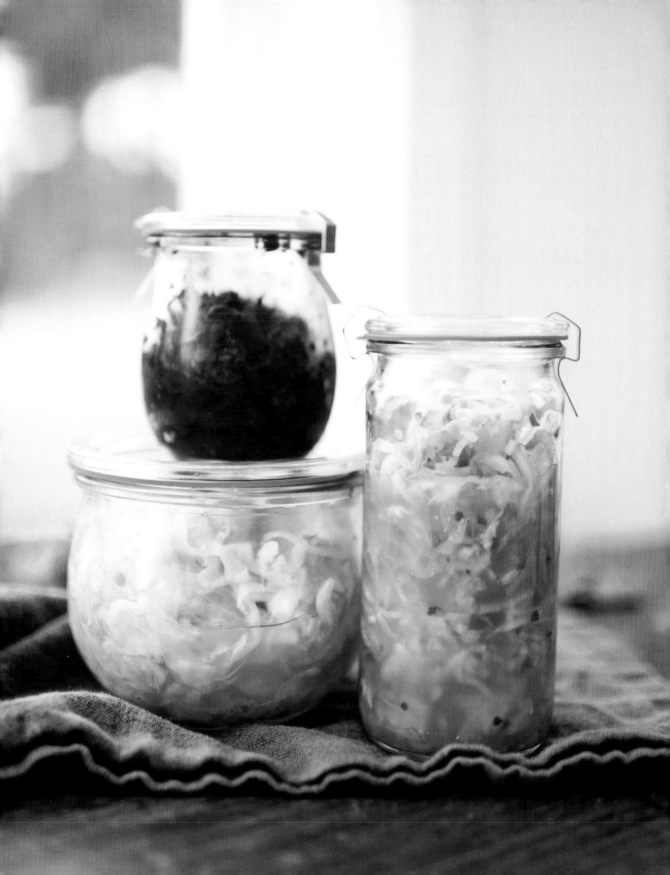

Mom's Dill Pickles

Ⓐ AUTOIMMUNE

Prep time: 15 minutes

Cook time: 7 to 10 days fermenting

Serves: 12

8 to 12 medium pickling cucumbers

2 bay leaves

2 cloves garlic

2 pinches black pepper (if tolerated)

1 (3-inch) piece horseradish or
3 tablespoons prepared horseradish

2 pinches allspice (if tolerated)

1 bunch fresh dill weed

2 cups purified (or boiled and then cooled) water

1 tablespoon sea salt or pink Himalayan sea salt

1 large cabbage leaf

This is my mom's yummy pickle recipe! Lacto-fermented pickles are a tasty way to get additional probiotics into your body. To make lacto-fermented pickles, you can use a traditional stoneware crock or a large glass jar. It is important to use either purified or sterilized (boiled) water, so that the pickles will be free of undesirable microbes. If you boil the water, be sure to let the water cool before you add the rest of the ingredients; hot water can destroy the beneficial microbes you are introducing! Be sure to store these pickles in the fridge after they've fermented to retain the beneficial microbes.

1. Wash and dry the cucumbers and place them tightly in a dry 1-quart jar.

2. Add the bay leaves, garlic, pepper, horseradish, and allspice to the jar and place the dill on top.

3. Mix the water with salt to create a brine and fill the jar to ½ inch above the top of the cucumbers.

4. Add a cabbage leaf to the top of the jar to hold the cucumbers in place, so they stay submerged.

5. Close the jar moderately tightly and store in a cool, dark place like a pantry, allowing it to ferment for 7 to 10 days.

6. Store in the fridge until ready to serve to ensure the survival of the beneficial microbes. Microbes will only stay active outside of the fridge for up to 2 weeks, but will stay alive for months if kept refrigerated.

Nutritional Analysis per Serving: Protein (g) 2.15; Fat (g) 0.37; Carbs (g) 12.02; B_{12} (mcg) 0; Iron (mg) 0.99; Iodine (mcg) 0; Magnesium (mg) 40.71; Potassium (mg) 472.83; Selenium (mcg) 0.98; Sodium (mg) 396.94

Bone Broth

Ⓐ AUTOIMMUNE

Prep time: 15 minutes

Cook time: 8 to 12 hours in a slow cooker; 8 to 12 hours on the stovetop; 90 minutes in an electric pressure cooker

Serves: Varies

4 to 5 chicken legs

1 tablespoon apple cider vinegar

2 stalks celery

1 onion

6 to 8 large carrots

Purified water

Sea salt or pink Himalayan sea salt to taste

Black pepper to taste (if tolerated)

Bone Broth offers amazing healing properties for your gut and immune system, and people who consume bone broth regularly report benefits such as shinier hair, clearer skin, and less joint pain. Who doesn't love a steaming hot mug of homemade Bone Broth? One of my favorite things in the world is waking up in the morning to the fragrance of fresh, delicious Bone Broth that has been slow-cooking all night in my kitchen while I'm sound asleep and resting my adrenals.

Here I've included three methods: slow cooker, stovetop, and electric pressure cooker. If you have a sensitivity to histamines, the pressure-cooker method is the way to go due to the reduction of histamines in the broth.

Slow Cooker:

1. Place the chicken, vinegar, and vegetables in a slow cooker.

2. Fill with water to 1 inch below the top of slow cooker, cover, and cook on high for 8 to 12 hours.

3. Season with salt and pepper to taste.

4. Strain, pour into Mason jars, and refrigerate.

Stovetop:

1. Place the chicken, vinegar, and vegetables in a stockpot.

2. Fill with water to 1 inch below the top of the stockpot.

3. Bring to a boil, reduce the heat to medium-low, and simmer for 8 to 12 hours.

4. Season with salt and pepper to taste.

5. Strain, pour into Mason jars, and refrigerate.

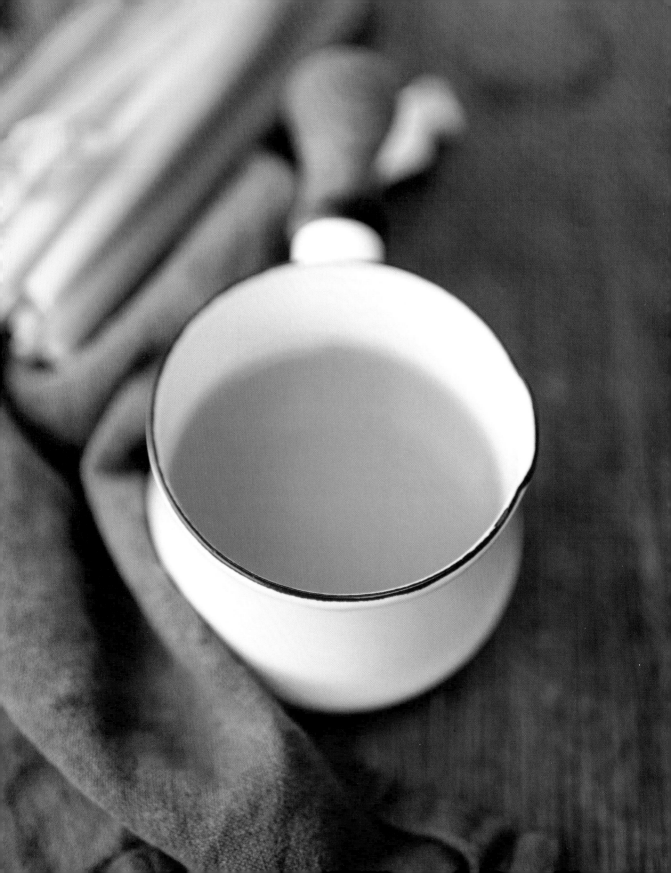

Electric Pressure Cooker:

1. Place the chicken, vinegar, and vegetables into the pot of the pressure cooker.

2. Fill two-thirds of the way up with water and secure the pressure cooker lid.

3. Press the Manual button, set the pressure on high, and set the timer for 90 minutes.

4. Season with salt and pepper to taste.

5. Strain, pour into Mason jars, and refrigerate.

Nutritional Analysis per Serving: Protein (g) 22.68; Fat (g) 6.88; Carbs (g) 4.84; B_{12} (mcg) 0.19; Iron (mg) 1.32; Iodine (mcg) 0; Magnesium (mg) 24.25; Potassium (mg) 298.58; Selenium (mcg) 22.51; Sodium (mg) 91.53

Everyday Dressing

Ⓐ AUTOIMMUNE

Prep time: 10 minutes

Serves: 4

¼ cup extra-virgin olive oil

¼ cup of lemon juice

1 tablespoon dried basil

One of the most common questions I receive from clients and readers who are starting to transition their lifestyle is, "What type of dressing can I use on my salad?" Many of our conventional packaged dressings are unfortunately filled with inflammatory oils and may even contain gluten and dairy. You can make your own tasty dressing in minutes! Everyday Dressing works well in place of Italian dressing and is packed with heart-healthy and anti-inflammatory olive oil, basil, and lemon juice.

1. Mix all ingredients together.

2. Refrigerate until ready to serve.

Nutritional Analysis per Serving: Protein (g) 0.3; Fat (g) 13.58; Carbs (g) 1.55; B$_{12}$ (mcg) 0; Iron (mg) 1.03; Iodine (mcg) 0; Magnesium (mg) 8.38; Potassium (mg) 43.46; Selenium (mcg) 0.05; Sodium (mg) 1.22

Fermented Coconut Water

Ⓐ AUTOIMMUNE

Prep time: 20 minutes

Cook time: 36 hours fermenting

Serves: 4

6 cups coconut water

1 teaspoon powdered high-quality lactobacillus-based probiotic/kefir starter or fermented coconut water

---

Nutritional Analysis per Serving: Protein (g) 2.59; Fat (g) 0.72; Carbs (g) 13.36; B_{12} (mcg) 0; Iron (mg) 1.04; Iodine (mcg) 0; Magnesium (mg) 90; Potassium (mg) 900; Selenium (mcg) 3.6; Sodium (mg) 378

Kefir is a beverage with multiple gut-health benefits because it contains beneficial bacteria. Unfortunately, traditional kefir is made with milk—not ideal for the 80 percent of people with Hashimoto's who have dairy sensitivity. Thankfully, one of my mentors, Donna Gates, introduced fermented coconut kefir to the world. Fermented Coconut Water can be consumed alone or used as a base for beverages like my Hashi-Mojito.

In order to ensure that the right type of bacteria are growing in your coconut water, you will need to use a starter of good bacteria. The starter bacteria can be sourced from a kefir starter, a high-quality probiotic powder, or another fermented coconut beverage. Just be sure that the starter you use is dairy free! In order to make sure the fermentation process happens correctly, you will need to watch the temperature of the beverage; I use a food thermometer.

1. Place the coconut water in a saucepan and gently heat until the temperature reaches 90°F (do not exceed 100°F).

2. Add the starter to the warmed coconut water and mix.

3. Pour the mixture into a 1-quart glass jar and cover.

4. Wrap the jar in a cloth and allow it to ferment at room temperature for 36 hours.

5. Once the coconut water has fermented, it should be fizzy and slightly tangy.

6. Store in fridge to preserve the activity of the bacteria.

7. Be sure to save 1 to 2 tablespoons of the remaining fermented coconut water for your next batch!

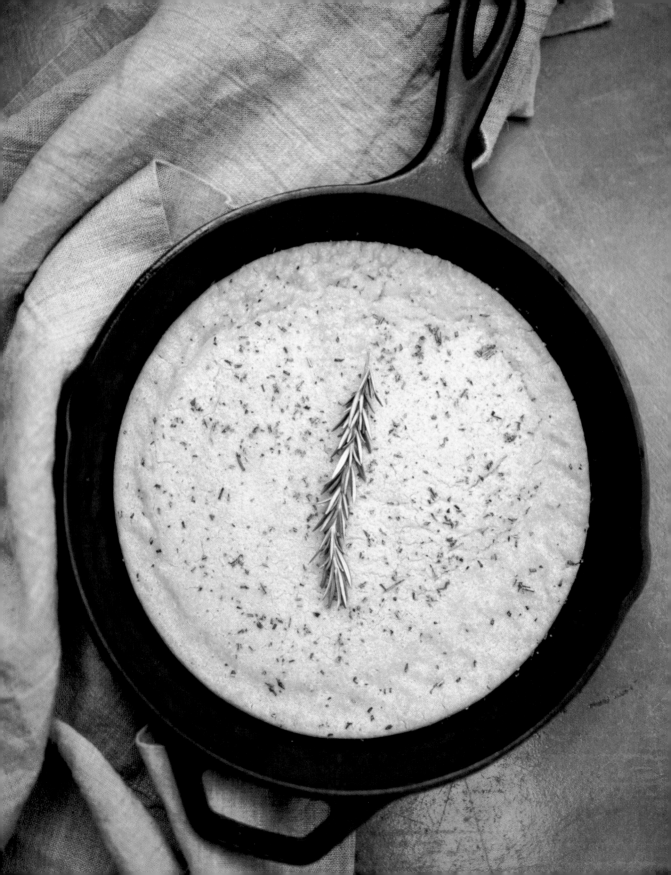

Farinata Bread

❶ INTRO

Prep time: 2 minutes

Cook time: 4 hours soaking,
10 to 12 minutes baking

Serves: 4

**Note: This bread is best eaten the
same day, warm.**

8 ounces garbanzo-bean flour

½ teaspoon sea salt or pink
Himalayan sea salt, plus ¼ teaspoon
for sprinkling

1½ cups water

2 tablespoons extra-virgin olive oil

1 teaspoon dried rosemary (optional)

Nutritional Analysis per
Serving: Protein (g) 7.57; Fat (g)
7.05; Carbs (g) 22.81; B$_{12}$ (mcg)
0; Iron (mg) 2.35; Iodine (mcg)
0; Magnesium (mg) 0.44;
Potassium (mg) 1.96; Selenium
(mcg) 0.01; Sodium (mg) 201.49

My husband and I discovered this delicious, gluten-free food while traveling to the Cinque-Terre region of Italy. Farinata Bread is an Italian pancake (or crepe) that's traditionally made from garbanzo-bean (chickpea) flour, which can improve digestion and is an exceptional plant-based protein. It's great served alongside a soup or stew, like my Creamy White Chicken Stew (p. 193).

1. In a medium-size mixing bowl, mix the bean flour and salt until combined.

2. Gently whisk the water into the dry ingredients until smooth and let sit, covered, for 4 hours. It's ready when the flour has separated from the water.

3. Preheat the oven to 550°F and position the oven rack in the middle of the oven.

4. Pour the olive oil into a 12-inch cast-iron skillet and swirl until the entire bottom of the pan is coated.

5. In the mixing bowl, skim off any foam from the water, mix the batter until combined, and pour into the cast-iron pan, swirling it around so the oil sits on top of the batter.

6. Mix the salt and rosemary together and sprinkle it evenly over the batter.

7. Shut the oven off and turn the broiler on low (if you have only one broil setting, turn the broiler on and adjust the oven rack so it's not too close to the broiler). Place the pan in the oven and bake for 10 to 12 minutes, checking periodically to ensure it does not burn. It is done when the middle no longer jiggles.

8. Remove from the oven and let rest.

9. Serve warm or at room temperature.

Hashi-Mayo

P PALEO

Prep time: 10 minutes

Serves: 20

Note: Hashi-Mayo should keep in the fridge for 5 to 7 days. If using olive oil, it is best to use a light-tasting olive oil, as extra-virgin olive oil can be very overpowering.

2 teaspoons lemon juice

*2 eggs (chicken or duck), at room temperature

½ teaspoon sea salt or pink Himalayan sea salt

1 cup olive or avocado oil

*Possible Modifications for Other Root Cause Diets: Use duck eggs if sensitive to chicken eggs.

Nutritional Analysis per Serving: Protein (g) 0.63; Fat (g) 11.36; Carbs (g) 0.07; B_{12} (mcg) 0.05; Iron (mg) 0.09; Iodine (mcg) 2.4; Magnesium (mg) 0.63; Potassium (mg) 7.42; Selenium (mcg) 1.54; Sodium (mg) 46.11

The ultimate comfort food, mayo can be a source of fat and help keep our appetite satisfied. Most grocery-store brands are made with soy and canola oil, both potential thyroid toxins. You can make your own mayo by creating an emulsion of either olive oil or avocado oil and eggs and adding a little acidity with lemon juice. Emulsification is a process of blending oil and water-based liquids to produce a semisolid form. We learned the art of emulsifications using a mortar and pestle during pharmacy school, but a high-speed blender or an immersion blender makes the process foolproof. Traditionally, raw eggs are used to make mayo, which may be a source of salmonella. If you feel confident in the source of your eggs, you can use them raw. If you are concerned with risk, you may choose to utilize pasteurized or lightly cooked eggs.

High-Speed Blender

1. Place the eggs, lemon juice, and salt in a high-speed blender and set on level 7.

2. Slowly add the oil into the blender to emulsify the eggs and oil; the process should take 2 to 3 minutes.

Immersion Blender

1. Place the eggs, lemon juice, salt, and oil, in that order, in a clear jar that the immersion blender can fit snugly into (or use the container it comes with if you have that option).

2. Start blending and watch the mixture. Once it starts to turn off-white at the bottom of the jar, slowly start to pull the blender upward. Once the entire mixture is off-white, it is emulsified.

3. Blend for about 30 to 45 seconds total.

Pizza Sauce

P PALEO

Prep time: 5 minutes

Cook time: 10 minutes

Makes 1 cup

6 ounces tomato paste

1 cup Bone Broth (p. 135) or water

¼ teaspoon dried oregano

¼ teaspoon dried parsley

¼ teaspoon dried basil

¼ teaspoon onion powder

¼ teaspoon garlic powder

⅛ teaspoon dried rosemary

Sea salt or pink Himalayan sea salt to taste

Black pepper to taste (if tolerated)

Making your own pizza sauce is so simple! The best part is that you get to create a version that includes only ingredients you can pronounce and doesn't contain any additives or preservatives. It's also super budget-friendly! The tomato paste is loaded with lycopene, which supports heart health, and the herbs and garlic help reduce inflammation.

1. In a saucepan, combine all ingredients and cook until the sauce is reduced and thickened, about 10 minutes. *Voilà!*

Nutritional Analysis per Serving: Protein (g) 13.68; Fat (g) 2.89; Carbs (g) 33.8; B_{12} (mcg) 0; Iron (mg) 5.71; Iodine (mcg) 0; Magnesium (mg) 77.27; Potassium (mg) 1948.03; Selenium (mcg) 9.31; Sodium (mg) 1855.41

Cashew Cream Cheese

P PALEO

Prep time: 8 hours soaking, 5 minutes prep

Serves: 4

1 cup raw cashews

1½ cups water

1 tablespoon lemon juice

1 tablespoon balsamic vinegar

2 tablespoons water

If you're looking for the flavor and texture of cream cheese, look no further than this Cashew Cream Cheese recipe! The nuts must soak overnight, so if you are eager to try this recipe, figure in the soaking time. Cashews are loaded with nutrients such as selenium, magnesium, and iron, which are essential in supporting thyroid health. Make sure to find a balsamic vinegar that is free of additives. The only ingredients should be red wine vinegar and grape must; any sulfites should be naturally occurring, not added.

1. The night before, soak 1 cup of raw cashews overnight in 1½ cups of water.

2. In the morning, drain the water from the soaked nuts, which should be soft.

3. Place the nuts, lemon juice, balsamic vinegar, and water in a high-speed blender.

4. Blend on low to combine ingredients. Then blend on high for 30 to 60 seconds until it reaches the consistency of cream cheese.

Nutritional Analysis per Serving: Protein (g) 5.84; Fat (g) 14; Carbs (g) 10.57; B_{12} (mcg) 0; Iron (mg) 2.16; Iodine (mcg) 0; Magnesium (mg) 93.84; Potassium (mg) 218.88; Selenium (mcg) 6.35; Sodium (mg) 4.78

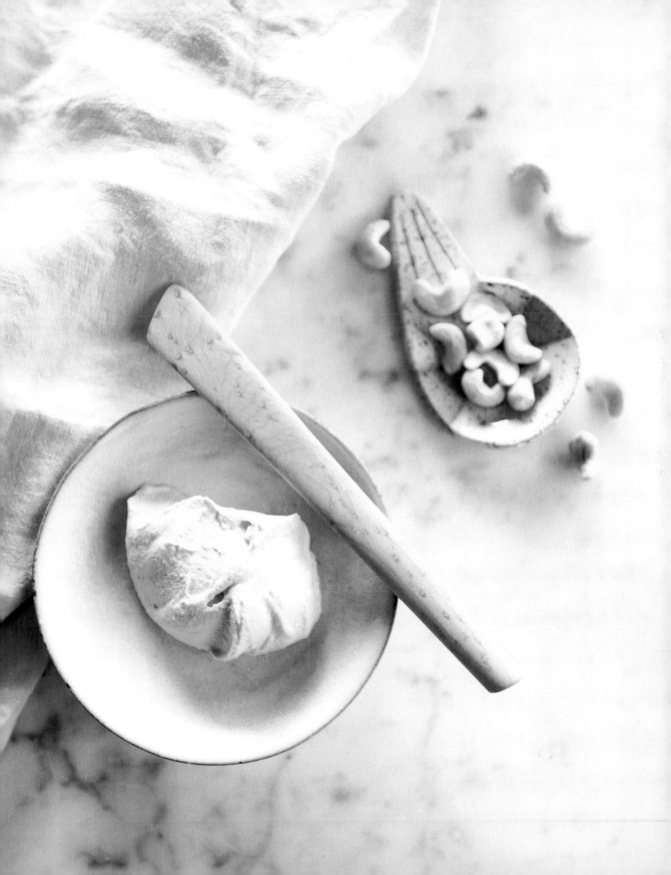

Chunky Applesauce

A AUTOIMMUNE

Prep time: 5 minutes

Cook time: 30 minutes

Serves: 6

1 cup water

4 fresh green apples, peeled, cored, and cut into wedges

½ teaspoon ground cinnamon

*½ teaspoon ground cardamom (if tolerated)

*Possible Modifications for Other Root Cause Diets: Remove the cardamom to make the applesauce compliant with the Autoimmune Diet.

Applesauce has long been known as a great gut-soothing food that can help you get diarrhea and other types of digestive distress under control. Apples are rich in pectin, and cooking them releases this wonderful substance that provides wonderful prebiotic food for beneficial bacteria, which in turn improves the gut barrier, and reduces gut-derived toxins (known as endotoxins).

1. Place the water and apple wedges in a small saucepan, cover, and bring to a boil.

2. Reduce the heat and simmer for 25 minutes, until the apples are soft and turn a light yellow color; if the pan becomes dry, add a bit more water.

3. Remove the apples from the saucepan, add cinnamon and cardamom, and then lightly mix or mash with a potato masher.

Variation

For a sweeter version, substitute gala apples for the green apples and nutmeg (if tolerated) for the cardamom, and you have a sweet treat low in sugar and high in fiber!

Nutritional Analysis per Serving: Protein (g) 0.51; Fat (g) 0.33; Carbs (g) 25.53; B_{12} (mcg) 0; Iron (mg) 0.28; Iodine (mcg) 0; Magnesium (mg) 9.84; Potassium (mg) 198.73; Selenium (mcg) 0.06; Sodium (mg) 1.89

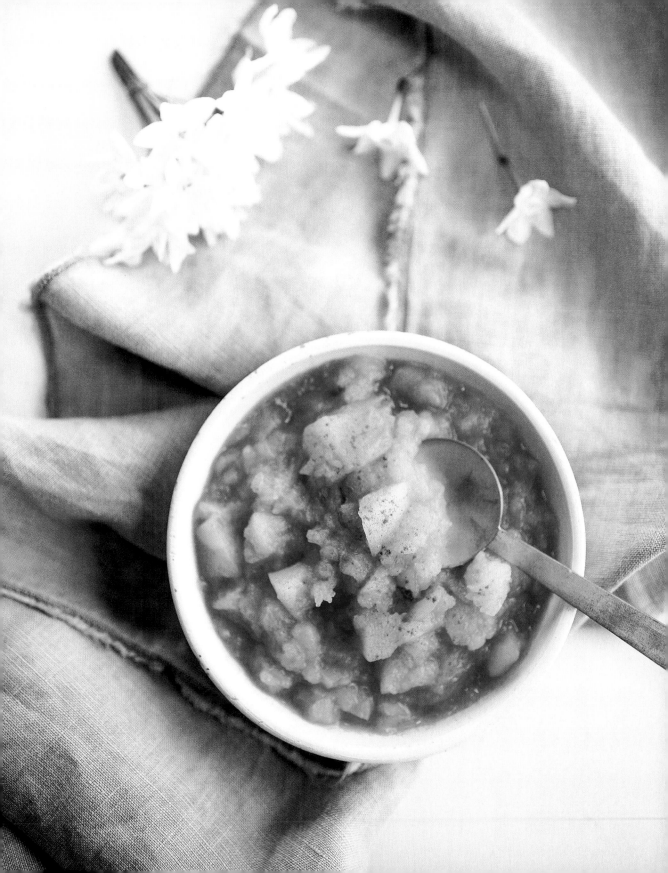

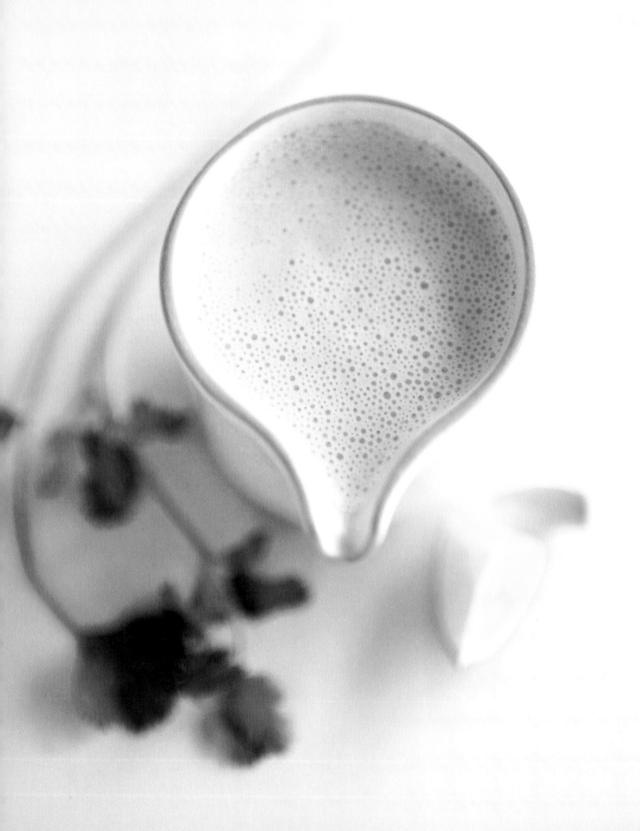

Goddess of Detox Dressing

Ⓐ AUTOIMMUNE

Prep time: 10 minutes

Serves: 4

1 cup loosely packed cilantro,
stems removed

½ cup plain Coconut Yogurt (p. 131)

¼ cup olive oil

2 tablespoons apple cider vinegar

1 medium clove garlic

Juice of 1 lime

Pinch of sea salt or pink Himalayan
sea salt

This delicious dressing contains plenty of health-promoting ingredients, including probiotic-rich coconut yogurt, digestion-supporting apple cider vinegar, and detoxifying cilantro! You can use it on salads in place of creamy dressings.

1. Place all ingredients in a high-powered blender and mix until a creamy consistency is formed.

2. Refrigerate until ready to serve.

Nutritional Analysis per Serving: Protein (g) 0.3; Fat (g) 14.41; Carbs (g) 3.19; B_{12} (mcg) 0.26; Iron (mg) 0.3; Iodine (mcg) 0; Magnesium (mg) 16.99; Potassium (mg) 35.08; Selenium (mcg) 0.15; Sodium (mg) 101.17

Tomato Sauce

P PALEO

Prep time: 10 minutes

Cook time: 30 to 45 minutes

Serves: 4

1 tablespoon avocado oil

1 small onion, diced

1 celery rib, diced

1 medium carrot, diced

2 garlic cloves, minced

1 (28-ounce) can diced tomatoes, or 4 large tomatoes, diced

1 teaspoon dried oregano

1 teaspoon dried parsley

1 bunch fresh basil

1 bay leaf

Sea salt or pink Himalayan sea salt to taste

Black pepper to taste (if tolerated)

Tomatoes contain lycopene, an important antioxidant that supports anti-aging and heart health. This is a simple chunky Tomato Sauce that can also be transformed into a smooth or a Bolognese version.

1. In a large saucepan, heat the oil on medium. Add the onions, celery, and carrots and cook until softened, about 10 minutes.

2. Add the garlic and sauté for 1 minute.

3. Add the tomatoes, dried herbs, and salt. Cook until the tomatoes release their juices, become soft, and can be mashed with a spoon, about 20 minutes.

4. Remove basil and bay leaf.

5. Serve over Spaghetti Squash Sauté (p. 301), zucchini noodles, or sweet potato noodles.

Variation: Smooth

1. Once the sauce has been cooked and the basil and bay leaf removed, pour the sauce into a blender and blend until smooth. (When working with a hot sauce, make sure the top of the blender is vented to let the steam escape.)

2. Pour back into the saucepan and cook until the sauce reduces slightly and becomes thick, about 15 minutes.

Nutritional Analysis per Serving: Protein (g) 2.62; Fat (g) 3.97; Carbs (g) 13.31; B_{12} (mcg) 0; Iron (mg) 1.13; Iodine (mcg) 0; Magnesium (mg) 33.42; Potassium (mg) 618.87; Selenium (mcg) 0.47; Sodium (mg) 420.55

Variation: Bolognese

1. Once the sauce has been cooked and the basil and bay leaf removed, pour the sauce into a blender and blend until smooth. (When working with a hot sauce, make sure the top of the blender is vented to let the steam escape.) Set aside.

2. Clean the saucepan out, and add 1 teaspoon of avocado oil.

3. Brown 1 pound of ground beef, and then pour the pureed sauce back into the pot.

4. Cook until the sauce is thick, about 15 minutes.

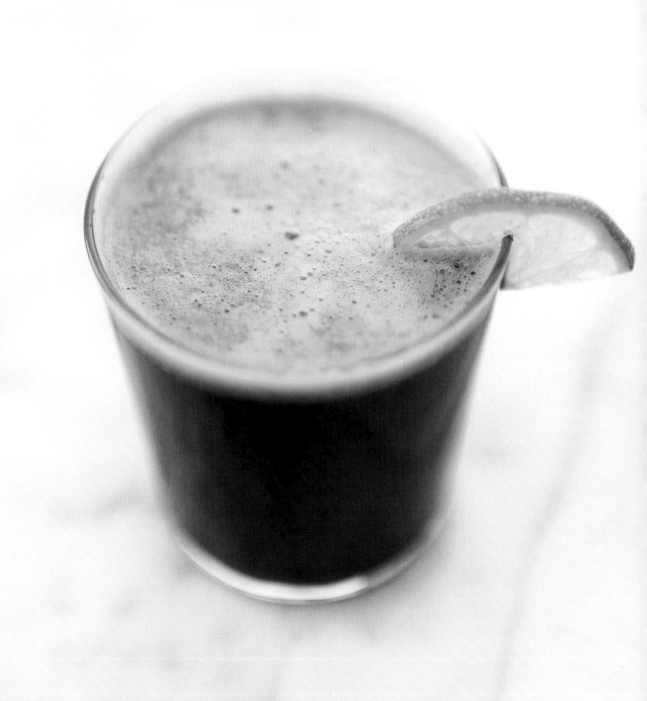

Green Juice

Ⓐ AUTOIMMUNE

Prep time: 10 minutes

Serves: 2

Note: You can keep leftover juice in a sealed glass container up to 24 hours in the fridge.

6 to 7 baby carrots

1 Granny Smith apple, cored and cut into wedges

3 to 4 stalks celery

1 small cucumber, sliced in half

3 cups finely chopped kale

1 lime, sliced in half

Sea salt or pink Himalayan sea salt to taste

1 to 2 tablespoons coconut oil or 1 avocado (optional)

Green juices are a fantastic way to get some nutrition into your system without having to stress your digestion. They are also full of chlorophyll, which has excellent detoxifying properties. If blood-sugar stabilization is an issue for you, go for the coconut oil or avocado!

1. Using a masticating juicer, slowly feed the vegetables and fruit (including the peels) into the juicer until all produce has been processed.

2. If using coconut oil or avocado, place it in a blender, add the juiced fruit and vegetables, and blend for 30 seconds.

Nutritional Analysis per Serving: Protein (g) 7.72; Fat (g) 11.77; Carbs (g) 38.82; B_{12} (mcg) 0; Iron (mg) 3; Iodine (mcg) 0; Magnesium (mg) 99.78; Potassium (mg) 1423.59; Selenium (mcg) 2.36; Sodium (mg) 333.6

Hashi-Mojito

℗ PALEO

Prep time: 10 minutes

Serves: 1

1 bunch fresh mint leaves

Juice of 1 lime

½ teaspoon ground ginger

1 cup fermented or plain coconut water

*Stevia to taste

*Possible Modifications for Other Root Cause Diets: Use maple syrup instead of stevia for Autoimmune Diet.

Imagine that you're sitting somewhere on a warm beach in Miami as you sip on this healthier version of the refreshing Mojito. Thanks to the mint and ginger, the Hashi-Mojito is a super gut-soothing and refreshing beverage you can enjoy in place of alcohol or soda!

1. Mash the mint leaves using a mortar and pestle to release the flavor.

2. In a glass, mix the mint with lime juice, ginger, coconut water, and sweetener. Alternatively, place all ingredients in a blender and blend.

Nutritional Analysis per Serving: Protein (g) 2.55; Fat (g) 0.72; Carbs (g) 12.85; B$_{12}$ (mcg) 0; Iron (mg) 1.78; Iodine (mcg) 0; Magnesium (mg) 77.45; Potassium (mg) 727.49; Selenium (mcg) 2.76; Sodium (mg) 258.34

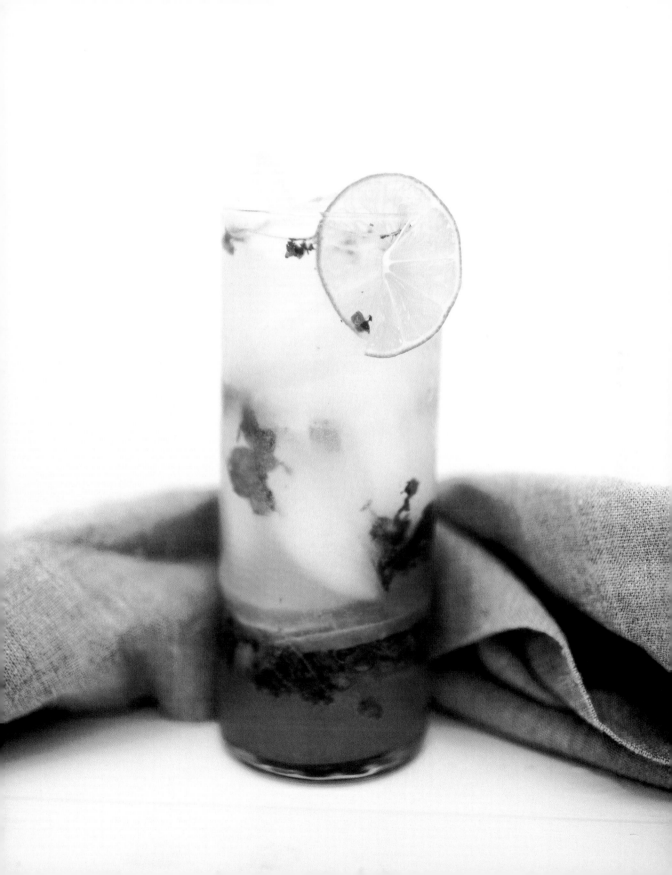

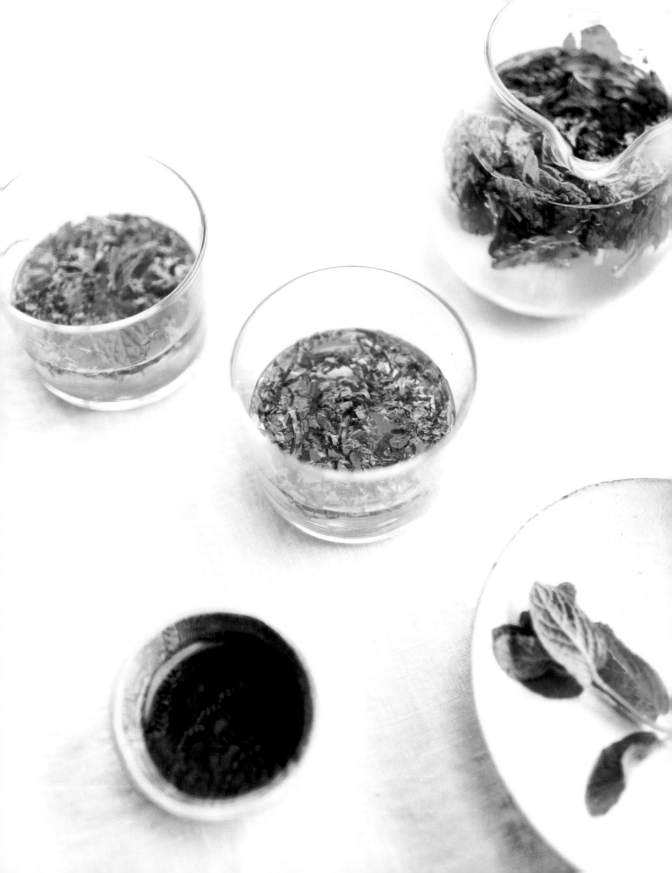

Mint Tea

Ⓐ AUTOIMMUNE

Prep time: 5 minutes

Serves: 1

1 tablespoon fresh mint leaves

1 cup boiling water

Maple syrup to taste

Mint is a soothing herb that can help with digestive issues and stimulate bile flow for healthy detoxification. Mint Tea is a popular, trendy drink found at most Amsterdam cafés, and it's so delicious and simple you'll want to make it every day. Peppermint oil has also been shown to be helpful for SIBO, so this simple recipe may be a good addition to your healing protocols.

1. Mash or chop the mint.

2. Add the mint to boiling water.

3. Sweeten to taste and enjoy!

Nutritional Analysis per Serving: Protein (g) 0.06; Fat (g) 0.02; Carbs (g) 4.71; B_{12} (mcg) 0; Iron (mg) 0.09; Iodine (mcg) 0; Magnesium (mg) 2.68; Potassium (mg) 23.23; Selenium (mcg) 0.04; Sodium (mg) 1.3

Maca Latte

P PALEO

Prep time: 5 minutes

Serves: 2

1½ cups hot water

1 cup coconut milk

2 teaspoons maca root powder

2 teaspoons maple syrup, honey, coconut nectar, or sweetener of your choice to taste

A Maca Latte hits the spot when you're trying to wean yourself off caffeine but are looking for something tasty. Maca, a yellow root vegetable originally grown in Peru, is an adaptogen (helps the body adapt to stress) and can help to stabilize our hormones and adrenals! Please note, some individuals may find maca too activating. If that is the case for you, reduce the amount or discontinue. I prefer using gelatinized maca powder. The gelatinization process removes the starch, making the maca less bitter and easier to digest, while retaining the hormone-balancing benefits.

1. Place all ingredients in a blender and blend for 30 seconds.

Nutritional Analysis per Serving: Protein (g) 2.75; Fat (g) 28.61; Carbs (g) 14.11; B_{12} (mcg) 0; Iron (mg) 2.63; Iodine (mcg) 0; Magnesium (mg) 45.8; Potassium (mg) 423.23; Selenium (mcg) 7.48; Sodium (mg) 19.6

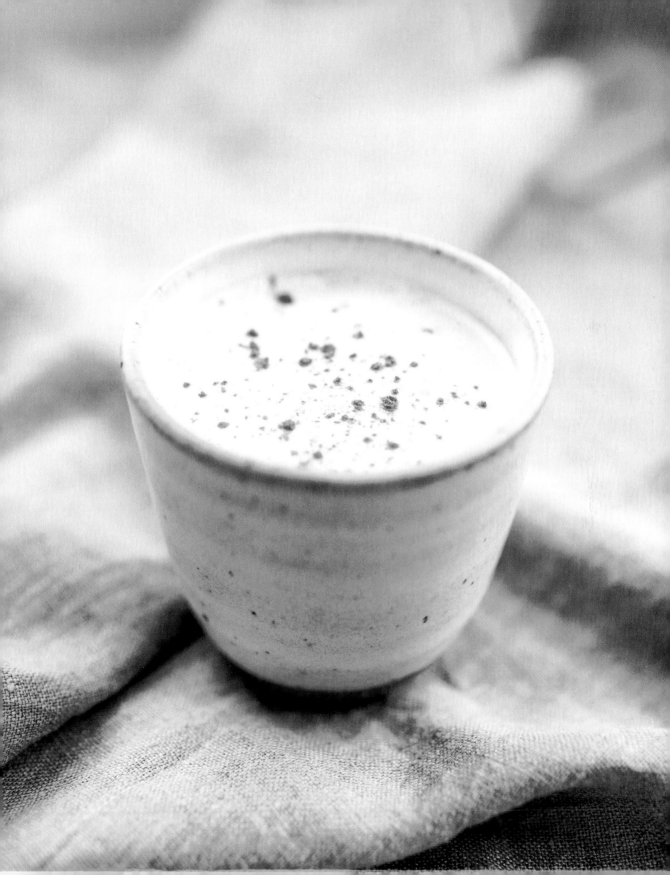

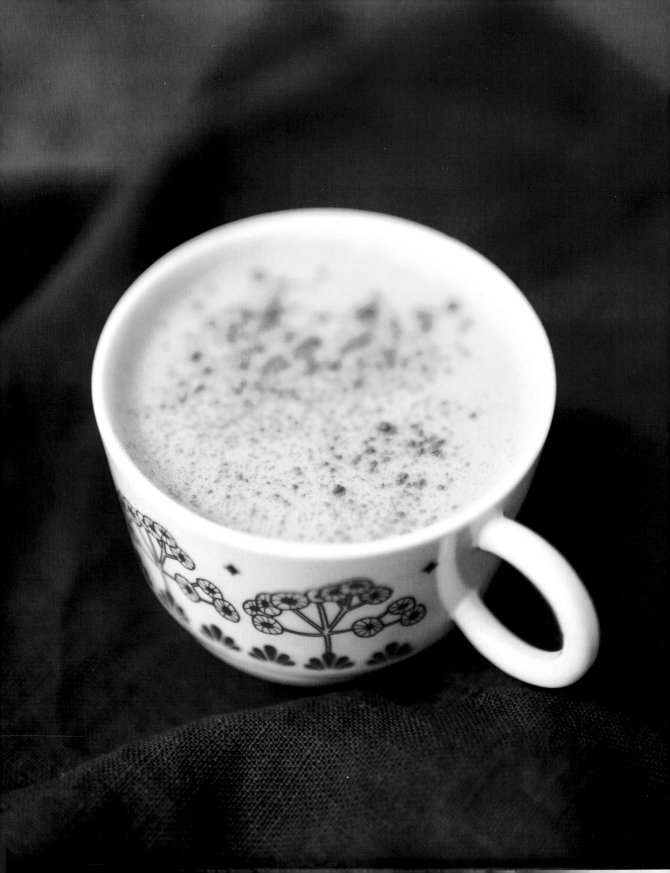

Pumpkin Maca Latte

Ⓟ PALEO

Prep time: 5 minutes

Serves: 1

1 cup boiling water

½ cup coconut milk

2 tablespoons canned organic pumpkin puree

2 teaspoons pumpkin pie spice (or AI Pumpkin Pie Spice, p. 95), plus 1 pinch for garnish

*1 teaspoon maca root powder (if tolerated)

1 teaspoon maple syrup

*Possible Modifications for Other Root Cause Diets: Maca is not Autoimmune friendly in the elimination phase, but may be able to be reintroduced during a later phase of the diet.

There's something magical about pumpkin pie spice. I know that whenever I smell the fragrant blend of cinnamon, ginger, lemon peel, and the other spices, I feel like celebrating. My Pumpkin Maca Latte will help you celebrate your great health by offering a caffeine-free, hormone- and blood sugar–balancing base of coconut milk, maca, and cinnamon. Plus, you'll get a boost of digestion support from the pumpkin puree and the spices in pumpkin pie spice. I prefer using gelatinized maca powder. The gelatinization process removes the starch, making the maca less bitter and easier to digest, while retaining the hormone-balancing benefits.

1. Place all ingredients in a blender and blend for 20 to 30 seconds until the color is uniform.

Nutritional Analysis per Serving: Protein (g) 3.28; Fat (g) 29.13; Carbs (g) 15.95; B_{12} (mcg) 0; Iron (mg) 3.07; Iodine (mcg) 0; Magnesium (mg) 57.47; Potassium (mg) 415.46; Selenium (mcg) 7.92; Sodium (mg) 22.1

Orange Cream Smoothie

Ⓐ AUTOIMMUNE

Prep time: 5 minutes

Serves: 2

1 cup coconut milk or Coconut Yogurt (p. 131)

¾ cup organic orange juice

*1 scoop Rootcology AI Paleo Protein

1 teaspoon vanilla

*Possible Modifications for Other Root Cause Diets: Use Rootcology Vanilla Paleo Protein if following the Paleo Diet.

Orange juice is a rich source of adrenal-healing vitamin C and can help digestion; however, drinking it straight can create blood-sugar swings. In the Orange Cream Smoothie, the fat from the coconut combined with the protein powder helps balance out the blood-sugar effect of the orange juice. This simple and delicious smoothie can be a great start to your day, a snack, or a dessert. This recipe can also be frozen in popsicle molds for a refreshing summer treat.

1. Place all ingredients in a high-powered blender and blend until smooth, 20 to 30 seconds.

Nutritional Analysis per Serving: Protein (g) 14.32; Fat (g) 5.11; Carbs (g) 20.61; B_{12} (mcg) 1.4; Iron (mg) 0.91; Iodine (mcg) 0; Magnesium (mg) 90.53; Potassium (mg) 189.11; Selenium (mcg) 0.09; Sodium (mg) 95.29

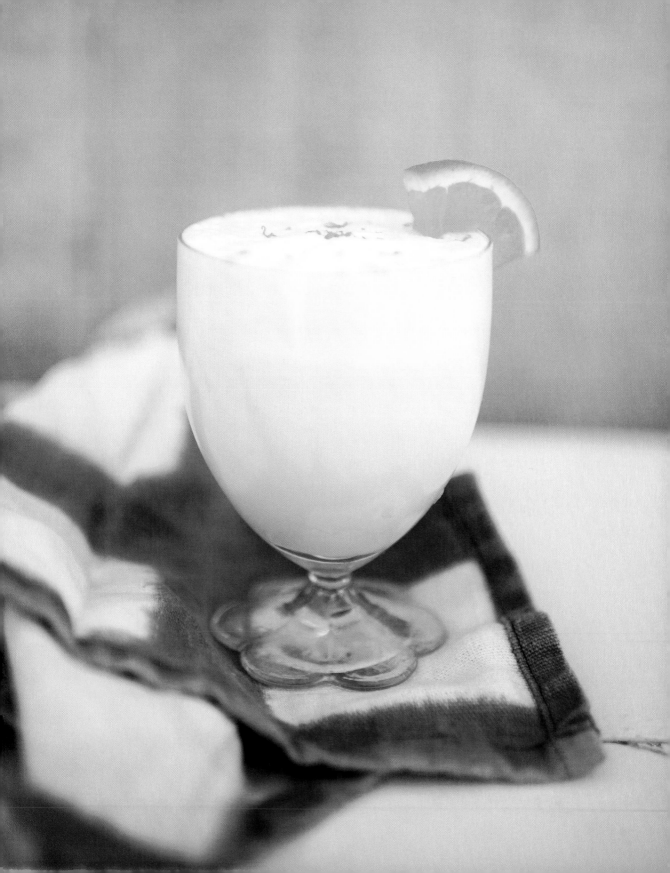

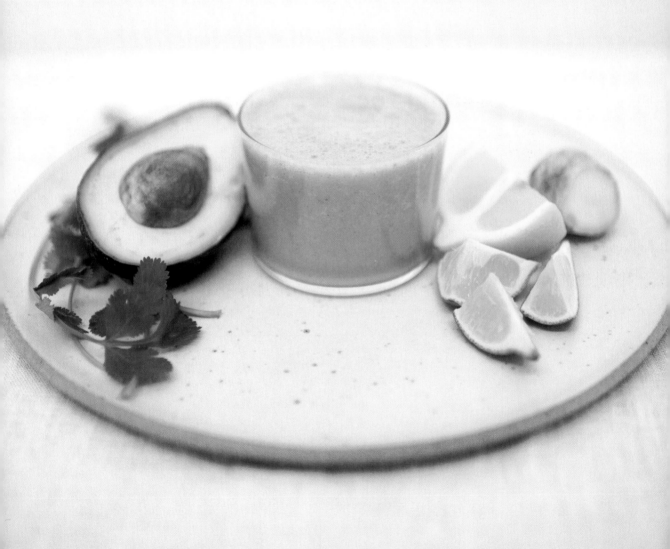

Cilantro-Citrus Cooler

Ⓐ AUTOIMMUNE

Prep time: 10 minutes

Serves: 1

1 cup coconut water

*1 scoop Rootcology AI Paleo
Protein

½ avocado

1 cup chopped cucumber

1 cup fresh cilantro, chopped

Juice of 1 lemon

Juice of 1 lime

½ teaspoon grated fresh ginger

*Possible Modifications for Other Root
Cause Diets: Use Rootcology Vanilla
Paleo Protein if following the Paleo
Diet.

The combination of coconut water, tangy citrus, cucumber, and cilantro in this Cilantro-Citrus Cooler creates a deeply refreshing and detoxifying beverage you can enjoy anytime!

1. Place all ingredients in a high-powered blender and blend until smooth.

Nutritional Analysis per Serving: Protein (g) 31.42; Fat (g) 11.78; Carbs (g) 25.49; B_{12} (mcg) 0; Iron (mg) 2.71; Iodine (mcg) 0; Magnesium (mg) 115.57; Potassium (mg) 1536.73; Selenium (mcg) 3.7; Sodium (mg) 476.38

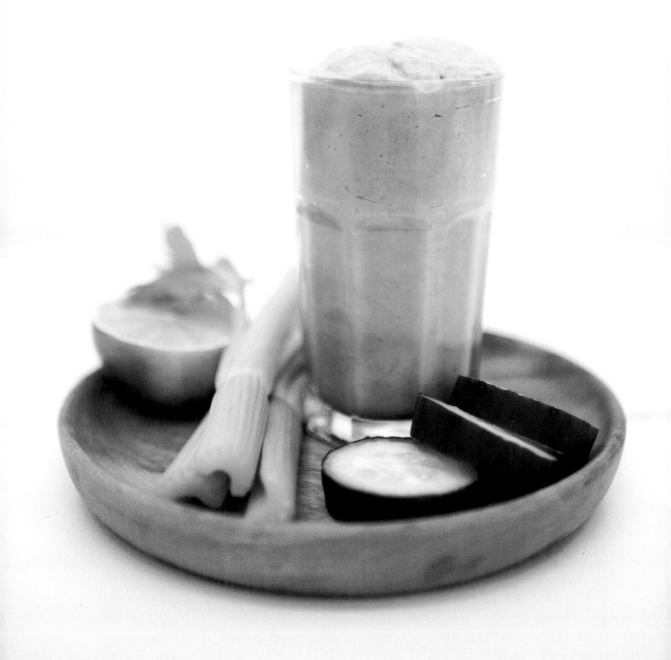

Root Cause Original Smoothie

(I) INTRO, (P) PALEO, OR (A) AUTOIMMUNE (DEPENDING ON PROTEIN POWDER)

Prep time: 10 minutes

Serves: 3

1 cup coconut milk

1 scoop Rootcology AI Paleo Protein
or Rootcology Paleo Protein

1 cup mixed baby greens

1 large carrot

1 ripe avocado

1 stick celery

1 cucumber

1 bunch fresh basil

Juice of 1 lime

Sea salt or pink Himalayan sea salt
to taste

OPTIONAL ADDITIONS

1 tablespoon camu powder
(vitamin C boost)

1 tablespoon cod liver oil
(anti-inflammatory boost,
omega-3 boost)

1 tablespoon Coconut Yogurt
(p. 131; probiotic boost)

1 tablespoon maca root powder
(hormone-balancing boost)

1 tablespoon turmeric powder
(anti-inflammatory boost)

*Possible Modifications for Other Root
Cause Diets: This recipe can be made
Paleo by using the Rootcology Paleo
Protein (Vanilla) or Autoimmune using
the Rootcology AI Paleo Protein.

This green smoothie, the Root Cause Original Smoothie, is packed with nutrition for your thyroid, helps reduce inflammation, and can help with detoxification. Coconut milk is hypoallergenic, helps reduce inflammation, and stabilizes blood sugar due to its (good) fat content. Optional boosts can be added to the basic recipe to increase the nutrient density of the smoothie. This smoothie makes a great breakfast each morning! People who have tried the Root Cause Green Smoothie have said that it helps them feel less hungry, more relaxed and calm, and full of energy. If needed, you can even double the recipe to make enough for lunch! While most people who have tried the green smoothie love it, some people (ahem, my husband, Michael) may not like the pudding-like consistency and the warmth of the smoothie. To create a thinner, milk-like consistency and a "cold and tropical flavor"—as my husband describes his ideal smoothie— you can make the following adjustments:

– Skip the avocado and add a tablespoon of chia seeds instead. Chia seeds are a less creamy source of good fat.

– Add the juice of one lemon or lime to make it more tropical and to support digestive juices.

– Blend the contents with a cup of ice cubes to make the smoothie cold and give it a more milky consistency.

1. Place all ingredients in a high-powered blender and blend until smooth, 20 to 30 seconds.

Nutritional Analysis per Serving: Protein (g) 12.79; Fat (g) 26.38; Carbs (g) 15.98; B_{12} (mcg) 0; Iron (mg) 2.28; Iodine (mcg) 0; Magnesium (mg) 67.44; Potassium (mg) 760.28; Selenium (mcg) 5.55; Sodium (mg) 233.47

Spa Water

A AUTOIMMUNE

Prep time: 10 minutes

Cook time: 15 minutes standing

Serves: 4

8 cups fluoride-free filtered water

8 strawberries, cut in half

8 mint leaves

1 small cucumber, cubed

Most of us are aware of the fact that we need to drink more water. Water flushes out toxins and keeps us hydrated. Drinking eight 8-ounce glasses of water a day is key to proper detox and body function. As a former caffeine and sugar junkie, I had a really tough time transitioning to water, because it didn't have any flavor. One of my friends introduced me to Spa Water, and I was hooked. I often make an entire pitcher of Spa Water in the morning and set it on my desk to remind myself to stay hydrated throughout the day. You can also make this recipe in smaller portions or in water bottles when you're on the go! You can use any fruits you prefer. Some of my favorites include strawberries, mint leaves, cucumbers, lemons, limes, and green apples. You'll love drinking Spa Water; it's so refreshing!

1. Place the strawberries, mint leaves, and cucumbers in a large water pitcher and pour in the cold filtered water.

2. Let the water stand for at least 15 minutes to allow the flavors to infuse the water.

Nutritional Analysis per Serving: As this is simply minty fruit-infused water, significant nutritional information is unavailable.

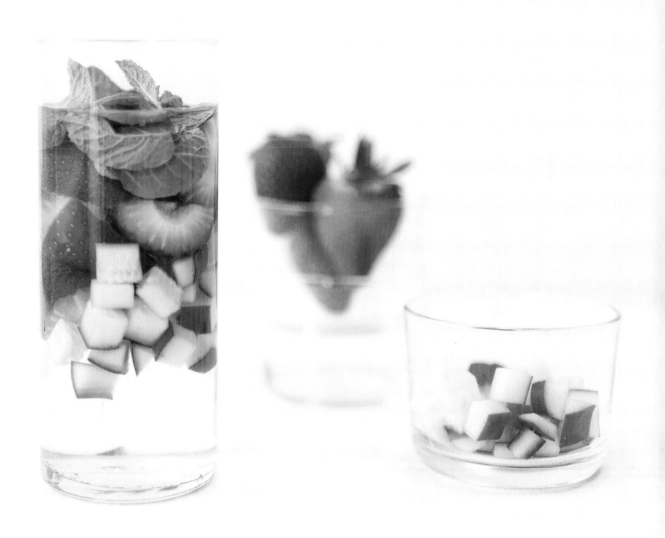

Hashi-Mojito Smoothie

Ⓐ AUTOIMMUNE

Prep time: 5 minutes

Serves: 1

½ cup mint

Juice of 2 limes

1 cup plain or fermented coconut water

1 (1-inch) piece fresh ginger, peeled

Maple syrup, honey, or dates to taste (optional)

1 scoop Rootcology AI Paleo Protein

Can you have mojitos on your healing journey? Sure! As long as they're Hashi-Mojitos. Using fermented or plain coconut water, you can create a satisfying and tasty beverage! Ginger and mint provide a wonderful blend of flavors as well as gut-soothing and healing properties to this Hashimoto's-friendly mojito.

1. Place all ingredients in a blender and blend for 20 to 30 seconds or until desired consistency.

Nutritional Analysis per Serving: Protein (g) 28.54; Fat (g) 1.16; Carbs (g) 17.21; B_{12} (mcg) 0; Iron (mg) 1.42; Iodine (mcg) 0; Magnesium (mg) 76.33; Potassium (mg) 761.76; Selenium (mcg) 2.47; Sodium (mg) 432.49

Root Cause Building Smoothie

Ⓟ PALEO

Prep time: 10 minutes

Serves: 2

1 cup coconut milk (150 calories)

1 scoop Rootcology AI Paleo Protein or Rootcology Paleo Protein (60 calories)

1 avocado (300 calories)

1 banana (100 calories)

1 cup cooked sweet potatoes (180 calories)

1 teaspoon vanilla extract, or to taste (optional)

*2 egg yolks, consider pasteurized or lightly cooked if concerned about salmonella (100 calories, if tolerated)

*Possible Modifications for Other Root Cause Diets: Remove the eggs and use the Rootcology AI Paleo Protein to make the smoothie Autoimmune Paleo compliant.

Although most people with Hashimoto's struggle with losing weight, some of my clients had a hard time gaining weight or lost too much weight when they began eating real food. As real foods are filling, in some cases it may be challenging to eat enough calories, so consuming the Root Cause Building Smoothie at the end of the day after all of your meals have been eaten can give you some extra calories to keep your weight on. Digestive-enzyme deficiencies, infections, and impaired adrenals can also be root causes of excess weight loss. This smoothie adds extra healthy fats thanks to the avocado, coconut milk, and eggs. The potassium-rich bananas lend a light sweetness that make this smoothie the perfect ending to your day. Although I don't normally advocate calorie counting for those with Hashimoto's, I've provided the calorie content of the ingredients for this smoothie for reference.

1. Place all ingredients in a high-powered blender and blend until smooth, 2 to 3 minutes.

Nutritional Analysis per Serving: Protein (g) 25.01; Fat (g) 44.14; Carbs (g) 39.52; B_{12} (mcg) 0.45; Iron (mg) 3.81; Iodine (mcg) 25.5; Magnesium (mg) 102.14; Potassium (mg) 1155.89; Selenium (mcg) 24.03; Sodium (mg) 219.19

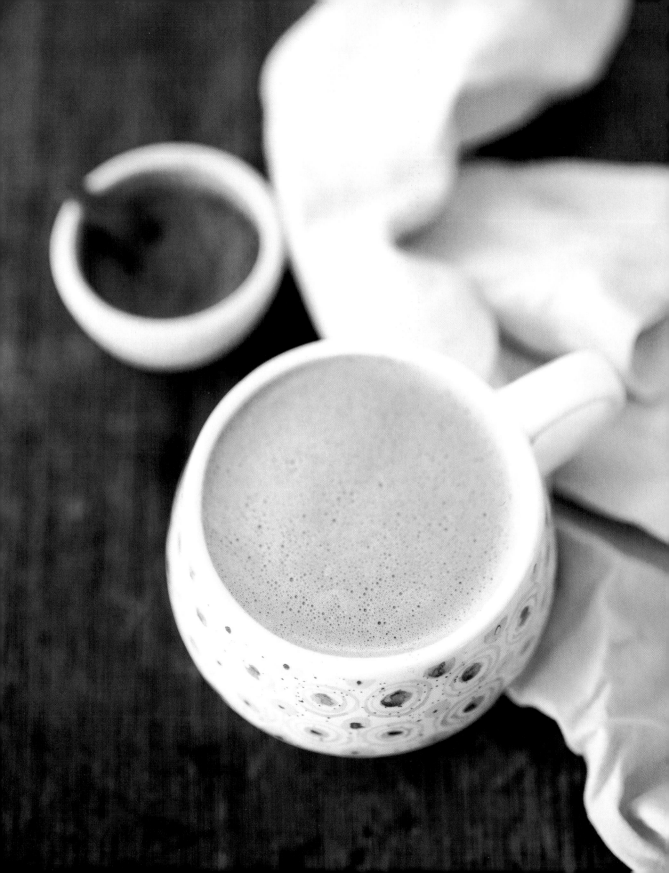

Hot Chocolate

Ⓟ PALEO

Prep time: 2 minutes

Cook time: 3 minutes

Serves: 1

Note: This is not your regular hot chocolate from a can or a packet; it tastes more like dark chocolate and therefore is not really kid friendly (unless your child likes dark chocolate).

1 (14-ounce) can full-fat coconut milk

*2 tablespoons cacao powder

1½ tablespoons maple syrup

1 tablespoon collagen powder or Rootcology AI Paleo Protein

OPTIONAL ADDITIONS, TO TASTE

Peppermint oil

Sea salt or pink Himalayan sea salt

Cinnamon

Nutmeg (if tolerated)

*Possible Modifications for Other Root Cause Diets: This recipe can be made Autoimmune compliant by substituting carob powder for the cacao powder.

This recipe for homemade hot chocolate is on the top of the list for a decadent treat and will be one that keeps you cozy on a cold winter night. It's rich and smooth, and the cacao powder is high in thyroid- and adrenal-supporting magnesium! If you're menstruating and always craving chocolate around that time, this could be why. Magnesium via food and supplements is important to consider.

1. In a saucepan, heat the coconut milk until simmering, but do not let it boil.

2. Add the cacao powder and whisk until combined.

3. Add the maple syrup and collagen or protein powder and whisk to combine.

4. Mix in your additions and serve warm.

Nutritional Analysis per Serving: Protein (g) 18.18; Fat (g) 43.91; Carbs (g) 23.14, B_{12} (mcg) 0; Iron (mg) 3.71; Iodine (mcg) 0; Magnesium (mg) 96.57; Potassium (mg) 587.11; Selenium (mcg) 12.02; Sodium (mg) 117.43

Beef Stew

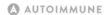 AUTOIMMUNE

Prep time: 5 minutes

Cook time: 8 hours in a slow cooker; 45 minutes in an electric pressure cooker

Serves: 8

Note: This stew is great for leftovers and frozen for prep meals.

2 pounds stewing beef

¼ cup arrowroot flour

Sea salt or pink Himalayan sea salt to taste

2 tablespoons coconut oil

2 large carrots, diced

1 large onion, sliced

3 stalks celery, chopped

2 parsnips, peeled and chopped

8 ounces mushrooms, sliced

1 teaspoon dried oregano

1 teaspoon dried parsley

½ teaspoon dried thyme

3 to 4 cups Bone Broth (p. 135)

When following the Autoimmune Diet, it's sometimes best to make one-pot meals in large batches, so that you have leftovers for a couple days. Because it is slow-cooked or cooked in a pressure cooker, the nutrients remain within the stew itself, so every mouthful is full of flavor and packed with vital nourishment. As a side bonus, this recipe is a crowd pleaser. It's even been approved by one of the toughest food critics I know—my dad!

1. Mix the arrowroot flour and salt together in a shallow bowl and dredge each piece of beef so it has a light coating of the flour mixture.

2. Heat the coconut oil on medium in a large skillet and brown the beef in batches.

3. Transfer the beef to a slow cooker and add the vegetables and spices.

4. Stir the meat and vegetables together until well mixed, and then pour the bone broth over the mixture until the liquid just covers the ingredients. (If you have leftover bone broth, heat it up and enjoy a warm mug!)

5. Cook on low for 8 hours.

6. Alternatively, sauté the beef in an electric pressure cooker on the sauté setting, and then add the vegetables and broth until the pot is two-thirds full. On Manual, set the pressure on high for 45 minutes.

Nutritional Analysis per Serving: Protein (g) 29.42; Fat (g) 9.18; Carbs (g) 11.67; B_{12} (mcg) 2.76; Iron (mg) 3.07; Iodine (mcg) 0; Magnesium (mg) 36.58; Potassium (mg) 776.28; Selenium (mcg) 32.61; Sodium (mg) 373.6

Chicken Soup

Ⓐ AUTOIMMUNE

Prep time: 5 minutes

Cook time: 30 minutes

Serves: 4

4 cups Bone Broth (p. 135)

2 large carrots, lightly chopped

2 celery stalks, lightly chopped on the diagonal

1 small onion, sliced

2 (6-ounce) boneless chicken breasts

Sea salt or pink Himalayan sea salt to taste

Black pepper to taste (if tolerated)

2 tablespoons chopped fresh parsley, for garnish

If you want to add some substance to your Bone Broth, turn it into Chicken Soup! Large chunks of carrot, celery, and onion plus shredded chicken make a great soup that is more than satisfying, even without noodles. If you'd like to have noodles, however, toss some zucchini noodles in the soup for extra fiber and nutrients.

1. In a medium-size pot, bring the broth to a boil, and then add the vegetables and chicken.

2. Bring back to a boil, then reduce to medium-low, and simmer for 25 to 30 minutes, or until vegetable chunks are tender and chicken can be easily broken apart with a fork.

3. Remove the chicken and shred with two forks.

4. Return the shredded chicken to the pot, season with salt, pepper, and parsley, and serve warm.

Nutritional Analysis per Serving: Protein (g) 19.57; Fat (g) 3.64; Carbs (g) 6.37; B_{12} (mcg) 0.12; Iron (mg) 0.54; Iodine (mcg) 0; Magnesium (mg) 25.88; Potassium (mg) 583.12; Selenium (mcg) 13.19; Sodium (mg) 282.27

Barszcz (Polish Beet Soup)

Ⓟ PALEO

Prep time: 1 hour

Cook time: 40 minutes

Serves: 8

6 cups Bone Broth (p. 135)

2 cups chopped red beets, or
3 medium whole beets

1 cup chopped sweet potatoes, or
1 medium whole sweet potato

1 cup chopped carrots, or 5 medium
whole carrots

1 cup chopped parsnips, or
5 medium whole parsnips

1 medium onion, chopped

3 allspice berries (if tolerated)

2 bay leaves

½ teaspoon garlic powder

1 tablespoon lemon juice or apple
cider vinegar

Sea salt or pink Himalayan sea salt
to taste

Black pepper to taste (if tolerated)

1 tablespoon lemon juice or apple
cider vinegar, or to taste

Barszcz is a traditional Polish soup made from beets. Beets are a rich source of betaine, a compound that supports detoxification, methylation, and digestion. This recipe has been adapted from my mom's world-famous Barszcz recipe. She prepares the traditional soup by peeling and chopping all of the root vegetables, but I lightly chop the onion, throw the root veggies in whole, and puree the soup in a high-powered blender. The pureed version is less time consuming and easier to digest, while the chopped version offers a variety of tastes and textures with each bite! In Poland, this soup is often served with a peeled boiled egg or a dollop of sour cream (you can use coconut cream for a similar effect).

1. Place the bone broth, beets, sweet potatoes, carrots, parsnips, onion, allspice, bay leaves, and garlic powder in a large stockpot and bring to a boil.

2. Reduce the heat to a simmer and add 1 tablespoon of lemon juice or apple cider vinegar. The lemon juice will bring out the beautiful red color of the beets.

3. Simmer for 40 minutes until all of the vegetables are cooked through.

4. If you did not chop your veggies, you can now mash them with a potato masher or put them in a high-powered blender to create a pureed soup. (When blending hot liquids, make sure the top of the blender is vented to let the steam escape.)

5. Season with salt, pepper, and lemon juice or apple cider vinegar to taste.

Nutritional Analysis per Serving: Protein (g) 3.64; Fat (g) 0.19; Carbs (g) 15.76; B_{12} (mcg) 0; Iron (mg) 0.82; Iodine (mcg) 0; Magnesium (mg) 25.66; Potassium (mg) 378.57; Selenium (mcg) 0.87; Sodium (mg) 151.53

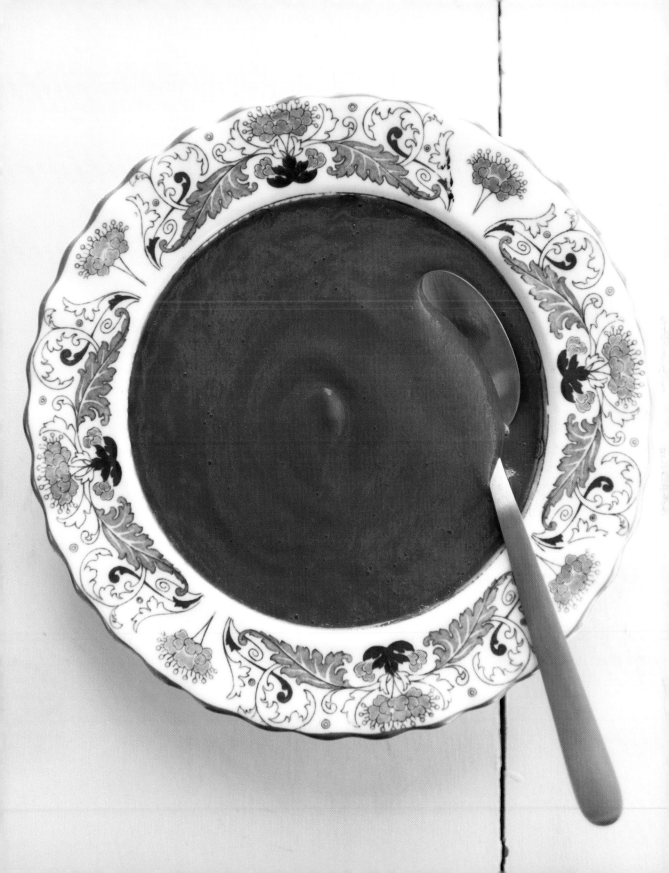

Chilly Day Chili

❶ INTRO

Prep time: 10 minutes

Cook time: 4 to 8 hours

Serves: 8

1 pound ground beef or turkey

1 (15-ounce) can white beans, rinsed and drained

1 (15-ounce) can red or black beans, rinsed and drained

30 ounces chopped fresh tomatoes, or 1 (28-ounce) can diced tomatoes, undrained

2 tablespoons cumin (if tolerated)

1 white onion, chopped

3 cloves garlic, finely minced

Sea salt or pink Himalayan sea salt to taste

Black pepper to taste (if tolerated)

The combination of ground meat, protein- and fiber-loaded beans, and lycopene-rich tomatoes creates the flavorful foundation of this simple yet satisfying iron- and ferritin-boosting slow-cooker chili! This recipe is one of my husband's favorites and one to enjoy on cold days! I try to keep a batch of this in my freezer to throw in the slow cooker whenever I don't have time to cook.

1. Place all ingredients in a slow cooker and cook on high for 4 hours or on low for 6 to 8 hours.

Nutritional Analysis per Serving: Protein (g) 19.43; Fat (g) 16.08; Carbs (g) 30.36; B_{12} (mcg) 1.5; Iron (mg) 5.07; Iodine (mcg) 0; Magnesium (mg) 92.5; Potassium (mg) 863.99; Selenium (mcg) 9; Sodium (mg) 175.89

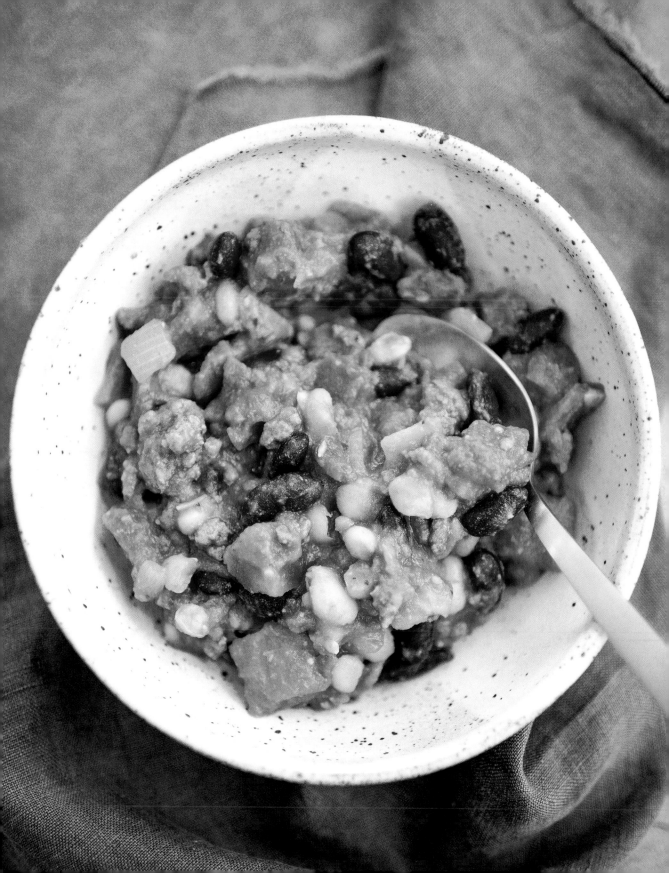

Polish Pea Soup

❶ INTRO

Prep time: 10 minutes

Cook time: 40 minutes

Serves: 6

Note: This recipe makes a large quantity of soup. You will have plenty to share or freeze for later use.

1 tablespoon coconut oil

1 small onion, chopped

2 garlic cloves, minced

6 cups Bone Broth (p. 135)

3 cups frozen organic peas

1 small sweet potato, chopped

4 cups broccoli florets

2 medium carrots, chopped

1 teaspoon dried oregano

Sea salt or pink Himalayan sea salt to taste

Black pepper to taste (if tolerated)

1 teaspoon chopped fresh parsley, for garnish

1 small avocado, diced, for garnish

Polish Pea Soup is another one of my mom's traditional Polish masterpieces. It is loaded with veggies that provide a wide variety of vitamins and minerals such as B, E, C, zinc, and calcium. The combination of veggies and Bone Broth (p. 135) makes this Polish Pea Soup a nutritional powerhouse that tastes amazing!

1. In a soup pot, heat the coconut oil on medium. Add the onion and sauté until softened, about 8 minutes.

2. Add the garlic, and cook 1 minute longer.

3. Add the bone broth, peas, sweet potato, broccoli, and carrots.

4. Bring to a boil, and then reduce the heat and simmer for 25 minutes.

5. Add the salt, pepper, and oregano and simmer for another 5 minutes.

6. Remove from the heat and let cool slightly.

7. In a high-speed blender, blend the soup in batches until smooth, about 1 minute per batch. (Make sure the top of the blender is vented to let the steam escape.) Return to the pot and keep warm.

8. Serve in bowls and garnish with avocado and parsley.

Nutritional Analysis per Serving: Protein (g) 11.96; Fat (g) 8.19; Carbs (g) 21.88; B_{12} (mcg) 0; Iron (mg) 1.67; Iodine (mcg) 3.55; Magnesium (mg) 45.84; Potassium (mg) 731.09; Selenium (mcg) 2.52; Sodium (mg) 224.65

Cuban Ropa Vieja

℗ PALEO

Prep time: 10 minutes

Cook time: 8 to 10 hours in a slow cooker; 50 minutes in an electric pressure cooker

Serves: 8

1½ pounds boneless beef or buffalo chuck steak

1 cup sliced onion

½ cup diced tomatoes

1 tablespoon tomato paste

1 tablespoon olive oil

1 tablespoon apple cider vinegar

1 tablespoon minced garlic

1 teaspoon ground cumin (if tolerated)

1 bay leaf

½ teaspoon sea salt or pink Himalayan sea salt

¼ cup pitted green olives

⅓ cup fresh cilantro

1 cup Bone Broth (p. 135)

I discovered this delicious Cuban recipe, Ropa Vieja, when I was looking for an easy-to-make gluten-free meal that I could serve for Sunday family gatherings. I serve this with my Mango Salsa (p. 296), plantains, grilled mahi mahi, and a nice salad with lots of avocados. You can also make rice and black beans to round out the meal and feed even more people. The steak slowly simmers in Bone Broth (p. 135), increasing its gut-healing properties.

1. Place all ingredients in a slow cooker and cook on low for 8 to 10 hours until the steak is very tender. (Alternatively, place all ingredients in an electric pressure cooker and, on Manual, set the pressure to high for 50 minutes.)

2. Remove the steak from the slow cooker (or pressure cooker) and shred with two forks.

3. If there is too much liquid in the pot, turn the slow cooker to high with the lid off to reduce the liquid (or use the sauté setting on the electric pressure cooker to reduce the liquid).

Nutritional Analysis per Serving: Protein (g) 19.7; Fat (g) 9.83; Carbs (g) 3.68; B_{12} (mcg) 2.14; Iron (mg) 1.91; Iodine (mcg) 0; Magnesium (mg) 27.28; Potassium (mg) 387.08; Selenium (mcg) 25.43; Sodium (mg) 304.89

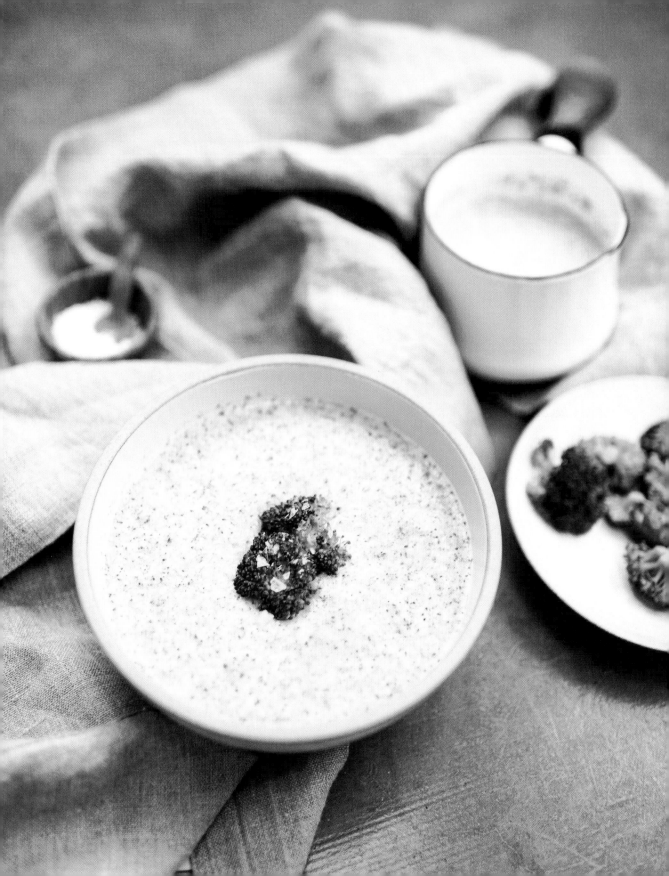

Cream of Broccoli Soup

Ⓐ AUTOIMMUNE

Prep time: 5 minutes

Cook time: 15 minutes

Serves: 4

2 tablespoons coconut oil

1 large leek, white parts only, chopped

1 tablespoon minced fresh ginger

1 garlic clove, minced

4 cups broccoli, tops and stalks, chopped

3 cups Bone Broth (p. 135)

1 (13½-ounce) can full-fat coconut milk

Sea salt or pink Himalayan sea salt to taste

Black pepper to taste (if tolerated)

Cream of Broccoli Soup is a wonderful comfort food that supports your detoxification pathways! Soups are such an easy and quick meal to make and full of wonderful nutrients. The broccoli provides plenty of fiber and B vitamins, and the coconut milk creates a delicious creamy base, full of beneficial fats.

1. Heat the coconut oil in a soup pot on medium. Add the leeks and cook until softened, about 6 minutes.

2. Add the ginger and garlic, and sauté until fragrant, about 1 minute.

3. Add the broccoli and broth and bring to a boil; reduce the heat and simmer for 5 minutes.

4. Add the coconut milk and simmer until heated through.

5. Remove from the heat and let cool slightly.

6. Puree the soup in batches in a high-speed blender until combined. (When blending hot liquids, make sure the top of the blender is vented to let the steam escape.)

7. Return to the pot, bring back to a simmer, and add salt and pepper (if tolerated) to taste.

8. Serve warm.

Nutritional Analysis per Serving: Protein (g) 9.49; Fat (g) 30.17; Carbs (g) 14.34; B_{12} (mcg) 0; Iron (mg) 2.64; Iodine (mcg) 0; Magnesium (mg) 59.09; Potassium (mg) 710.31; Selenium (mcg) 8.09; Sodium (mg) 333.03

Moroccan Lamb Stew

Ⓐ AUTOIMMUNE

Prep time: 20 minutes

Cook time: 1¾ hours

Serves: 4

2 pounds lamb stew meat, cut into 1-inch cubes

Sea salt or pink Himalayan sea salt to taste

Black pepper to taste (if tolerated)

½ teaspoon ground cinnamon

2 tablespoons coconut oil

1 small onion, chopped

4 cloves garlic, minced

1 (2-inch) piece fresh ginger, peeled and minced

2 tablespoons chopped fresh rosemary

1 tablespoon apple cider vinegar

½ cup Bone Broth (p. 135)

½ cup water

2 small oranges, zested and juiced

4 cups chopped carrots

2 tablespoons minced fresh dates

½ cup chopped fresh cilantro, for garnish (optional)

This fragrant Moroccan Lamb Stew is perfect on a cold day—or on any day when you're in need of a boost of flavor. As an added bonus, the cinnamon aids in balancing blood sugar. Garnish with cilantro to add a little detox to your day!

1. In a medium-size bowl, season the meat evenly with the salt, pepper, and cinnamon.

2. In a large cooking pot on medium, heat the coconut oil and brown the meat, 2 to 3 minutes per side.

3. Add the onion and cook for 3 minutes, or until it begins to brown slightly.

4. Add the garlic, ginger, and rosemary and cook until fragrant, another couple of minutes.

5. Add the apple cider vinegar, bone broth, water, orange zest and juice, carrots, and dates and bring to a boil.

6. Reduce the heat to medium-low, cover, and cook for about 1½ hours, or until the lamb reaches the desired tenderness.

7. Serve warm garnished with cilantro.

> Nutritional Analysis per Serving: Protein (g) 47.48; Fat (g) 33; Carbs (g) 23.31; B$_{12}$ (mcg) 4.54; Iron (mg) 3.69; Iodine (mcg) 18; Magnesium (mg) 74.48; Potassium (mg) 1295.33; Selenium (mcg) 5.56; Sodium (mg) 694.43

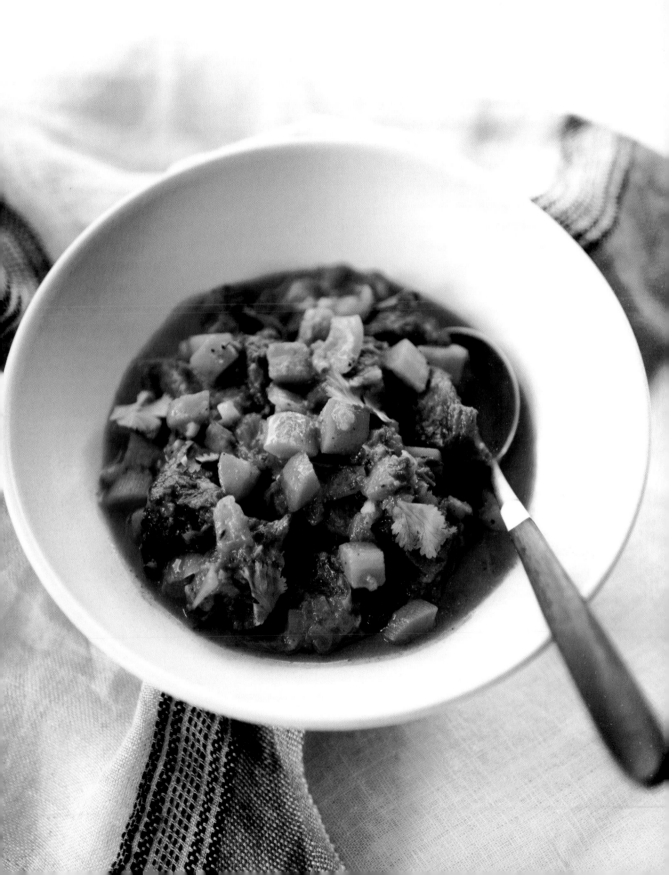

Carrot-Ginger-Pear Soup

Ⓐ AUTOIMMUNE

Prep time: 5 minutes

Cook time: 30 minutes

Serves: 4

2 tablespoons coconut oil

4 medium carrots, chopped

1 small onion, diced

1 pear (peeled if not organic), diced

4 cups Bone Broth (p. 135)

1 (1-inch) piece fresh ginger, peeled and grated

Sea salt or pink Himalayan sea salt to taste

Black pepper to taste (if tolerated)

Coconut milk, for garnish

Carrot-Ginger-Pear Soup is sure to warm you up and be a treat for your taste buds. The ginger provides some immune-boosting properties, while the carrots provide you with carotenoids and vitamin A and the pear adds a bright, flavorful punch of fiber!

1. Heat the oil in a soup pot on medium. Add the carrots and onions and cook until onions are translucent, about 10 minutes.

2. Add the pear and cook until softened, about 5 minutes.

3. Add the bone broth and bring to a boil; reduce the heat and simmer for 15 minutes or until carrots are tender.

4. Add the grated ginger and blend in a blender in batches (when blending hot liquids, make sure the top of the blender is vented to let the steam escape) or with an immersion blender.

5. Return to the pot (if using a blender); season to taste with salt and pepper.

6. Serve warm with a dollop of coconut milk (optional).

Nutritional Analysis per Serving: Protein (g) 7.75; Fat (g) 16; Carbs (g) 16.75; B$_{12}$ (mcg) 0; Iron (mg) 0.83; Iodine (mcg) 0; Magnesium (mg) 24.95; Potassium (mg) 560.4; Selenium (mcg) 2.12; Sodium (mg) 265.83

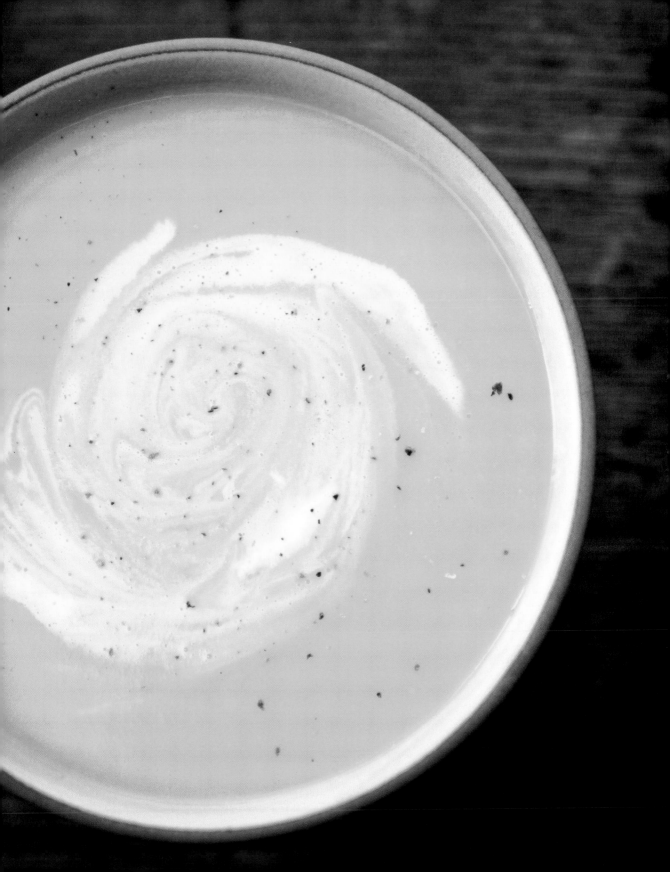

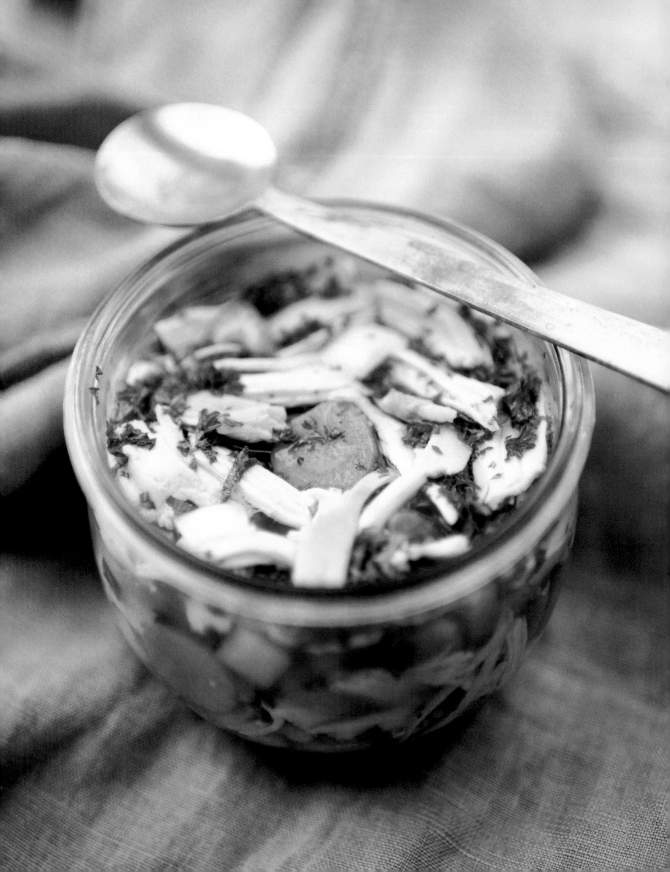

Galaretka (Polish Gelatin Broth)

Ⓐ AUTOIMMUNE

Prep time: 15 minutes

Cook time: Bone Broth (p. 135) cooking time, plus 2 to 4 hours chilling

Serves: 4

3 chicken drumsticks

1 cup diced or chopped carrots

1 cup chopped celeriac or celery

1 cup chopped onion

2 bay leaves

½ teaspoon black peppercorns (if tolerated)

¼ cup chopped fresh parsley

Sea salt or pink Himalayan sea salt to taste

1 tablespoon gelatin

Galaretka is a delicious and upgraded version of gut-healing Bone Broth (p. 135) that is made into a gelatin dish! This is my Aunt Halina's traditional Polish recipe that is a surprise hit with all of my American friends and family members! The traditional version is often made with chicken feet or pig feet in addition to chicken. Galaretka tastes like chicken soup and the gelatin-like consistency makes it supereasy to transport. The broth, extra gelatin, and collagen will support your body's healing capacities!

1. Make bone broth from the chicken legs, carrots, celeriac or celery, onion, bay leaves, peppercorns, parsley, and salt. See Bone Broth, p. 135, for cooking options.

2. When the broth is done, remove and discard the peppercorns and bay leaves.

3. Strain the chicken legs and vegetables out of the broth. Remove the meat from the bones.

4. Place 1 cup of the meat and 1 cup of the cooked vegetables into a medium-size glass bowl.

5. Add 2 cups of the strained bone broth to the chicken and veggies.

6. Add the gelatin to the broth, meat, and veggies in the bowl and mix.

7. Let stand in the fridge for 2 to 4 hours, until the gelatin is set.

8. Serve cold.

Nutritional Analysis per Serving: Protein (g) 12.3; Fat (g) 4.71; Carbs (g) 7.93; B$_{12}$ (mcg) 0; Iron (mg) 1.13; Iodine (mcg) 0; Magnesium (mg) 13.35; Potassium (mg) 247.26; Selenium (mcg) 1; Sodium (mg) 280.99

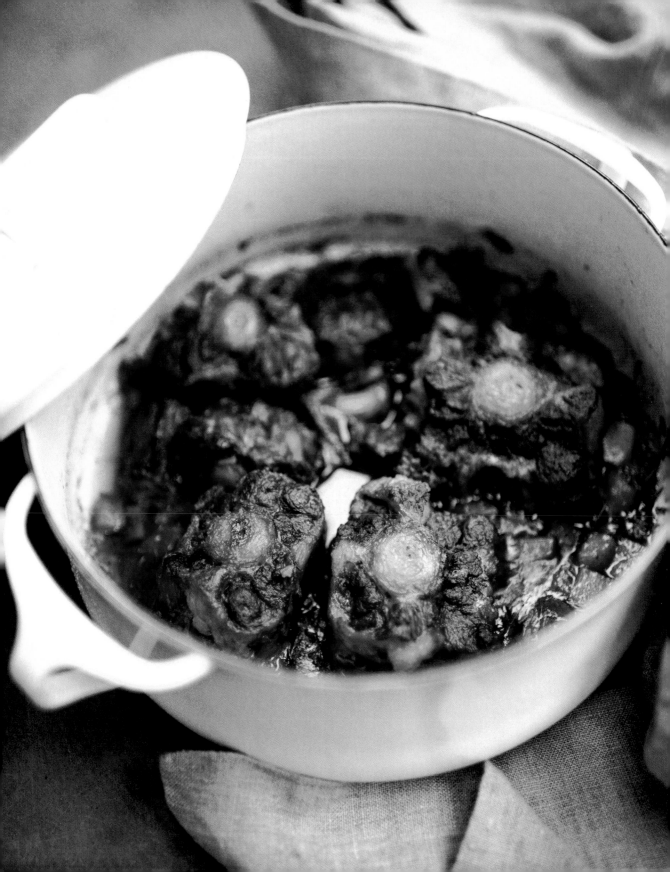

Winter Oxtail Stew

P PALEO

Prep time: 30 minutes

Cook time: 6 hours in a slow cooker

Serves: 6

2 pounds beef oxtails
(or 2 pounds short ribs)

Sea salt or pink Himalayan sea salt
to taste

Black pepper to taste (if tolerated)

1 tablespoon coconut oil

2 large onions, diced (about 3 cups)

2 large carrots, diced
(about 1½ cups)

4 cloves garlic, minced

1 (1-inch) piece fresh ginger,
peeled and minced

2 cups Bone Broth (p. 135)

1 teaspoon ground allspice
(if tolerated)

3 tablespoons dried thyme

This hearty, robust stew provides an excellent meal during the cold winter months. The distinctive aroma of immune-boosting garlic, ginger, and thyme will fill the house as Winter Oxtail Stew slowly simmers on the stove. Bathed in Bone Broth (p. 135), the oxtail is a great source of vitamins and nutrients, perfect for nourishing your body and mind. This is one of my hubby's favorites.

1. On a cutting board, season the oxtails with salt and pepper and set aside.

2. In a large pan on medium-high, heat the oil and brown the oxtails on all sides. Remove from the pan and place in a slow cooker.

3. Add the onions, carrots, garlic, and ginger to the pan and cook 4 to 5 minutes, or until the onions are translucent.

4. Transfer the contents of the pan to the slow cooker.

5. Add the bone broth, allspice, and thyme to the slow cooker.

6. Cover and cook on high for 6 hours or until the oxtails reach the desired tenderness.

7. Before serving, remove the bones from the meat and season with salt.

8. Serve warm.

Nutritional Analysis per Serving: Protein (g) 35.9; Fat (g) 24.77; Carbs (g) 12.92; B_{12} (mcg) 0.45; Iron (mg) 6.91; Iodine (mcg) 0; Magnesium (mg) 46.66; Potassium (mg) 689.11; Selenium (mcg) 0.84; Sodium (mg) 338.27

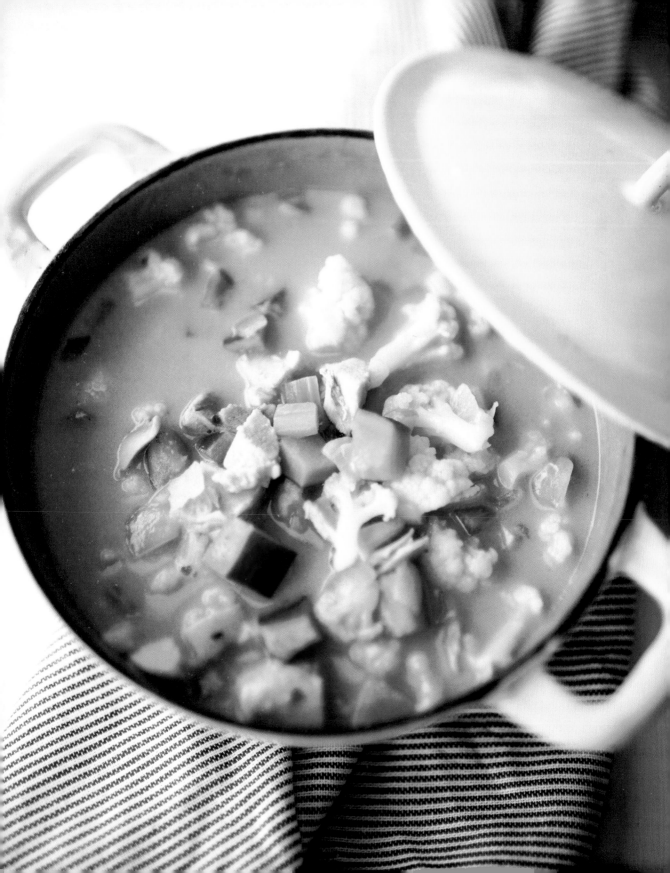

Creamy White Chicken Stew

Ⓐ AUTOIMMUNE

Prep time: 30 minutes

Cook time: 20 to 25 minutes

Serves: 6

1 tablespoon coconut oil

2 large leeks, chopped

2 cloves garlic, minced

1 pound boneless chicken breast, cut into ½-inch cubes

3 cups Bone Broth (p. 135)

2 (13½-ounce) cans coconut cream

Sea salt or pink Himalayan sea salt to taste

Black pepper to taste (if tolerated)

1 tablespoon lemon zest

1 large stalk celery, chopped

2 cups cauliflower florets

2 medium sweet potatoes, diced

Creamy White Chicken Stew is one of my all-time favorite recipes! This stew is perfect for a cold day when you just want to cuddle up in your jammies and receive the healing benefits of a hearty stew. The cooked cauliflower combined with coconut adds a nice potato soup–like consistency without all of the starch!

1. In a large pot on medium, heat the coconut oil. Add the leeks, garlic, and chicken and cook for 5 minutes until tender.

2. To the leek mixture, add the broth, coconut cream, salt, pepper, and lemon zest. Cover and bring to a boil.

3. Add the celery, cauliflower, and sweet potatoes and reduce the heat to low. Cover and simmer for 10 to 15 minutes, until chicken is cooked through and vegetables are tender.

4. Serve warm.

Nutritional Analysis per Serving: Protein (g) 27.02; Fat (g) 53.93; Carbs (g) 24.31; B$_{12}$ (mcg) 0.159; Iron (mg) 4.53; Iodine (mcg) 0; Magnesium (mg) 80.78; Potassium (mg) 1026.02; Selenium (mcg) 17.97; Sodium (mg) 206.63

Pork Curry Stew

P PALEO

Prep time: 10 minutes

Cook time: 1½ hours

Serves: 6

2 pounds pork shoulder, cut into 1-inch cubes

Sea salt or pink Himalayan sea salt to taste

Black pepper to taste (if tolerated)

2 teaspoons coconut oil

1 large sweet potato, peeled and diced (about 1½ cups)

4 small tomatoes, diced (about 2 cups)

3 cloves garlic, minced

1 teaspoon ground turmeric

1 teaspoon garlic powder

½ teaspoon ground ginger

½ cup water

Loaded with veggies such as lycopene-rich tomatoes and vitamin-loaded sweet potatoes, Pork Curry Stew helps fight inflammation and support digestion. The immune-boosting spices ginger, turmeric, and garlic lend an earthy, aromatic fragrance to this simple yet satisfying stew the entire family is sure to love!

1. On a large cutting board, season the pork with salt and pepper and set aside.

2. In a large pot on medium, heat the coconut oil and cook the pork for 10 to 12 minutes, stirring occasionally.

3. Reduce the heat to medium-low. Add the sweet potato and cook, uncovered, for 10 minutes without stirring.

4. Add the tomatoes, garlic, turmeric, garlic powder, ginger, and water, stir to combine, and simmer on medium-low for 1 hour, or until desired tenderness.

5. Serve warm.

Nutritional Analysis per Serving: Protein (g) 29.41; Fat (g) 10.34; Carbs (g) 7.94; B_{12} (mcg) 1.38; Iron (mg) 2.35; Iodine (mcg) 0; Magnesium (mg) 47.18; Potassium (mg) 752.23; Selenium (mcg) 43.17; Sodium (mg) 178.94

Golden Raisin Chicken Salad

Ⓟ PALEO

Prep time: 5 minutes

Serves: 4

1½ cups cooked and shredded chicken breast

*1 medium bell pepper, diced

⅓ cup toasted almonds

¼ cup golden raisins

1 medium stalk celery, chopped (about ½ cup)

1 large avocado, peeled, pitted, and mashed

Sea salt or pink Himalayan sea salt to taste

Black pepper to taste (if tolerated)

1 tablespoon lime juice

4 large romaine lettuce leaves, for serving

*Possible Modifications for Other Root Cause Diets: Remove the bell pepper and almonds from this recipe to make it Autoimmune.

A healthy substitute for traditional chicken salad, Golden Raisin Chicken Salad uses creamy mashed avocados instead of mayonnaise. Adding raisins provides a sweet flavor and packs even more vitamins into the already nutritious chicken salad, while the almonds can help lower blood-sugar levels and add just the right amount of crunch.

1. In a large bowl, place the chicken, bell pepper, almonds, raisins, celery, avocado, salt, pepper, and lime juice.

2. Stir until combined.

3. Spoon the chicken salad onto lettuce leaves and serve.

Nutritional Analysis per Serving: Protein (g) 19.26; Fat (g) 10.94; Carbs (g) 14.83; B_{12} (mcg) 0.18; Iron (mg) 1.36; Iodine (mcg) 0; Magnesium (mg) 53.72; Potassium (mg) 522.26; Selenium (mcg) 15.06; Sodium (mg) 149.38

Jar Salad

① INTRO

Prep: 20 minutes

Serves: 1

2 tablespoons salad dressing

1 cup chopped firm vegetables

½ cup whole small veggies and/or fruit

¼ cup carbs, if using

1 tablespoon nuts or seeds

1 cup greens and herbs

DAY-OF-USE ADDITIONS (OPTIONAL)

¼ cup fresh vegetables

3 ounces protein

¼ cup chopped fruit

Nutritional Analysis per Serving: Protein (g) 6.03; Fat (g) 22.20; Carbs (g) 17.22; B$_{12}$ (mcg) 0; Iron (mg) 2.87; Iodine (mcg) 0; Magnesium (mg) 69.64; Potassium (mg) 696.2; Selenium (mcg) 8.54; Sodium (mg) 115.43

Jar Salads were essential to helping me make healthy food a part of my routine. When I first started making them, I was working 9:00 a.m. to 9:00 p.m. at a pharmacy, and I only had about fifteen minutes to eat lunch. At the time, I slept for eleven or twelve hours each night. So I would wake up at 8:30, throw on my clothes and white coat, and rush out the door to get to work. I never had time for breakfast and spent the whole morning drinking caffeine to get myself going. By the time lunch came around, I was starving. I had a tuna sandwich from the sub shop with chips and a large soda every day.

And then I discovered Jar Salads. I started prepping five salads on Sunday nights and grabbing one from the fridge each workday morning. When my life was nothing but working and sleeping and I had no time to make healthy foods, these convenient nutrient powerhouses were a lifesaver. Jar Salads will keep for 5 days in the fridge. This recipe is for one Jar Salad, but it is more efficient to make several at a time.

1. Put the dressing in the bottom of a quart-size Mason jar.

2. Add chopped firm veggies and pack them at the bottom.

3. Next, add whole small veggies and/or fruit.

4. Next, put in a carb source, if using.

5. The next layer is nuts or seeds.

6. Top the jar with lettuce, greens, and herbs.

7. Put the lid on and place in the fridge.

8. One the day you are going to eat the salad, open the lid and place any additional ingredients on top or pack in a separate container.

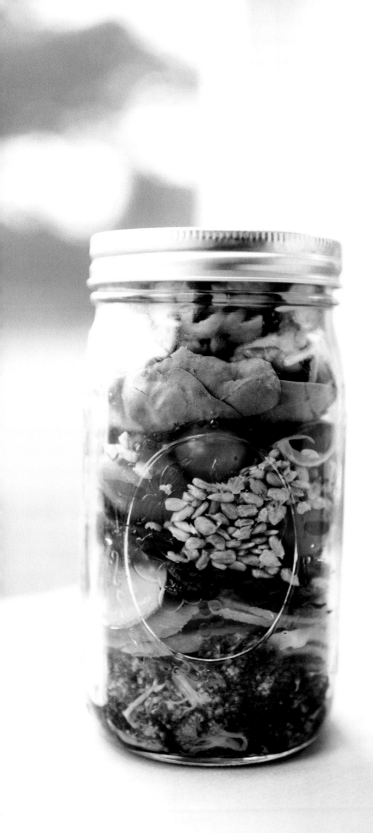

JAR SALAD OPTIONS

Salad dressing: Everyday Dressing (p. 138), Goddess of Detox Dressing (p. 149), or simply 1 tablespoon olive oil and 1 tablespoon lemon juice

Chopped firm vegetables: cucumbers, carrots, peppers, radishes, broccoli, onions, or any combination

Whole small vegetables or fruits: olives, cherry tomatoes, blueberries, grapes

Carb source (if using): non-GMO beans, corn, quinoa, rice

Nuts or seeds: almonds, pumpkin seeds, sunflower seeds, flax seeds, chia seeds, walnuts, pecans

Chopped greens: lettuce, spinach, kale, chard, arugula, herbs

Day-of-use additions: fresh fruit and vegetables: cooked beets, chopped tomatoes avocados, diced apples, mangoes, pears, peaches; Protein: tuna, salmon, hard-boiled eggs, chicken, turkey, bacon, or steak

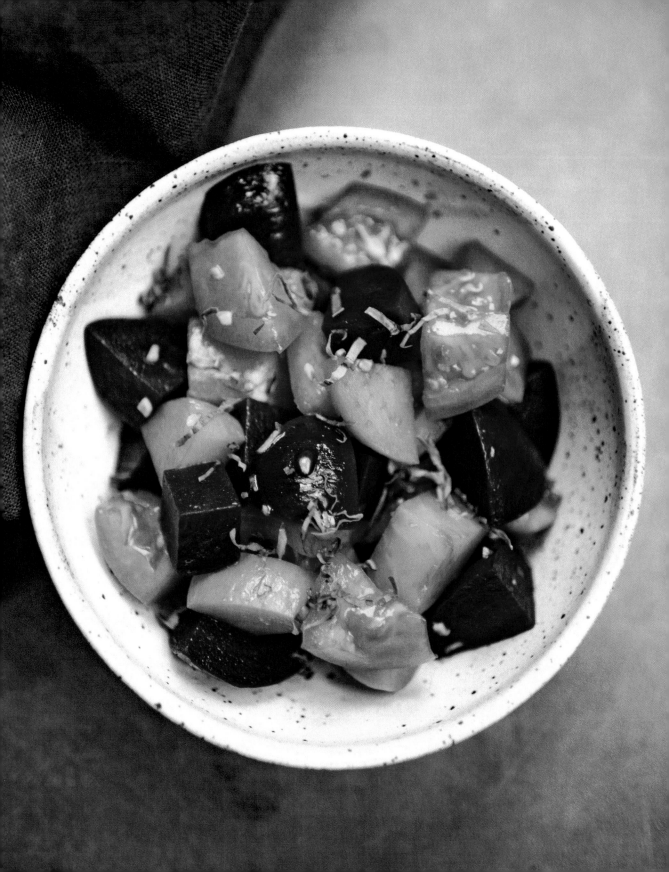

Heirloom Tomato and Beet Salad

P PALEO

Prep time: 15 minutes

Cook time: 40 to 60 minutes

Serves: 6

2 tablespoons olive oil, *divided*

2 large beets (1 golden, 1 Chioggia, or any combo you like)

3 large ripe heirloom tomatoes, chopped

3 tablespoons fresh basil, cut into thin strips

1 large clove garlic, minced superfine

3 tablespoons balsamic vinegar

Sea salt or pink Himalayan sea salt to taste

Black pepper to taste (if tolerated)

Beets are a rich source of betaine, an amino-acid derivative that can be a powerful ally in breaking down inflammation and supporting digestion. Roasting beets creates a rich and delightful sweetness. Paired with the mildly smoky flavor of antioxidant-rich heirloom tomatoes, this salad is one of my all-time favorites!

1. Preheat the oven to 375°F.

2. Rub 1 tablespoon olive oil over the whole beets and roast in the oven for 40 minutes to 1 hour until just tender when pierced; set aside to cool for 10 minutes.

3. Toss the tomatoes with the basil, remaining 1 tablespoon olive oil, garlic, and balsamic vinegar in a salad bowl.

4. Peel and chop cooked beets and add to salad bowl, tossing to coat with dressing.

Nutritional Analysis per Serving: Protein (g) 1.36; Fat (g) 4.72; Carbs (g) 8.03; B_{12} (mcg) 0; Iron (mg) 0.62; Iodine (mcg) 0; Magnesium (mg) 18.45; Potassium (mg) 301.2; Selenium (mcg) 0.4; Sodium (mg) 168.66

Katy's Greek Salad

Ⓟ PALEO

Prep time: 10 minutes

Serves: 4

1 cup pitted Kalamata olives

1 large cucumber, diced small

1 avocado, diced

2 tomatoes, diced

1 green pepper, seeded and finely diced

½ red onion, minced

½ cup chopped fresh cilantro (optional)

½ cup chopped fresh parsley (optional)

1 tablespoon lemon juice (or the juice of ½ lemon)

1 tablespoon extra-virgin olive oil

1 tablespoon dried basil

I love Greek salad. I got this recipe from my sister-in-law, Katy, and made it Hashimoto's friendly by removing the feta cheese. Last summer, my mom and I made this almost every day with heirloom tomatoes from her garden. This recipe is a great crowd pleaser for parties! Including cilantro and parsley in the salad will boost its detoxification power, and if you're in need of protein, you can always add some nuts, chicken, or salmon!

1. Mix the olives, cucumber, avocado, tomatoes, green pepper, and red onion together in a bowl.

2. Add the cilantro and parsley, if using, and mix.

3. In a small dish, combine the lemon juice with the extra-virgin olive oil and basil; dress the salad with the desired amount.

Nutritional Analysis per Serving: Protein (g) 3.05; Fat (g) 12.55; Carbs (g) 14.5; B_{12} (mcg) 0; Iron (mg) 3.42; Iodine (mcg) 0; Magnesium (mg) 45.99; Potassium (mg) 624.19; Selenium (mcg) 0.86; Sodium (mg) 266.03

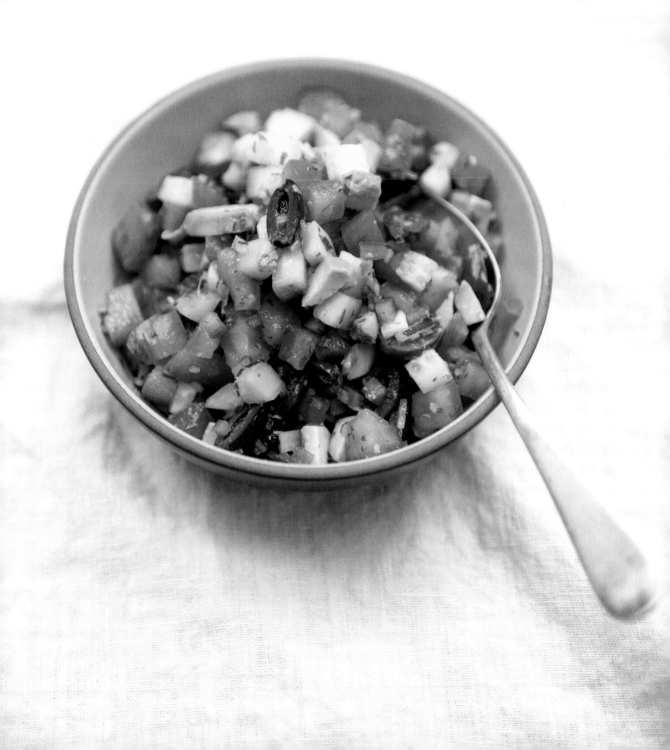

Bibimbap Bowl (Korean Mixed Veggie Bowl)

① INTRO

Prep time: 45 minutes

Serves: 1

*1 cup cooked rice (or lentils or "riced" cauliflower)

½ cup roasted vegetables (sweet potato, beets, carrots, parsnips, or butternut squash)

1 cup sautéed greens (spinach, broccoli, or swiss chard)

3 ounces grilled protein (beef, chicken, pork, bison, or venison)

*1 cooked chicken or duck egg (sunny-side up or poached; optional)

1 tablespoon coconut aminos

¼ large avocado, peeled, pitted, and chopped

Sea salt or pink Himalayan sea salt to taste

*Possible Modifications for Other Root Cause Diets: This recipe can be made into an Autoimmune version by using riced cauliflower instead of rice and omitting the egg.

When Michael and I were newlyweds living in Los Angeles, we used to love eating at a place called Destiny Cafe, where we were introduced to bibimbap. Some of the traditional ingredients, like soy sauce (which may contain gluten), now prevent me from ordering this meal at restaurants, so I love making it at home with safe and thyroid-nourishing ingredients like coconut aminos.

Coconut aminos is a sauce made from the sap of coconut trees that is gluten, dairy, and soy free and is rich in amino acids. Amino acids play a vital role in brain and nervous system function and are a great alternative to soy sauce. You can find coconut aminos in most health-food stores or online.

The beauty of Bibimbap Bowls is that you can batch-cook them ahead of time. You can freeze the cooked ingredients in premeasured bowls for thawing and reheating later, when you will add the egg or other toppings. You can create your own bowl of deliciousness by combining my suggested ingredients with various other ingredients that you love.

1. Place the rice in a large bowl. Add the roasted vegetables, sautéed greens, and grilled protein.

2. Top it off with a cooked egg, if using.

3. Season with coconut aminos, avocado, and salt.

4. Mix the bowl ingredients and enjoy!

Nutritional Analysis per Serving: Protein (g) 17.08; Fat (g) 11.95; Carbs (g) 25.84; B$_{12}$ (mcg) 1.06; Iron (mg) 3.56; Iodine (mcg) 6; Magnesium (mg) 90.71; Potassium (mg) 785.36; Selenium (mcg) 15.58; Sodium (mg) 250.52

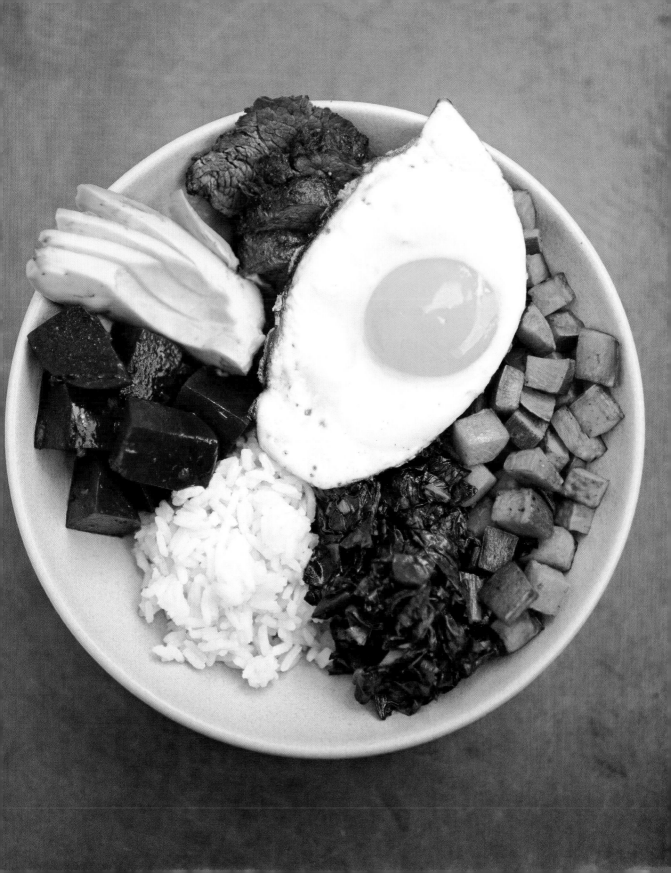

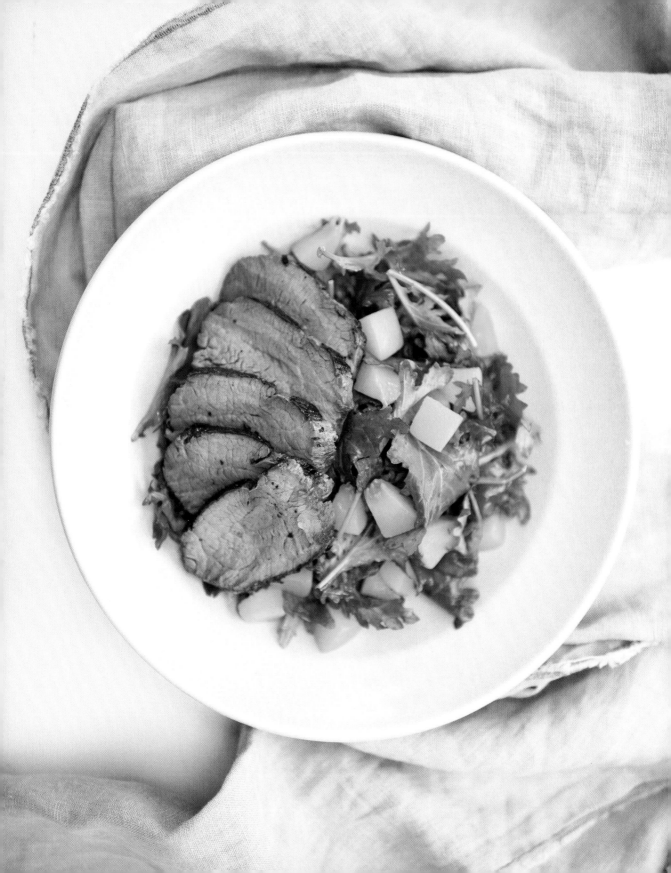

Peaches and Steak

Ⓐ AUTOIMMUNE

Prep time: 10 minutes

Cook time: 20 minutes

Serves: 4

4 tablespoons coconut oil

4 (4-ounce) filet mignons

4 large peaches, peeled and diced (about 4 cups)

6 cups chopped baby kale

4 tablespoons olive oil

Sea salt or pink Himalayan sea salt to taste

Black pepper to taste (if tolerated)

2 tablespoons apple cider vinegar

Iron-rich filet mignons are selected for this recipe because of their tenderness and exceptional taste. When served atop the refreshing peach and kale salad, you won't believe this melt-in-your-mouth meal supports both your immune system and heart health.

1. In a large skillet on medium-high, heat the coconut oil and cook the filets 5 minutes per side, or until desired doneness.

2. Remove from the skillet, set aside, and keep warm.

3. Add the peaches to the heated skillet and cook for 5 to 8 minutes, or until slightly softened. Remove the pan from the heat.

4. In a large bowl, toss the kale with the cooked peaches along with the olive oil, salt, pepper, and apple cider vinegar.

5. Divide the salad among four plates, top each with a filet, and serve immediately.

Nutritional Analysis per Serving: Protein (g) 30.89; Fat (g) 36.45; Carbs (g) 23.82; B_{12} (mcg) 1.36; Iron (mg) 3.84; Iodine (mcg) 0; Magnesium (mg) 88.08; Potassium (mg) 1178.73; Selenium (mcg) 29.89; Sodium (mg) 493.2

Crunchy Arugula Salad

Ⓐ AUTOIMMUNE

Prep time: 8 minutes

Serves: 4

3 cups arugula

30 seedless grapes, cut in half

6 radishes, chopped

⅓ cup unsweetened coconut flakes

½ cup chopped hearts of palm

⅓ cup coconut milk

Juice of 2 limes

1 tablespoon honey or maple syrup

Crunchy Arugula Salad is another one of my favorite summertime salads—it has the perfect blend of crunch, sweetness, and flavor. The sweet crunch factor from the grapes and coconut and the mellowness from the radishes pair nicely with the kick you get from the arugula. Enjoy the salad on its own or topped with some grilled shrimp to create a satisfying island-inspired treat!

1. Place the arugula in the bottom of a large salad bowl and top with the grapes, radishes, coconut flakes, and hearts of palm; set aside while you make the dressing.

2. In a high-speed blender, blend the coconut milk, lime juice, and sweetener on high for 30 seconds, or until combined.

3. Pour the dressing over the salad and carefully mix.

Nutritional Analysis per Serving: Protein (g) 2.91; Fat (g) 7.5; Carbs (g) 13.47; B_{12} (mcg) 0; Iron (mg) 2.1; Iodine (mcg) 0; Magnesium (mg) 47.35; Potassium (mg) 417.18; Selenium (mcg) 2.3; Sodium (mg) 101.1

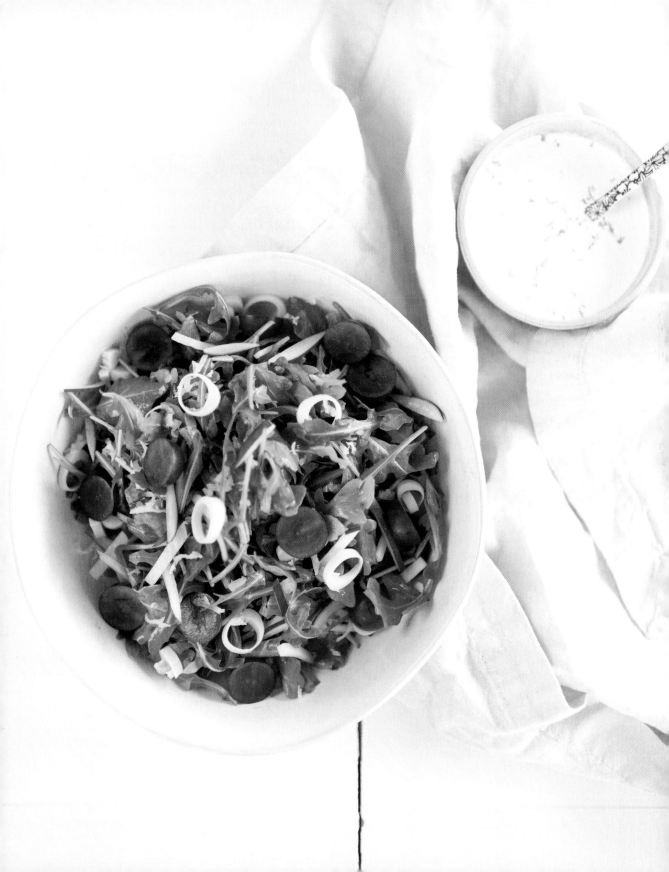

Duck Salad

P PALEO

Prep time: 15 minutes

Cook time: 15 minutes

Serves: 6

8 to 12 ounces boneless duck (or chicken) breasts, cut into ½-inch cubes

1 tablespoon coconut oil

1 tablespoon garlic powder

½ cup chopped carrots

½ cup chopped celery

½ cup chopped onions

½ cup chopped green apple

½ cup grapes, cut in half

½ cup chopped walnuts (optional)

½ cup Hashi-Mayo (p. 142)

Sea salt or pink Himalayan sea salt to taste

Black pepper to taste (if tolerated)

Like traditional chicken salad, this Duck Salad combines protein, fat, sweetness, and crunch. I like to use boneless duck (or chicken) breasts that are pan fried in coconut oil; however, this recipe is also a fantastic way to use leftovers from a whole roasted duck or chicken. To save time, I purchase carrots, celery, and onions that are prechopped whenever they're available at the grocery store!

1. Heat the coconut oil in a large pan on medium. Add the cubed duck, season with garlic powder, and pan fry until lightly browned and fully cooked through, about 4 to 5 minutes per side. Let cool.

2. While the duck is cooling, mix the carrots, celery, onions, apple, grapes, and walnuts, if using, with the Hashi-Mayo in a bowl.

3. Once cooled, chop the duck by hand or in a food processor and add into the mixture. Add salt and pepper to taste.

Nutritional Analysis per Serving: Protein (g) 13.39; Fat (g) 20.02; Carbs (g) 9.22; B_{12} (mcg) 0.42; Iron (mg) 3.11; Iodine (mcg) 0; Magnesium (mg) 33.66; Potassium (mg) 314.38; Selenium (mcg) 8.63; Sodium (mg) 221.7

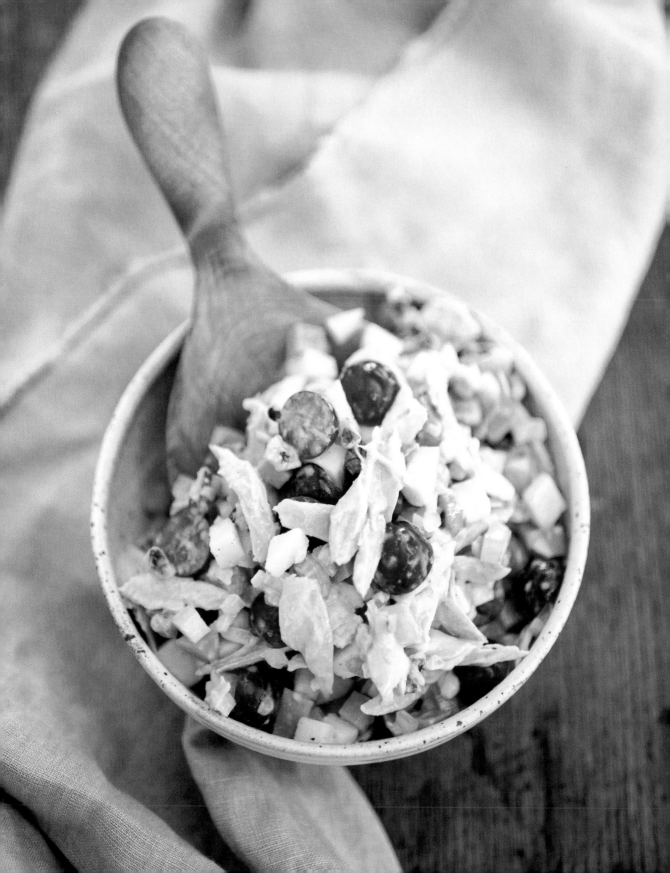

Cucumber-Fig Salad

Ⓐ AUTOIMMUNE

Prep time: 10 minutes

Serves: 4

1 pound boneless chicken breast, cooked and cubed

½ cup sliced cucumber

2 heads romaine lettuce, chopped

2 large figs, sliced

3 tablespoons avocado oil or melted coconut oil

¼ cup apple cider vinegar

1 tablespoon finely chopped leek or green onion

1 tablespoon chopped fresh dill or 1 teaspoon dried dill weed

Sea salt or pink Himalayan sea salt to taste

Black pepper to taste (if tolerated)

Cucumber-Fig Salad, an easy and versatile salad, is one of my hubby's favorites. If you are making this ahead, be sure to store the chicken and dressing separately from the salad. If figs are not in season, red plums are a tasty alternative.

1. In a large bowl combine the chicken, cucumber, lettuce, and figs.

2. In a small bowl, whisk the oil, vinegar, leek, and dill.

3. Pour the dressing over the salad, season with salt and pepper, toss, and serve.

Nutritional Analysis per Serving: Protein (g) 35.59; Fat (g) 14.37; Carbs (g) 5.85; B_{12} (mcg) 0.39; Iron (mg) 1.52; Iodine (mcg) 0; Magnesium (mg) 41.27; Potassium (mg) 392.28; Selenium (mcg) 31.43; Sodium (mg) 183.15

Taco the Town Salad

ⓘ INTRO

Prep time: 10 minutes

Cook time: 7 to 8 minutes

Serves: 4

4 (4-ounce) boneless chicken breasts

1 teaspoon garlic powder

1 teaspoon sea salt or pink Himalayan sea salt

2 tablespoons olive oil

¼ cup sliced black olives

1 avocado, peeled, pitted, and diced

2 heirloom tomatoes, seeded and diced

*1 cup canned black beans, drained and rinsed well

1 red bell pepper, diced

1 red onion, thinly sliced

1 bunch fresh cilantro, chopped

¼ cup Goddess of Detox dressing (p. 149)

*Possible Modifications for Other Root Cause Diets: This recipe can be easily converted to Paleo by omitting the black beans.

Taco the Town Salad is not your typical Tex-Mex fare. It's packed with liver-loving cilantro and healthy fats. Note: You must love cilantro to enjoy this salad!

1. Season both sides of the chicken breasts with garlic powder and salt.

2. Heat the olive oil in a skillet on medium and fry the chicken breasts 3 to 4 minutes on each side, or until cooked through.

3. Place the chicken in a bowl and let cool slightly, then shred with two forks or in a blender. Set aside.

4. In a large bowl, mix the olives, avocado, tomatoes, beans, bell pepper, onion, and cilantro.

5. Toss the dressing with the beans and vegetables and mix until combined.

6. Add the chicken and serve.

> Nutritional Analysis per Serving: Protein (g) 31.76; Fat (g) 19.97; Carbs (g) 22.51; B_{12} (mcg) 0.3; Iron (mg) 2.63; Iodine (mcg) 0; Magnesium (mg) 94.78; Potassium (mg) 1065.34; Selenium (mcg) 27.12; Sodium (mg) 559.16

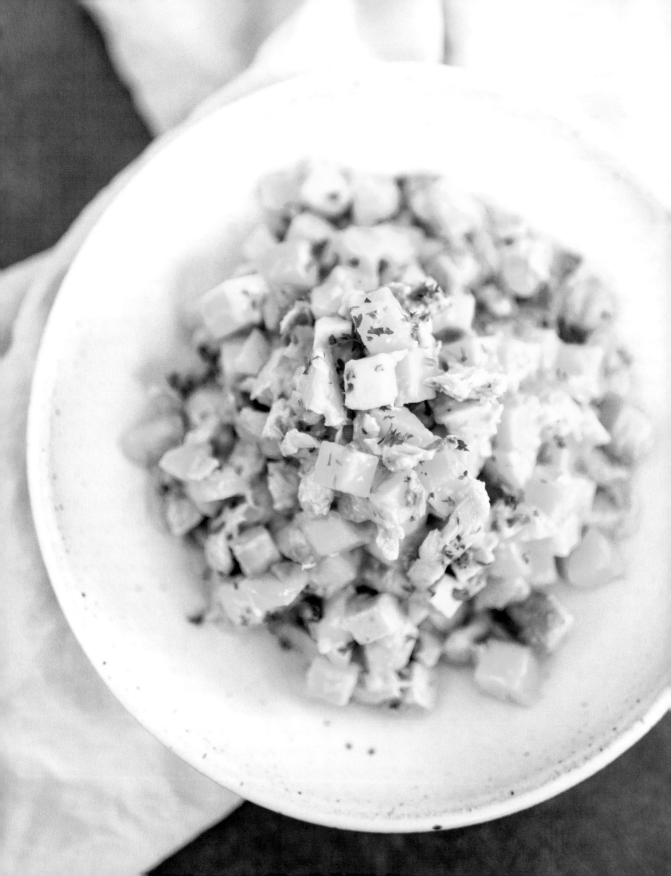

SAM Salad

Ⓐ AUTOIMMUNE

Prep time: 10 minutes

Cook time: 6 to 10 minutes

Serves: 2

1 ripe mango, diced

1 ripe avocado, diced

1 teaspoon coconut oil

1 (6-ounce) salmon fillet

¼ cup **Goddess of Detox Dressing** (p. 149)

I had a salad similar to my SAM Salad at a café in Switzerland, and I could not believe how tasty and filling it was! I added my own twist with my favorite dressing, Goddess of Detox Dressing! If you're feeling fancy, you can make this recipe using pan-fried salmon and Goddess of Detox Dressing as suggested below. If you're on the go or traveling, you can always use precooked salmon and dress the salad with lemon juice and olive oil.

1. In a large bowl, gently mix the mango and avocado. Set aside.

2. Heat the coconut oil in a large skillet on medium-high and place the fish skin-side up in the pan.

3. Cook until the fish becomes golden brown, about 3 to 5 minutes.

4. Flip the fish onto the skin side and cook for another 3 to 5 minutes until the fish feels firm.

5. Flake the salmon, add to the avocado and mango, and combine.

6. Lightly dress with the desired amount of dressing.

Nutritional Analysis per Serving: Protein (g) 19.18; Fat (g) 25.62; Carbs (g) 22.89; B_{12} (mcg) 2.84; Iron (mg) 1.41; Iodine (mcg) 10.5; Magnesium (mg) 62.96; Potassium (mg) 947.15; Selenium (mcg) 32; Sodium (mg) 94.8

Chopped BLT Salad

P PALEO

Prep time: 30 minutes

Cook time: 15 minutes

Serves: 6

8 bacon slices, cooked and diced (about ½ cup)

2½ cups chopped purple cabbage (about 8 ounces)

1 large bunch hearts of romaine, chopped (about 6 cups)

¼ cup chopped onion

¼ cup extra-virgin olive oil

1 medium tomato, chopped (about ¾ cup)

1 teaspoon celery salt

Sea salt or pink Himalayan sea salt to taste

Black pepper to taste (if tolerated)

An updated twist on the classic sandwich, the Chopped BLT Salad is gluten free and dairy free. It offers a delightful mix of antioxidant-rich purple (often referred to as red) cabbage and romaine lettuce topped with savory bacon pieces and tomatoes and drizzled with rich olive oil.

1. In a large bowl, combine all ingredients.

2. Serve immediately.

Nutritional Analysis per Serving: Protein (g) 7.65; Fat (g) 29.35; Carbs (g) 5.82; B$_{12}$ (mcg) 0.25; Iron (mg) 1.03; Iodine (mcg) 0; Magnesium (mg) 20.4; Potassium (mg) 346.86; Selenium (mcg) 10.59; Sodium (mg) 673.54

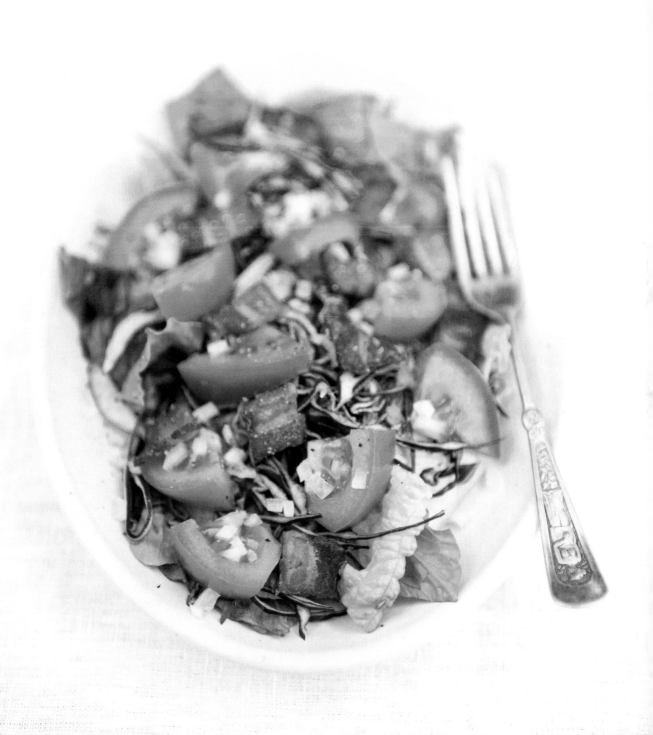

Frittata with Ham and White Sweet Potato

P PALEO

Prep time: 5 minutes

Cook time: 20 minutes

Serves: 4

8 eggs

¼ cup water

1 tablespoon coconut oil

4 ounces cooked ham, diced

1 small onion, thinly sliced

1 small steamed but firm white sweet potato, or regular sweet potato, diced

1 teaspoon minced garlic

1 small tomato, seeded and diced

Sea salt or pink Himalayan sea salt to taste

Black pepper to taste (if tolerated)

Even though we often think of a frittata as a breakfast or brunch meal, you can enjoy this protein-rich Frittata with Ham and White Sweet Potato any time of the day. It's hearty and filling and is great paired with a side salad or a side of bacon.

1. Break the eggs in a bowl, whisk them with the water, and set aside.

2. Preheat the broiler.

3. Heat the coconut oil in a 12-inch cast-iron skillet or other oven-proof skillet on medium. Add the ham, onion, and potatoes, and sauté until the onions are soft and the potatoes and ham are slightly browned, about 10 minutes.

4. Add the garlic and cook for 1 more minute.

5. Add the egg mixture to the skillet and swirl the pan to distribute the eggs evenly.

6. Cook the frittata for about 3 to 4 minutes, or until the edges start to set. The middle should still be undercooked.

7. Sprinkle the tomatoes over the frittata and place under the broiler for 5 minutes or until cooked through, watching carefully to keep it from burning.

8. Season to taste with salt and pepper.

Nutritional Analysis per Serving: Protein (g) 20.07; Fat (g) 15.38; Carbs (g) 11.69; B_{12} (mcg) 1.09; Iron (mg) 2.52; Iodine (mcg) 48; Magnesium (mg) 32.81; Potassium (mg) 477.74; Selenium (mcg) 36.78; Sodium (mg) 535

Duck with Date Sauce

Ⓐ AUTOIMMUNE

Prep time: 15 minutes

Cook time: 90 minutes

Serves: 4

Note: Store-bought herbes de Provence may contain fennel, which is not permitted on the Autoimmune Diet. Alternatively, you could make a modified herbes de Provence blend (p. 95).

1 (4- to 5-pound) whole duck, interior organ packet removed

1 cup dates

1 cup water

1 teaspoon allspice (if tolerated)

1 teaspoon cardamom (if tolerated)

1 teaspoon maple syrup

1 teaspoon AI Herbes de Provence (p. 95)

Sea salt or pink Himalayan sea salt to taste

2 tablespoons duck fat

Duck may seem like an intimidating and fancy dish, but in reality Duck with Date Sauce is a really simple and tasty recipe you can make in a roasting pan. Pairing the duck with Date Sauce adds a healthy source of sugar and fiber with a flavor you can't resist! I love adding the extra duck fat from a jar to make this dish all the more savory. The duck fat is also delicious in baked vegetables.

1. Preheat the oven to 375°F.

2. In a high-powered blender, blend the dates with the water, allspice, cardamom, maple syrup, and herbes de Provence until a paste is formed. Rub half of the paste on the top and sides of the duck, and reserve the other half of the paste.

3. Place the duck breast-side up in a roasting pan.

4. Roast for 90 minutes or until the duck is browned and the internal temperature in the thickest portion of the thigh measures 180°F on a meat thermometer.

5. Remove duck from oven and serve with the remaining date paste as a dipping sauce.

Nutritional Analysis per Serving: Protein (g) 13.39; Fat (g) 20.02; Carbs (g) 9.22; B_{12} (mcg) 0.42; Iron (mg) 3.11; Iodine (mcg) 0; Magnesium (mg) 33.66; Potassium (mg) 561.68; Selenium (mcg) 8.63; Sodium (mg) 72.81

Bigos (Polish Hunter's Stew)

ⓟ PALEO

Prep time: 10 minutes

Cook time: 6 to 8 hours in a slow cooker

Serves: 6

2 (24-ounce) jars sauerkraut, or 1 large cabbage, shredded (about 6 cups)

2 cups shredded vegetables like celery, broccoli, and/or carrot (optional)

16 ounces boneless chicken breast, cubed

1 pound ground turkey, beef, or pork

1 tablespoon dried basil

1 tablespoon dried paprika (if tolerated)

1 teaspoon sea salt or pink Himalayan sea salt

1 bay leaf

1 cup water

Bigos, also known as Hunter's Stew, is considered a Polish national dish and is often served in cold winter months. This hearty dish is naturally Paleo, with vegetables and meats all in one pot. Enjoy it whenever you need an extra nutrient boost! In Poland, every family has its own version of this recipe—some include wild meats like rabbit, others include plums—but it always consists of various meats, vegetables, and spices that are stewed with cabbage, one of the key ingredients. Traditionally, Bigos is made on the stovetop, but I make mine in a slow cooker; I love the fact that I can make a big batch and eat it for a few days. Bigos often tastes better the longer you let the flavors meld.

1. Place all ingredients in a slow cooker, mix, and cook on low for 6 to 8 hours.

Nutritional Analysis per Serving: Protein (g) 32.38; Fat (g) 17.8; Carbs (g) 8.43; B_{12} (mcg) 1.92; Iron (mg) 2.87; Iodine (mcg) 0; Magnesium (mg) 40.09; Potassium (mg) 475.58; Selenium (mcg) 26.12; Sodium (mg) 1258.62

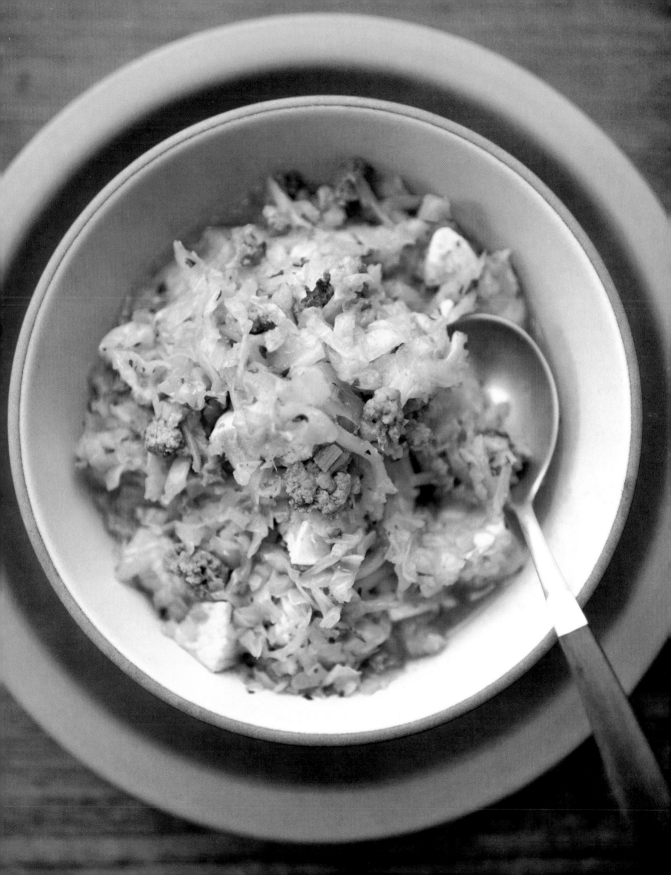

Shrimp Ceviche

Ⓐ AUTOIMMUNE

Prep time: 7 minutes

Cook time: 6 hours marinating

Serves: 6

1 teaspoon coconut oil

1 pound raw shrimp, peeled, deveined, and diced

1 clove garlic, minced

1 cup avocado, diced (1 to 1½ avocados)

2 small lemons, juiced

2 small limes, juiced

¼ cup chopped fresh cilantro

Sea salt or pink Himalayan sea salt to taste

Black pepper to taste (if tolerated)

1 lemon, sliced, for garnish

2 tablespoons chopped fresh parsley, for garnish

In Shrimp Ceviche, a popular Latin American seafood dish, shrimp is marinated in a combination of lemon and lime juices, both high in the detoxifying nutrient limonene. Add that to the combination of immune-boosting garlic and heart-healthy avocados, and this ceviche provides an incredibly healthy meal with minimal effort. Citrus juices are traditionally used to "cook" the raw seafood that is used in ceviches. However, while the juices do tenderize the meat, they do not kill bacteria that may be present. Unless your shrimp is superfresh, you may want to lightly cook it before putting it in the juice to kill any potentially pathogenic bacteria.

1. Add coconut oil and shrimp to a frying pan and cook for 1 to 2 minutes on high (optional).

2. Combine all ingredients in a large bowl.

3. Cover, making sure all shrimp are submerged in the juice, and refrigerate for 6 hours or until the shrimp have gone from translucent to opaque.

4. Serve chilled.

Nutritional Analysis per Serving: Protein (g) 11.29; Fat (g) 6.75; Carbs (g) 6.59; B_{12} (mcg) 0.84; Iron (mg) 0.57; Iodine (mcg) 20.83; Magnesium (mg) 31.44; Potassium (mg) 337; Selenium (mcg) 22.66; Sodium (mg) 498

Sweet and Sour Chicken Skewers with Broccoli Salad

A AUTOIMMUNE

Prep time: 2 hours

Cook time: 20 minutes

Serves: 4

CHICKEN SKEWERS

1 pound boneless chicken thighs, cut into ½-inch-wide strips

¼ cup coconut aminos

2 teaspoons lemon zest

1 teaspoon molasses

1 teaspoon honey

Sea salt or pink Himalayan sea salt to taste

Black pepper to taste (if tolerated)

8- to 12-inch) wooden skewers soaked in water for 30 minutes

BROCCOLI SALAD

3 cups packaged broccoli slaw, or 5 broccoli stalks

¼ cup raisins

1 tablespoon minced shallot

2 tablespoons canned full-fat coconut milk

1 tablespoon honey

2 tablespoons lime juice

Sea salt or pink Himalayan sea salt to taste

Black pepper to taste (if tolerated)

Marinated in a mixture of coconut aminos, lemon zest, iron-boosting molasses, and honey, Sweet and Sour Chicken Skewers are a perfect meal for the grill. Enjoy with a side of immune-boosting Broccoli Salad, the perfect complement to this Asian-inspired dish.

1. Place the chicken in a large resealable bag.

2. In a small bowl, whisk together coconut aminos, lemon zest, molasses, honey, salt, and pepper and pour the mixture into the bag.

3. Seal the bag, press a few times to distribute the marinade, and place chicken in the fridge for at least 2 hours.

4. Peel and shred the broccoli if not already done.

5. In a large bowl, toss the slaw, raisins, and shallot with the coconut milk, honey, lime juice, salt, and pepper. Refrigerate until serving time.

6. Preheat the grill to medium.

7. Thread the chicken evenly onto the skewers.

8. Place skewers on the grill and cook for 5 to 10 minutes on each side until chicken is cooked through and no longer pink inside.

9. Serve the chicken with the salad.

Nutritional Analysis per Serving: Protein (g) 26.9; Fat (g) 4.83; Carbs (g) 23.5; B_{12} (mcg) 0.24; Iron (mg) 0.92; Iodine (mcg) 0; Magnesium (mg) 43.79; Potassium (mg) 520.33; Selenium (mcg) 26.8; Sodium (mg) 783.76

Citrus Bison Meatballs

Ⓐ AUTOIMMUNE

Prep time: 25 minutes

Cook time: 18 minutes

Serves: 6

MEATBALLS

4 tablespoons coconut oil, *divided*

¾ cup minced onion

3 cloves garlic, minced

1 teaspoon ground ginger

2 pounds ground bison

1 tablespoon chopped fresh thyme

Sea salt or pink Himalayan sea salt to taste

Black pepper to taste (if tolerated)

½ cup fresh orange juice

¼ cup coconut aminos

NOODLES

2 large sweet potatoes, peeled

4 tablespoons coconut oil, *divided*

In Citrus Bison Meatballs, the meatballs get a punch of flavor from the thyme and ginger, and when paired with the glaze, they have an Asian-meets-Western flair. To save time, you can buy your spiralized sweet potato noodles from the grocery store—just be sure there are no additives! This would also taste good with zucchini noodles.

1. In a large skillet, heat 2 tablespoons coconut oil on medium. Add the onion and cook, stirring, for 8 minutes or until translucent.

2. Add the garlic and ginger and cook, stirring, for 1 minute, just until fragrant.

3. Remove from the heat and place onion mixture in a bowl. Set aside to cool for a few minutes.

4. When the onion mixture has cooled, add it to a large mixing bowl with the ground bison, thyme, salt, and pepper. Gently mix with your hands until well incorporated. Form into 1½-inch meatballs.

5. Add the remaining 2 tablespoons oil to the skillet used for the onions and heat on medium. Add the meatballs and brown for 3 minutes on one side; flip and add the orange juice and coconut aminos. Cook covered, for 10 minutes, or until cooked through. Remove the meatballs from the pan and set aside.

6. Leave the remaining juices in the pan and turn up the heat to medium-high. Let the sauce reduce to about half the amount, about 5 to 10 minutes. Return the meatballs to the sauce and keep warm.

7. Using a vegetable peeler, peel the sweet potatoes into long, flat ribbons, or spiralize them with a vegetable spiralizer.

8. In another skillet, heat 1 tablespoon coconut oil on medium-high. Add half of the sweet potatoes. Cook, stirring occasionally, for about 10 minutes, being sure not to stir them too often, so that they brown on the bottom. Remove the first batch; then add the remaining oil and repeat with the second batch of sweet potatoes.

9. Serve the glazed meatballs on a bed of crispy sweet potato noodles.

Nutritional Analysis per Serving: Protein (g) 31.79; Fat (g) 29.15; Carbs (g) 15.57; B_{12} (mcg) 2.93; Iron (mg) 4.72; Iodine (mcg) 0; Magnesium (mg) 48.67; Potassium (mg) 726.07; Selenium (mcg) 31; Sodium (mg) 409.63

Lentil Shepherd's Pie

❶ INTRO

Prep time: 25 minutes

Cook time: 40 minutes

Serves: 6

FILLING

1 tablespoon coconut oil

1 medium onion, finely chopped

2 carrots, finely chopped

1 celery stalk, finely chopped

1 cup finely chopped mushrooms

1 teaspoon chopped garlic

1 cup chopped kale

¾ cup cooked lentils

1 teaspoon dried parsley

½ teaspoon dried thyme

½ teaspoon sea salt or pink Himalayan sea salt

Black pepper to taste (if tolerated)

1 tablespoon coconut aminos

TOPPING

3 medium white sweet potatoes, scrubbed

1 tablespoon coconut oil

6 tablespoons plain Coconut Yogurt (p. 131)

Sea salt or pink Himalayan sea salt to taste

Black pepper to taste (if tolerated)

Lentil Shepherd's Pie is filled with veggies and lentils, and no meat! Although I believe that animal protein is essential for healing, adding a different source of protein, such as lentils, can provide other important nutrients and mix up flavors. Lentils are also a great source of fiber and folate! If you cannot find white sweet potatoes, then substitute regular sweet potatoes.

1. Preheat the oven to 350°F.

2. In a skillet, heat the coconut oil on medium and add the onions, carrots, and celery; cook until onions are translucent and carrots are soft, about 6 minutes.

3. Add the mushrooms and garlic, and cook for 2 minutes.

4. Add the kale, lentils, parsley, thyme, salt, pepper, and coconut aminos and cook until the lentils are warmed and the kale is wilted.

5. Press the lentil mixture into a 9-inch square casserole dish and set aside.

6. Steam the white sweet potatoes in a steamer basket for 10 to 12 minutes or until cooked.

7. When the potatoes are steamed, remove them from the basket and let cool slightly.

8. Peel the skins off and place the sweet potatoes in a mixing bowl.

9. Add the coconut oil, coconut yogurt, salt, and pepper and whip until combined and fluffy.

10. Place the whipped potatoes on top of the lentil mixture and spread evenly across the top.

11. Cover the casserole dish with aluminum foil and bake for 25 minutes, or until the lentil mixture is bubbling.

12. Remove from the oven, let cool slightly, and serve.

Nutritional Analysis per Serving: Protein (g) 8; Fat (g) 4.87; Carbs (g) 35.74; B_{12} (mcg) 0; Iron (mg) 3.07; Iodine (mcg) 0; Magnesium (mg) 28.71; Potassium (mg) 559.26; Selenium (mcg) 2.28; Sodium (mg) 264.88

Turkey and Pepper Avocado Boats

P PALEO

Prep time: 10 minutes

Serves: 4

4 ounces cooked ground turkey

1 tablespoon chopped red onion

1 small red or yellow bell pepper, seeded and diced

1 tablespoon chopped fresh cilantro

2 tablespoons fresh lime juice

2 teaspoons honey

Sea salt or pink Himalayan sea salt to taste

Black pepper to taste (if tolerated)

2 large avocados, halved and pitted

In Turkey and Pepper Avocado Boats, savory turkey is mixed with sweet bell peppers and honey and served in a fun, kid-friendly avocado boat. Avocados have heart-healthy monounsaturated fatty acids and are high in fiber. A splash of fresh lime juice and chopped onion finish off this simple, healthy meal the entire family will enjoy. These also make a perfect snack!

1. In a large bowl, combine the turkey, onion, bell pepper, cilantro, lime juice, honey, salt, and pepper.

2. Spoon the turkey mixture into the avocados.

3. Serve immediately.

> Nutritional Analysis per Serving: Protein (g) 17.46; Fat (g) 15.31; Carbs (g) 10.96; B_{12} (mcg) 1.82; Iron (mg) 1.23; Iodine (mcg) 0; Magnesium (mg) 35.5; Potassium (mg) 625.79; Selenium (mcg) 4.55; Sodium (mg) 249.63

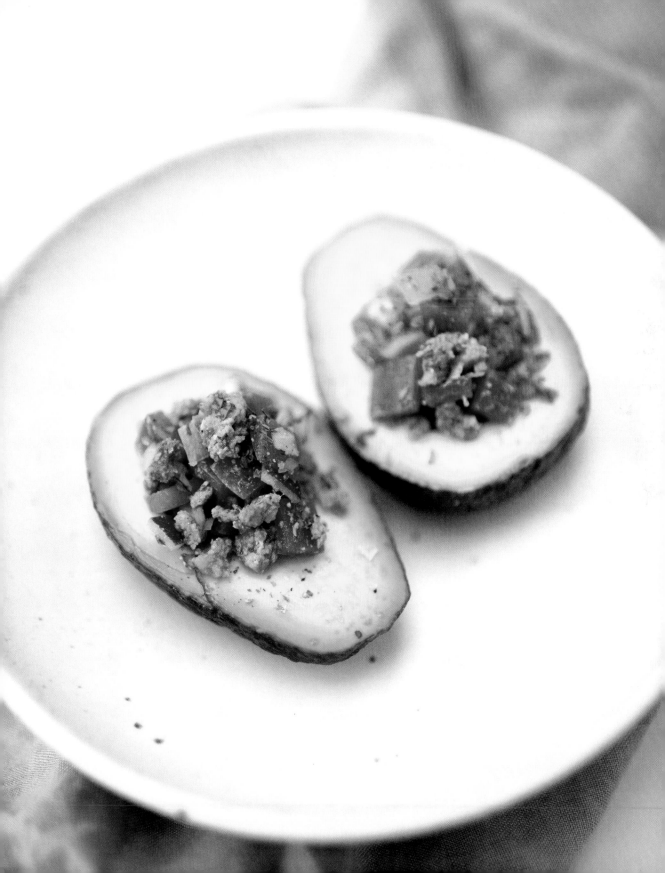

Hubby's Carnitas

Ⓟ PALEO

Prep time: 5 minutes

Cook time: 3 to 3¾ hours

Serves: 8

3 to 5 pounds boneless pork shoulder

1 teaspoon sea salt or pink Himalayan sea salt

½ teaspoon black pepper (if tolerated)

*1 teaspoon ground cumin (if tolerated)

½ teaspoon dried oregano

*½ teaspoon paprika (if tolerated)

1 bay leaf

4 garlic cloves, sliced

1 onion, chopped

Water to cover

*Possible Modifications for Other Root Cause Diets: To make the dish Auto-immune, remove the cumin and paprika.

My wonderful hubby makes these mouthwatering carnitas on the weekends, and we enjoy them for days on end! This is a great recipe to make on a meal-prepping day. Enjoy with eggs and spaghetti squash sautéed in olive oil in the morning, with a salad at lunch, and with veggies for dinner!

1. Preheat the oven to 350°F.

2. Place the meat in a Dutch oven or other braising pot with a cover.

3. Mix the salt, pepper, cumin, oregano, and paprika together in a small bowl and rub the mixture on the meat on all sides.

4. Add the bay leaf, garlic, and onion on top of the meat.

5. Pour in enough water to almost cover the meat.

6. Braise for 3 to 3½ hours, mixing the meat and turning it over every hour or so. You'll know the meat is done when the water is mostly evaporated and the meat is slightly brown, tender, and easy to shred with a fork.

7. When most of the water is gone and the pork turns slightly brown, shred the pork, discard the fat, and mix the meat with the pan juices.

8. Place the pot back into the oven, uncovered, and cook for an additional 10 minutes.

Nutritional Analysis per Serving: Protein (g) 49.73; Fat (g) 35.13; Carbs (g) 2.16; B_{12} (mcg) 2.58; Iron (mg) 3.5; Iodine (mcg) 0; Magnesium (mg) 60.22; Potassium (mg) 938.65; Selenium (mcg) 74.59; Sodium (mg) 369.33

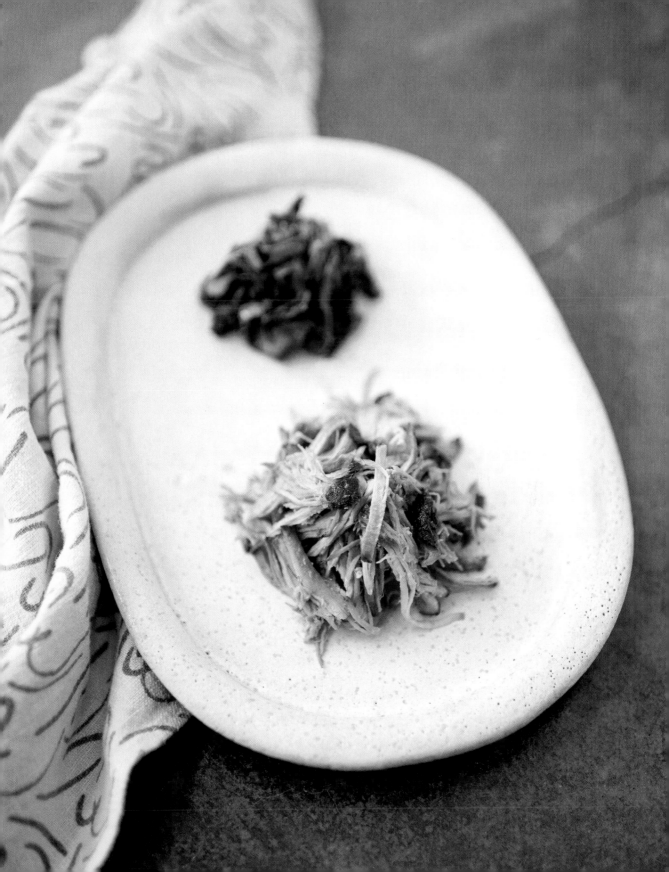

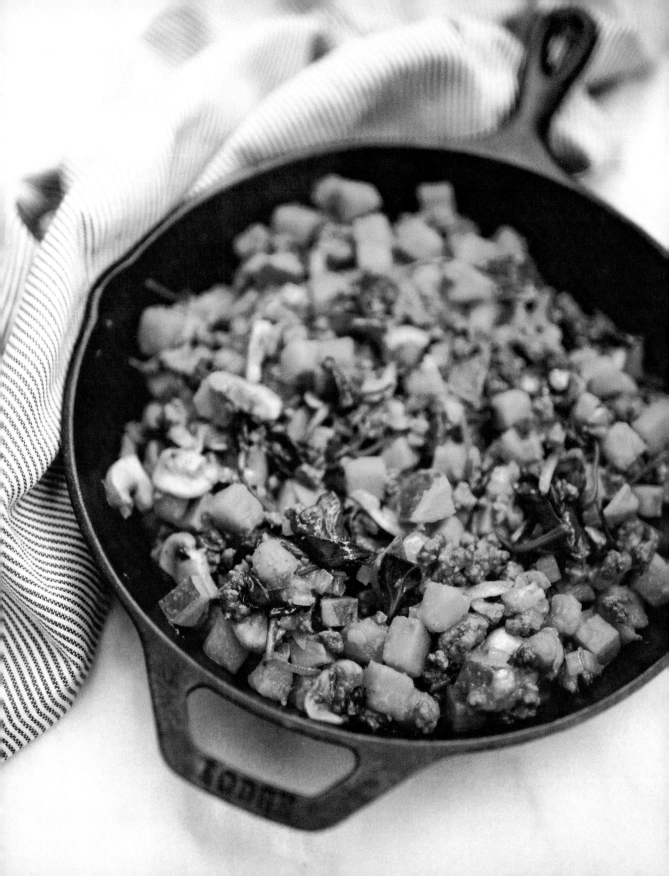

Hashi Hash Hash

Ⓐ AUTOIMMUNE

Prep time: 5 minutes

Cook time: 20 minutes

Serves: 2

1 large sweet potato, finely diced

5 ounces cremini mushrooms

½ white onion, finely diced

1 pound ground turkey or bison

1 handful baby spinach

Sea salt or pink Himalayan sea salt to taste

My hubby came up with this delicious Hashi Hash Hash recipe, which has so much nutritious goodness to offer. Sweet potatoes and spinach are extremely high in vitamin A, and when you make this meal in a cast-iron skillet (bonus: it's naturally nonstick!), you will also bump up the iron content. I love it when he wakes me up on the weekends with his cooking!

1. Preheat a large cast-iron skillet over medium-high heat.

2. Place the diced sweet potatoes in the skillet. Cook until they are halfway done, somewhere between soft and firm (they should feel spongy to the touch)

3. Add the sliced mushrooms and diced onions. Cook, stirring, for 1 to 2 minutes.

4. Add the ground turkey or bison, breaking it up with a spatula and distributing it somewhat evenly around the skillet.

5. Cover and cook until meat is fully cooked.

6. Stir in a handful of spinach and cook until the spinach is wilted.

7. Add salt to taste and serve.

Nutritional Analysis per Serving: Protein (g) 24.58; Fat (g) 8.82; Carbs (g) 16.48; B_{12} (mcg) 1.14; Iron (mg) 2.25; Iodine (mcg) 0; Magnesium (mg) 56.73; Potassium (mg) 593.59; Selenium (mcg) 27.42; Sodium (mg) 115.1

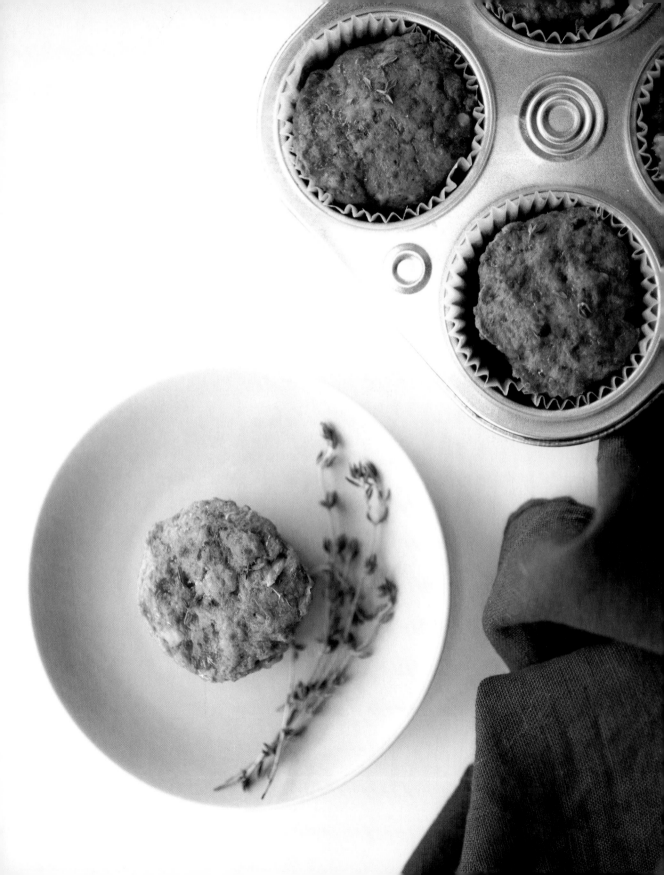

Maple Meatloaf Muffins

Ⓐ AUTOIMMUNE

Prep time: 45 minutes

Cook time: 20 minutes for each batch

Serves: 12

2 cups water

2 cups diced sweet potatoes

5 ounces bacon, cooked and chopped

1 tablespoon chopped fresh thyme, or 1 teaspoon dried

½ teaspoon garlic powder

Sea salt or pink Himalayan sea salt to taste

Black pepper to taste (if tolerated)

4 tablespoons maple syrup

2 pounds ground beef or bison

Nutritional Analysis per Serving: Protein (g) 15.25; Fat (g) 20.34; Carbs (g) 9.24; B_{12} (mcg) 1.83; Iron (mg) 1.58; Iodine (mcg) 0; Magnesium (mg) 22.45; Potassium (mg) 312.75; Selenium (mcg) 14.45; Sodium (mg) 179.95

Maple Meatloaf Muffins is one of my favorite recipes to batch-cook! I like to make these muffins with white sweet potatoes, which are starchier and less sweet than their orange counterparts. If you can't find white sweet potatoes, you can use regular sweet potatoes. I use a 24-cup muffin pan, so that I can enjoy two dozen cupcake-size burgers—they make a perfect snack any time of day!

1. Preheat the oven to 350°F.

2. Place the water and a steamer basket in a medium-size cooking pot over high heat. Bring the water to a boil.

3. Place sweet potatoes in the basket, cover, and steam for 10 to 12 minutes, or until the potatoes easily break apart with a fork. Drain remaining water. Let potatoes cool.

4. In a food processor, place the cooked sweet potatoes, bacon, thyme, garlic powder, salt, pepper, and maple syrup. Process into a thick paste.

5. Place the meat in a large bowl, add the sweet potato mixture, and combine well.

6. Gently spoon ⅓ cup of the meatloaf mixture into each of 12 muffin cups.

7. Bake on the middle rack for 15 to 20 minutes or until cooked through.

8. Remove cooked meatloaf muffins and repeat with remaining meatloaf mixture.

Chicken Tandoori

P PALEO

Prep time: 10 minutes

Cook time: 6 to 8 hours in a slow cooker

Serves: 4 to 6

1 chicken, cut into pieces, or 8 chicken drumsticks

1 teaspoon turmeric

1 teaspoon paprika (if tolerated)

1 teaspoon curry powder (if tolerated, or AI Curry Powder, p. 95)

1 teaspoon garlic powder

1 teaspoon sea salt or pink Himalayan sea salt

½ teaspoon black pepper (if tolerated)

2 cups coconut milk

This delicious version of Chicken Tandoori is so easy to make that it's become my go-to recipe for busy work days as well as for big dinner parties. The curcumin, found in turmeric and curry, can help protect the intestinal barrier from bacterial infections, help heal a leaky gut, and improve liver function and has even shown tumor-inhibiting activity in thyroid cancer. Plus, it has anti-inflammatory benefits! Although dietary curcumin leaves the body rather quickly when compared to supplemental curcumin, consuming it along with pepper can actually extend the time it stays in the body.

1. Place all ingredients in a slow cooker and cook on low for 6 to 8 hours.

Nutritional Analysis per Serving: Protein (g) 33.80; Fat (g) 35.61; Carbs (g) 2.39; B_{12} (mcg) 0.32; Iron (mg) 3.34; Iodine (mcg) 0; Magnesium (mg) 65.58; Potassium (mg) 689.16; Selenium (mcg) 20.64; Sodium (mg) 127.27

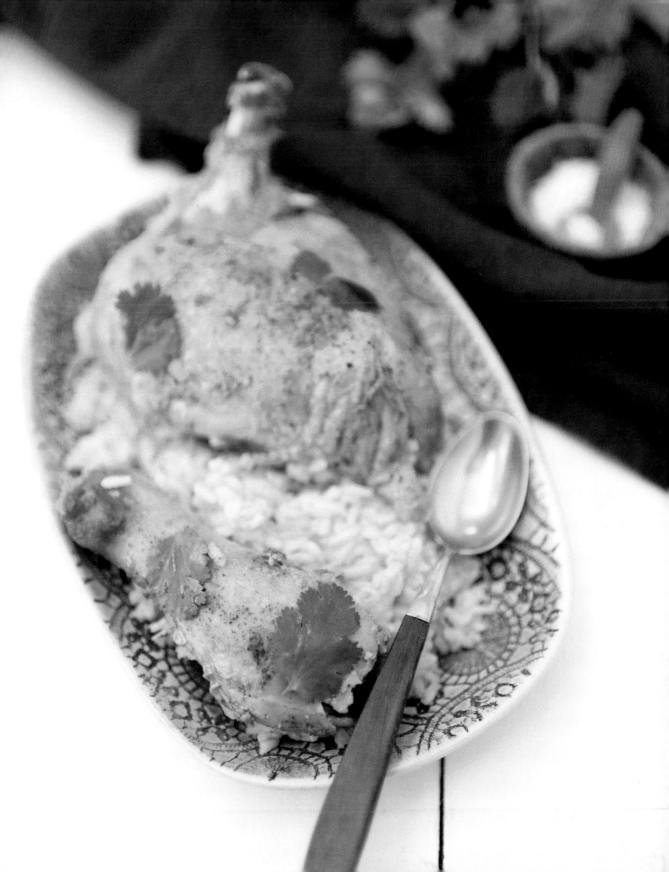

Tropical Grilled Chicken Skewers

Ⓐ AUTOIMMUNE

Prep time: 12 minutes

Cook time: 27 minutes

Serves: 4

MARINADE

Juice of 1 lemon

Juice of 1 lime

1 tablespoon olive oil

1 teaspoon minced garlic

½ teaspoon dried thyme

SKEWERS

½ pound boneless chicken breast, cut in 1-inch cubes

1 large zucchini, sliced in ½-inch rounds

1 large pineapple, cut in 1-inch chunks

8 ounces button mushrooms, stems removed

½ red onion, cut in 1-inch chunks

12 (8- to 12-inch) wooden skewers soaked in water for 30 minutes

Here is an easy weeknight dinner dish that can also be prepared the night before. If you do prep the Tropical Grilled Chicken Skewers ahead of time, simply pop them into the oven when you are ready to make dinner. Enjoy with a quick side salad, like my Crunchy Arugula Salad (p. 206).

1. Combine the marinade ingredients in a medium-size bowl, add the chicken cubes, and refrigerate for 1 hour.

2. Preheat the oven to 350°F.

3. Remove the chicken cubes from the marinade. Thread the meat, fruit, and vegetables on the skewers, placing one chicken cube between each vegetable or fruit piece. Discard the marinade.

4. Place the skewers on a rimmed baking sheet and bake for 12 minutes on each side.

5. Preheat the broiler.

6. Broil for 3 minutes on each side until cooked through and vegetables are slightly brown.

7. Alternatively, you can grill the skewers 5 to 10 minutes on each side, until cooked through.

Nutritional Analysis per Serving: Protein (g) 16.56; Fat (g) 5.48; Carbs (g) 22.15; B_{12} (mcg) 0.15; Iron (mg) 1.32; Iodine (mcg) 0; Magnesium (mg) 48.09; Potassium (mg) 682.37; Selenium (mcg) 19.14; Sodium (mg) 133.15

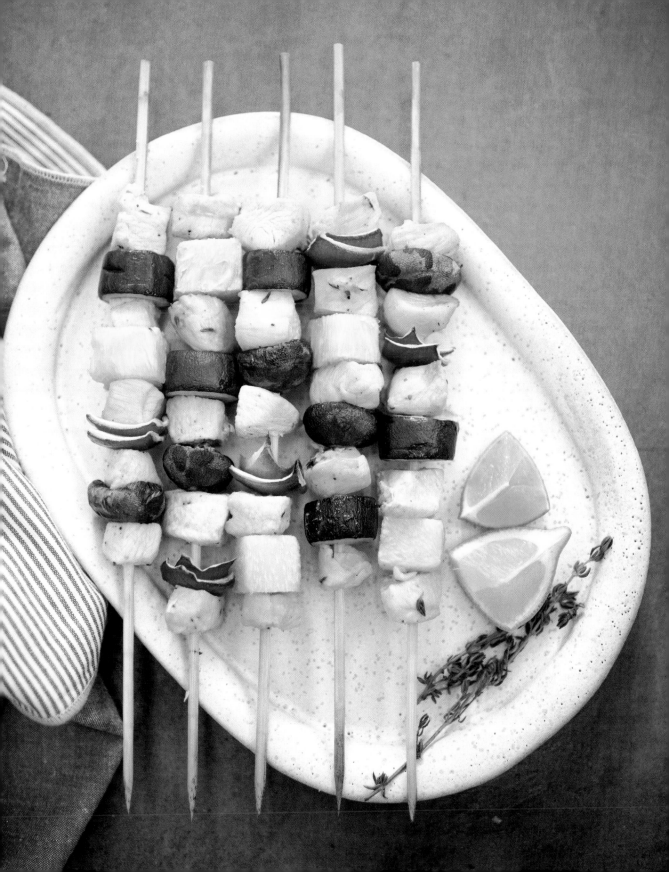

Salmon-Parsnip Cakes

P PALEO

Prep time: 12 minutes

Cook time: 20 minutes

Serves: 8

SALMON CAKES

3 cups cooked and flaked salmon

1 large egg, beaten

Sea salt or pink Himalayan sea salt to taste

Black pepper to taste (if tolerated)

1 cup shredded parsnips

2 tablespoons almond flour

1 tablespoon chopped fresh parsley

1 medium shallot, minced

½ teaspoon garlic powder

1 tablespoon coconut oil

LEMON-OIL DRESSING

¼ cup lemon juice

3 tablespoons olive oil

1 clove garlic, minced

2 teaspoons honey

1 teaspoon dried dill weed

Here is my twist on crab cakes—instead of using crab, I like to use omega-3-rich salmon! Serve these Salmon-Parsnip Cakes as a lunch with a side salad or make them smaller and serve them as appetizers with the lemon-oil dressing; they are sure to be a crowd pleaser!

1. Preheat the oven to 350°F.

2. In a large bowl, mix the salmon, egg, salt, pepper, parsnips, almond flour, parsley, shallot, and garlic powder. Form the salmon mixture into patties about the size of the palm of your hand (smaller if you are making appetizers).

3. In a large skillet on medium, heat the coconut oil. Add the salmon patties and brown on each side for 5 minutes until golden, taking care to flip the patties gently so they don't break apart.

4. Place the browned salmon cakes in a large baking dish and bake for 10 minutes, until the centers of the cakes are warm.

5. For the lemon-oil dressing, whisk together the dressing ingredients or place in a blender and blend until combined. Serve alongside the salmon cakes or drizzle on top.

Nutritional Analysis per Serving: Protein (g) 36.83; Fat (g) 27.11; Carbs (g) 11.95; B_{12} (mcg) 5.52; Iron (mg) 2.31; Iodine (mcg) 27; Magnesium (mg) 73.66; Potassium (mg) 1070.95; Selenium (mcg) 67.12; Sodium (mg) 196.5

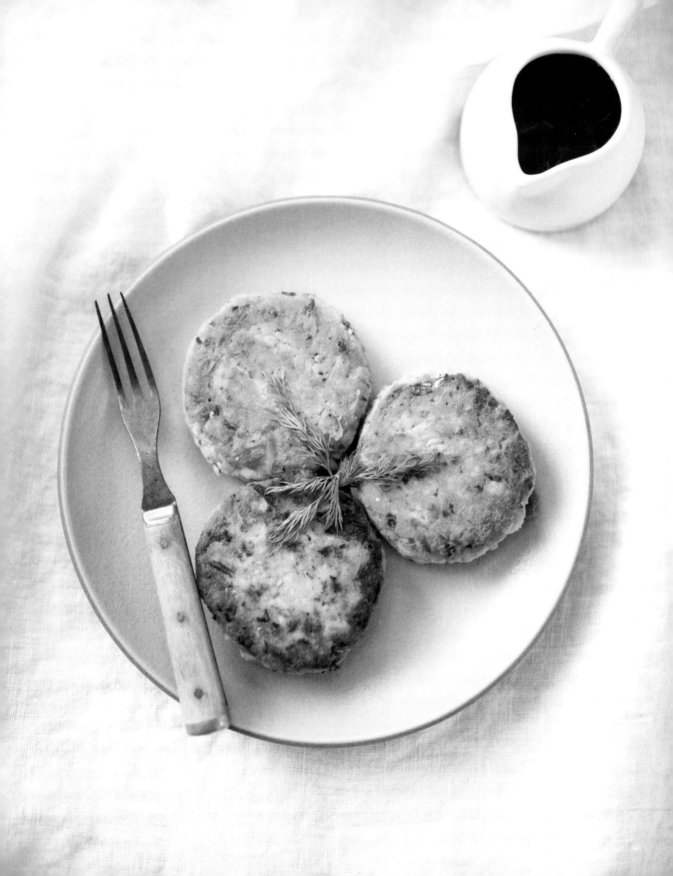

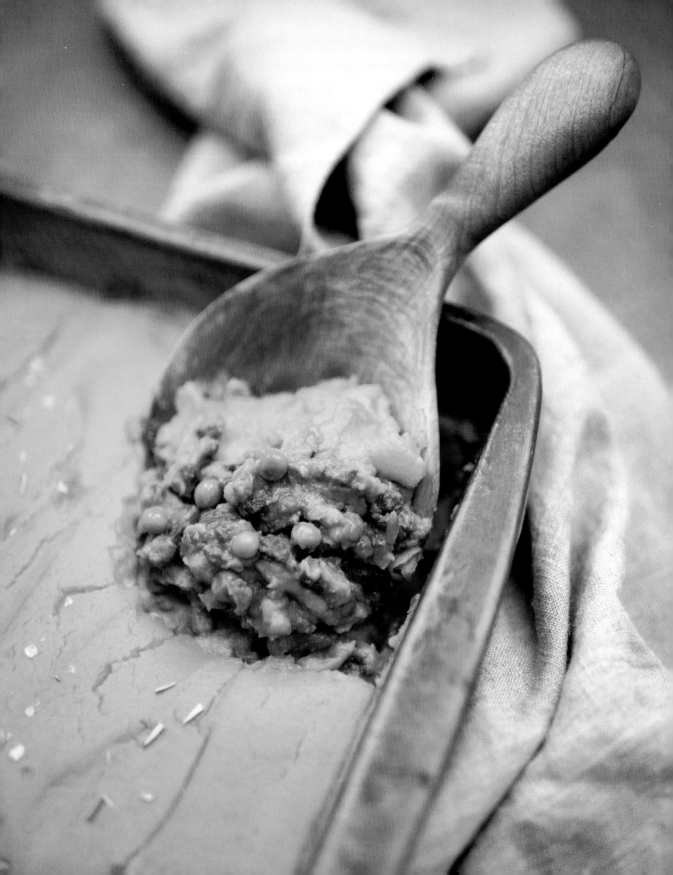

Shepherd's Pie

Ⓟ PALEO

Prep time: 15 minutes

Cook time: 10 to 15 minutes

Serves: 4 to 6

FILLING

1 tablespoon coconut oil

1 medium yellow onion, diced

2 large carrots, peeled and diced

3 cloves garlic, chopped

2 cups coarsely chopped mushrooms

8 ounces ground beef

8 ounces ground lamb

3 tablespoons tomato paste

¾ cup water or Bone Broth (p. 135)

1¼ cups frozen peas

2 tablespoons fresh rosemary

Sea salt or pink Himalayan sea salt to taste

Black pepper to taste (if tolerated)

TOPPING

3 large sweet potatoes, peeled and cut into large chunks

½ cup or more canned full-fat coconut milk

Sea salt or pink Himalayan sea salt to taste

Black pepper to taste (if tolerated)

Nutritional Analysis per Serving: Protein (g) 8.36; Fat (g) 20.82; Carbs (g) 25.56; B_{12} (mcg) 1.78; Iron (mg) 3.1; Iodine (mcg) 1.48; Magnesium (mg) 59.14; Potassium (mg) 832.45; Selenium (mcg) 17.79; Sodium (mg) 174.04

Unlike traditional shepherd's pie, this recipe uses the blood sugar–balancing power of sweet potatoes and creamy coconut milk to top a divine mixture of beef, lamb, peas, carrots, and mushrooms. I hope that this Shepherd's Pie will become a new family favorite for you!

1. Preheat the oven to 350°F.

2. In the oil in a heavy-bottomed skillet over medium heat, sauté the onions, carrots, peas, and garlic for 5 to 6 minutes.

3. Add the mushrooms and cook until softened.

4. Add the meats, breaking them up with a wooden spoon, and cook until well browned.

5. When the carrots are tender, add the tomato paste and water or Bone Broth and simmer for 3 to 4 minutes.

6. Remove from the heat. Add the rosemary, salt, and pepper.

7. Spread the filling in 9 × 9-inch glass baking dish.

8. Steam the sweet potatoes for 10 to 12 minutes or until soft (this can be started while the filling is cooking).

9. While the potatoes are still warm, place in a bowl and whip, adding coconut milk a bit at a time until smooth and spreadable. Season with salt and pepper.

10. Spread the whipped potatoes evenly on top of the filling.

11. Bake for 10 to 15 minutes.

12. Let rest 5 minutes before serving.

Beef Fried Rice

ⓘ INTRO

Prep time: 10 minutes

Cook time: 20 minutes

Serves: 6

2 tablespoons coconut oil

1 cup chopped onion

1 teaspoon minced garlic

1 pound ground beef

2 teaspoons garlic powder

1 cup finely chopped carrots

1 cup finely chopped celery

1 cup frozen peas

2 cups cooked rice or riced cauliflower

4 large eggs, beaten

1 cup coconut aminos

Sea salt or pink Himalayan sea salt to taste

Black pepper to taste (if tolerated)

Beef Fried Rice is one of the ultimate comfort foods in my book. You can make your own cleaner version of this dish by substituting coconut aminos for soy sauce. You can take this meal from Intro to Paleo by substituting riced cauliflower for the cooked rice. Riced cauliflower is a wonderful grain-free substitute for rice that replicates the taste and texture of cooked rice and has the added benefit of delivering a dose of detoxifying crucifers to your meal. Already "riced" cauliflower can be found in some grocery stores, or you can make your own by pulsing cauliflower florets in a food processor until they resemble rice.

1. Heat the oil in a wok or 12-inch cast-iron skillet on medium-high. Add the onion and garlic and cook for 3 minutes or until the onion starts to soften.

2. Add the ground beef and garlic powder and cook for 3 to 5 minutes until browned.

3. Add the carrots, celery, and peas to the skillet and cook for 3 minutes. Then stir in the rice or cauliflower.

4. Clear a circle in the center of the pan and pour in the beaten eggs. Stir to scramble the eggs and combine them with the other ingredients.

5. Cook for 5 to 10 minutes or until the meat and veggies are cooked through.

6. Add coconut aminos and combine. Season with salt and pepper to taste.

7. Serve warm.

Nutritional Analysis per Serving: Protein (g) 19.46; Fat (g) 28.08; Carbs (g) 18.62; B_{12} (mcg) 2.3; Iron (mg) 2.6; Iodine (mcg) 17.18; Magnesium (mg) 36.9; Potassium (mg) 537.08; Selenium (mcg) 20.92; Sodium (mg) 1060.01

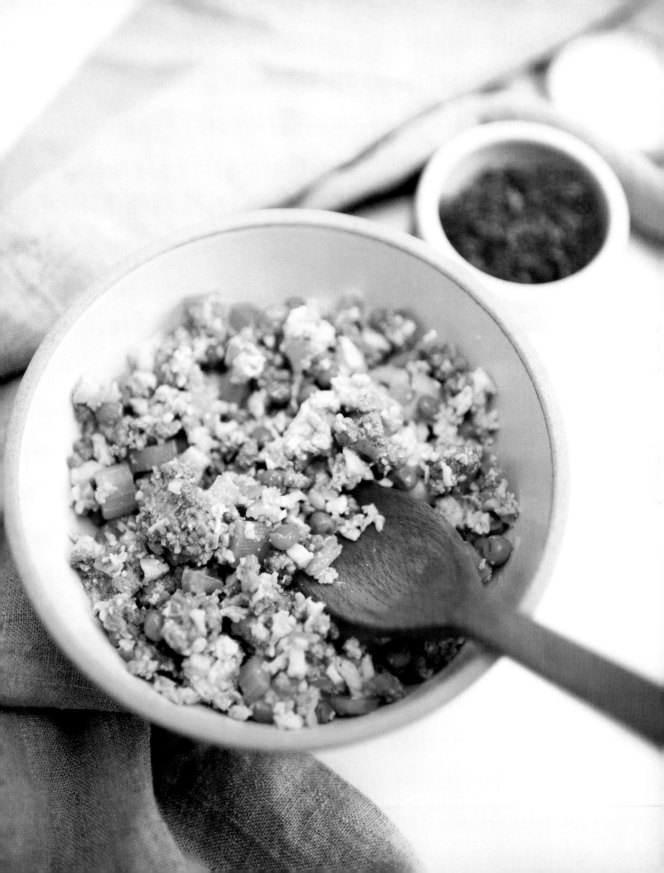

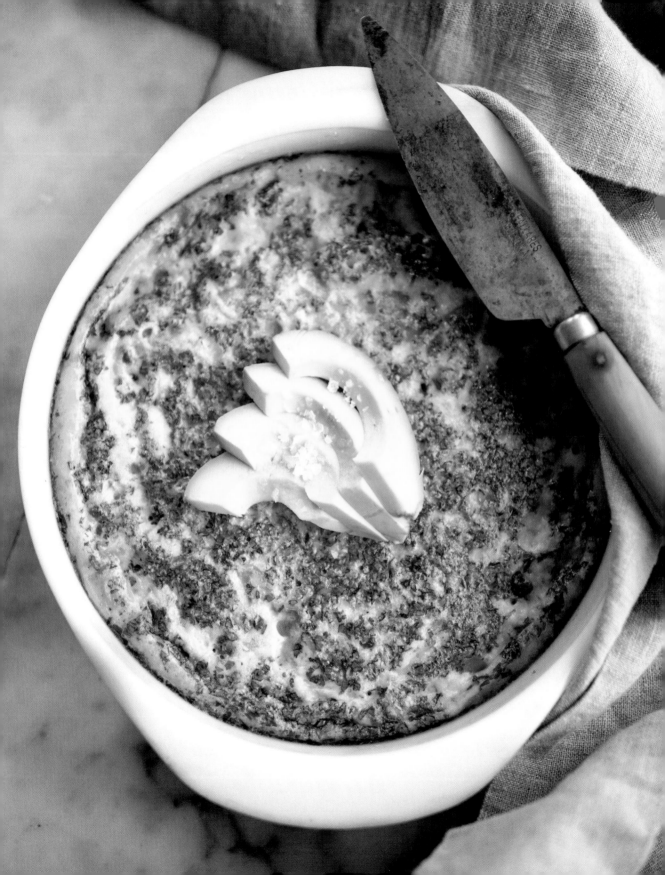

Mexican Quiche

ⓟ PALEO

Prep time: 15 minutes

Cook time: 20 minutes

Serves: 4

1 tablespoon coconut oil

1 pound ground beef

½ medium onion, diced

1 large yellow bell pepper, seeded and diced

1 teaspoon garlic powder

8 large eggs, beaten

¼ cup unsweetened coconut milk

Black pepper to taste (if tolerated)

¼ cup chopped fresh cilantro

1 large avocado, pitted and sliced

Sea salt or pink Himalayan sea salt to taste

This easy and delicious crustless Mexican Quiche is a great dish to start your day, or it can be enjoyed with a side salad for lunch or dinner. I love to make this dish for brunches with friends and family.

1. Preheat the oven to 375°F.

2. In the oil in a large skillet over medium heat, sauté the beef, onion, bell pepper, and garlic powder for 10 minutes, or until the beef is cooked through and vegetables are tender-crisp.

3. Place the beef mixture in a 9 x 13-inch baking dish and spread evenly.

4. In a large bowl, whisk the eggs, coconut milk, pepper, and cilantro and pour over the beef mixture.

5. Bake for 15 to 20 minutes, or until the eggs have set. Allow the quiche to cool, then top with avocados, season with salt to taste, and serve.

Nutritional Analysis per Serving: Protein (g) 21.97; Fat (g) 32.24; Carbs (g) 5.74, B_{12} (mcg) 2.58, Iron (mg) 2.87; Iodine (mcg) 32, Magnesium (mg) 35.37, Potassium (mg) 505.96; Selenium (mcg) 30.44; Sodium (mg) 356.27

Broccoli and Chicken Quiche

P PALEO

Prep time: 5 minutes

Cook time: 25 minutes

Serves: 4

1 tablespoon coconut oil

8 ounces boneless chicken breast, chopped

1 small leek, chopped

1 cup sliced mushrooms

2 cups broccoli florets (about three-quarters of medium head of broccoli)

6 eggs, beaten

¼ cup unsweetened almond milk

Sea salt or pink Himalayan sea salt to taste

Black pepper to taste (if tolerated)

1 teaspoon minced fresh rosemary

Broccoli and Chicken Quiche makes a perfect meal that everyone in the family will love. With the combination of protein-rich chicken, selenium-packed mushrooms, and folate-filled broccoli, this quiche is infused with an abundant amount of nutrients. Mix in high-quality protein from the eggs, and this quiche is sure to satisfy everyone's appetite.

1. Preheat the oven to 375°F.

2. In the coconut oil in a 12-inch ovenproof skillet over medium heat, brown the chicken for 5 minutes.

3. Add the leek, mushrooms, and broccoli and cook for 5 minutes until chicken is cooked through and vegetables are starting to get tender.

4. In a large bowl, whisk the beaten eggs with almond milk, salt, pepper, and rosemary. Pour over the chicken mixture in the skillet.

5. Place the skillet in the oven and bake for 20 minutes or until eggs have set. Alternatively, if you don't have an ovenproof skillet, transfer the chicken and vegetable mixture to a 9 x 9-inch baking dish, pour the egg mixture on top, and bake.

6. Slice and serve.

Nutritional Analysis per Serving: Protein (g) 21.64; Fat (g) 11.97; Carbs (g) 7.65; B$_{12}$ (mcg) 0.77; Iron (mg) 2.35; Iodine (mcg) 36; Magnesium (mg) 29.68; Potassium (mg) 364.8; Selenium (mcg) 35.18; Sodium (mg) 251.66

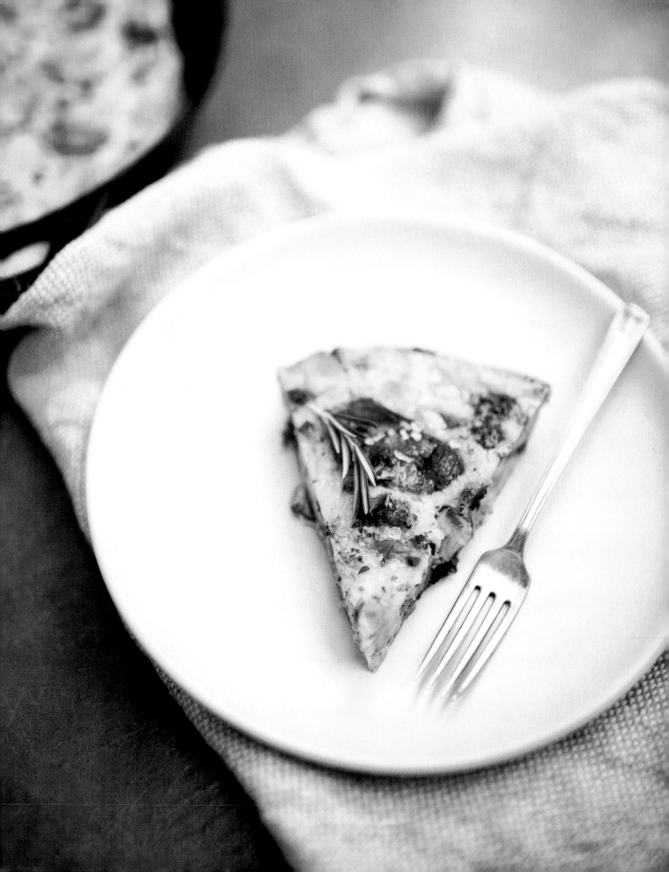

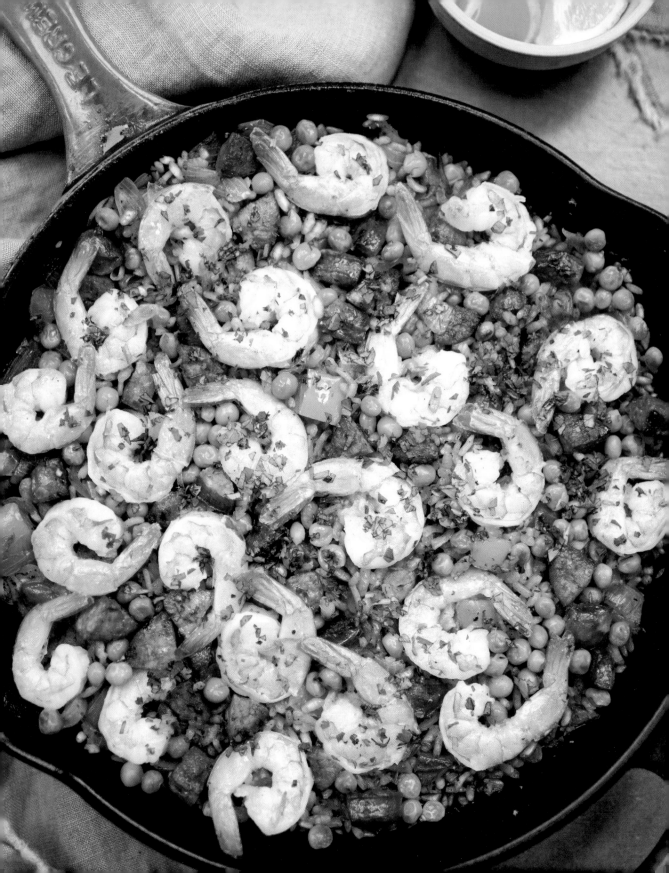

Paella

❶ INTRO

Prep time: 30 minutes

Cook time: 30 to 40 minutes

Serves: 8

2 cups Calasparra rice (traditional paella rice) or other short-grained rice, such as arborio

4 cups water

4 cups Bone Broth (p. 135)

1 tablespoon olive oil

1 pound seafood (shrimp, calamari, bay scallops, or a combination), thawed

2 cups diced preservative-free, gluten-free, dairy-free sausage, precooked (optional)

1⅓ cups frozen peas

½ green pepper, seeded and diced (about ½ cup)

½ orange pepper, seeded and diced (about ½ cup)

½ teaspoon saffron

Sea salt or pink Himalayan sea salt to taste

2 lemons, cut into quarters

Nutritional Analysis per Serving: Protein (g) 21.7; Fat (g) 7.79; Carbs (g) 7.88; B$_{12}$ (mcg) 0.84; Iron (mg) 1.24; Iodine (mcg) 24.51; Magnesium (mg) 47.72; Potassium (mg) 361.17; Selenium (mcg) 23.07; Sodium (mg) 648.95

I visited Spain with my husband a few years ago and was thrilled to learn that Paella is naturally gluten and dairy free. My husband makes this surprisingly simple recipe at home whenever we want to feel as though we're in Barcelona again or if we want to impress our friends. Cooking the Paella in a cast-iron skillet will infuse this dish with extra iron, a mineral commonly deficient in those with Hashimoto's. This dish makes great leftovers; just reheat in the oven in an oven-safe bowl.

1. Place rice, water, and bone broth in a large paella pan or 12- to 15-inch cast-iron skillet on high heat and bring to boil. Then turn the heat turn down and let it simmer for 18 to 20 minutes until cooked through, stirring every 5 to 7 minutes to prevent sticking.

2. While the rice is cooking, place the olive oil and seafood in a second pan and cook for 5 to 7 minutes until the seafood becomes less translucent.

3. If using sausage, add it to seafood pan and sauté for 2 to 3 minutes until warmed.

4. Add peas and diced peppers to the pan with seafood and sauté until the vegetables are cooked through.

5. Add the contents of the sauté pan to the rice pan, and mix.

6. Add saffron, salt to taste (we use about 2 teaspoons), and mix.

7. Once everything is mixed together, transfer the paella pan or cast-iron skillet directly to middle rack of oven and broil for 5 to 7 minutes.

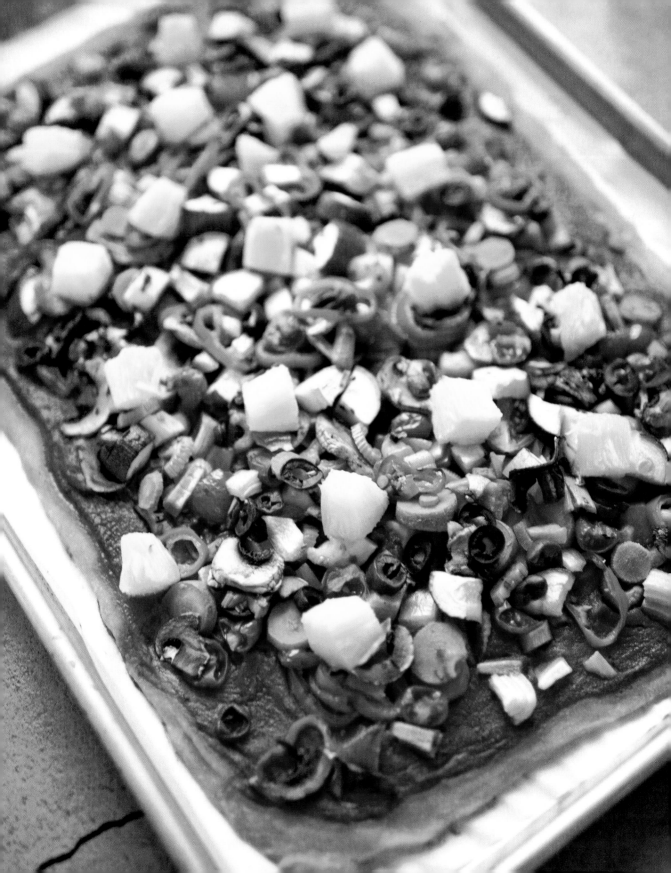

Paleo Pizza

P PALEO

Prep time: 15 minutes

Cook time: 20 to 25 minutes

Serves: 6

Note: The pizza is flexible; it bends and moves and can be rolled up like a wrap!

CRUST

4 green plantains, peeled and diced

1 cup water

⅓ cup extra-virgin olive oil

3 cloves garlic

1 teaspoon sea salt or pink Himalayan sea salt

1 teaspoon arrowroot powder

1 teaspoon apple cider vinegar

TOPPINGS

Pasta or tomato sauce (an organic store-bought version or homemade; see Pizza Sauce, p. 143)

1 tablespoon dried oregano

Chopped vegetable and fruit toppings: tomatoes, peppers, celery, black olives, red onions, mushrooms, chives, zucchini, carrots, pineapple

Additional toppings to increase protein content: pepperoni; bacon; ground pork, beef, or turkey; sausage

My husband loves pizza! Before I went gluten free and dairy free, he and I would split a pizza every Friday night. I used to call him my Teenage Mutant Ninja Turtle.

Although my husband doesn't have an autoimmune condition, he's an athlete and feels better eating Paleo. I made this Paleo Pizza recipe for him. The texture of the plantain crust somehow hits the spot for both deep dish and cheese for this Chicago-raised girl. I hope you like it as much as we do!

1. Preheat the oven to 400°F.

2. Place all crust ingredients in a high-speed blender and blend until a smooth mixture forms.

3. Pour the mixture onto a parchment paper-lined baking sheet or rimmed pizza stone and spread until the mixture is ⅓ inch thick.

4. Spoon pasta sauce onto the plantain mixture.

5. Top evenly with chopped vegetables, and protein, if using.

6. Top with oregano.

7. Bake for 20 to 25 minutes until the crust is slightly brown.

Nutritional Analysis per Serving: Protein (g) 9.06; Fat (g) 30.19; Carbs (g) 10.82; B_{12} (mcg) 0.2; Iron (mg) 1.71; Iodine (mcg) 0; Magnesium (mg) 46.42; Potassium (mg) 609.43; Selenium (mcg) 9.2; Sodium (mg) 695.91

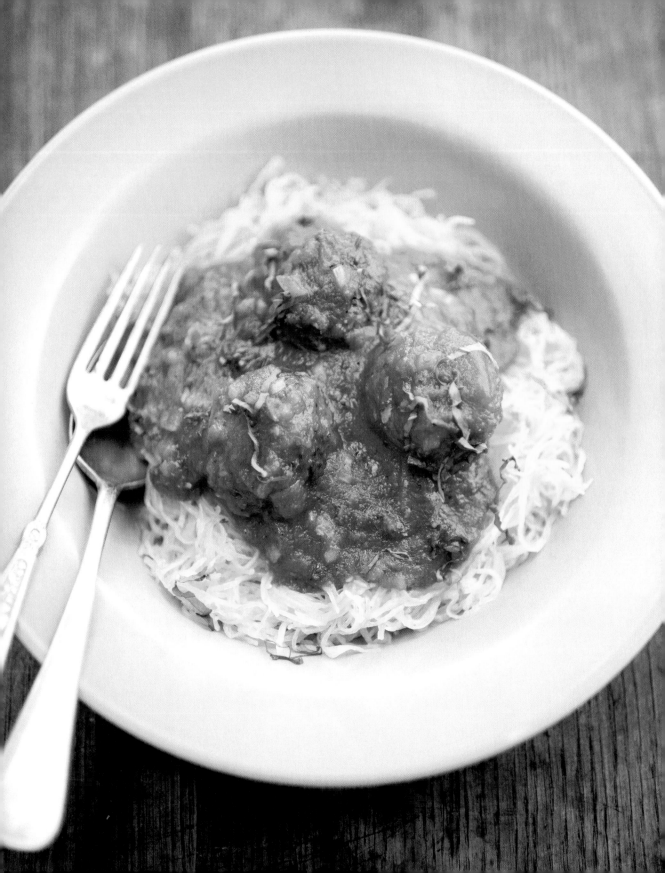

Squashghetti and Meatballs

P PALEO

Prep time: 10 minutes

Cook time: 1¼ hours

1 large spaghetti squash

2 cups water

1 pound ground beef or turkey

1 egg (optional)

1 teaspoon dried basil

1 teaspoon minced garlic

Sea salt or pink Himalayan sea salt to taste

Black pepper to taste (if tolerated)

1 batch Tomato Sauce (p. 150)

1 tablespoon olive oil

Nutritional Analysis per Serving: Protein (g) 24.64; Fat (g) 30.29; Carbs (g) 9.34; B_{12} (mcg) 2.77; Iron (mg) 3.91; Iodine (mcg) 6; Magnesium (mg) 63.69; Potassium (mg) 949.49; Selenium (mcg) 23.3; Sodium (mg) 423.41

Sometimes you just want to have some spaghetti and meatballs. The good news is that, unlike the traditional version, mine won't leave you in a food coma! You can use spaghetti squash or spiralized zucchini. Some stores even sell spiralized zucchini. This is one of my first Paleo recipes!

1. Preheat the oven to 350°F.

2. Cut the spaghetti squash lengthwise, scoop out the seeds and stringy stuff, and place the halves cut side down in a baking dish filled halfway with water. Place in the oven and bake for 1 hour. (Alternatively, to an electric pressure cooker add 1 cup of water, use the high-pressure setting on Manual, and cook for 7 minutes.)

3. Combine the ground meat, egg, basil, garlic, salt, and pepper in a bowl and mix until the seasoning is distributed throughout. Roll into meatballs and place in a baking pan.

4. When the squash is cooked, remove it from the oven (or pressure cooker) and set aside to cool slightly.

5. Put the meatballs in the oven and bake for 40 minutes, or until browned and cooked through.

6. Heat the sauce in a large saucepan and, when warm, add the cooked meatballs to the sauce.

7. Scoop the flesh out of the spaghetti squash and set aside.

8. Heat a large pan on medium-low and add the olive oil. Add the squash and sauté slightly until warm. Season with salt and pepper.

9. Place the sautéed spaghetti squash into a serving bowl and ladle the sauce and meatballs over the top.

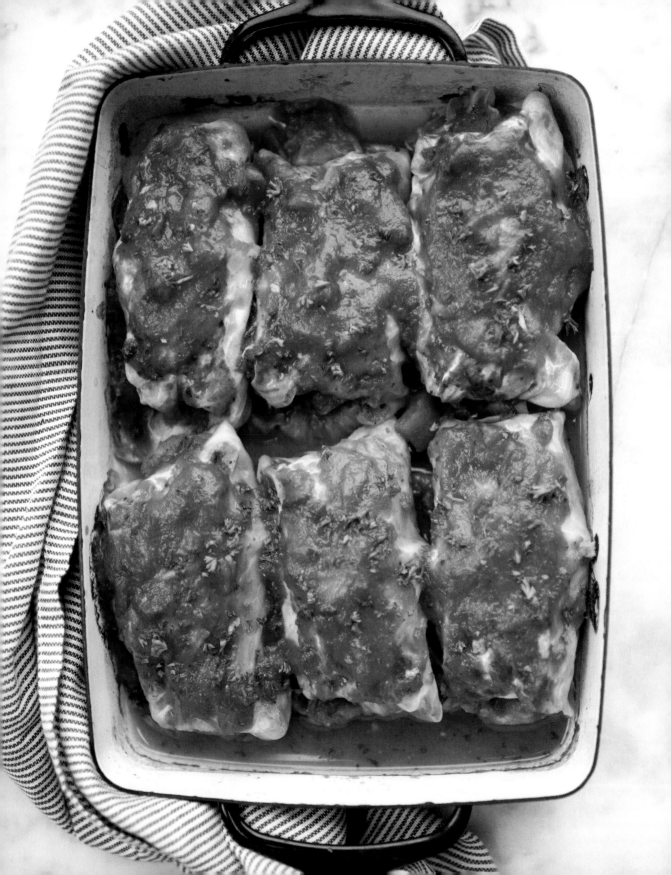

Gołąbki (Polish Stuffed Cabbage Rolls)

❶ INTRO

Prep time: 40 minutes

Cook time: 1 hour

Serves: 6

SAUCE

1¾ cups Tomato Sauce (p.150)

6 cups Bone Broth (p. 135)

½ teaspoon dried oregano

½ teaspoon paprika (if tolerated)

1 teaspoon arrowroot starch

CABBAGE ROLLS

3 cups cooked rice

2 pounds ground turkey, beef, or bison

½ teaspoon sea salt or pink Himalayan sea salt

¼ teaspoon black pepper (if tolerated)

2 eggs (optional)

1 medium-size cabbage

This is one of my favorite recipes from when I was growing up. In Poland, this recipe is known as Gołąbki, or "Pigeons," because when rolled up, the cabbage rolls are about the size of a pigeon! Legend has it that a Polish king fed his army Gołąbki before a key battle to give them plenty of energy. The traditional recipe uses rice. However, you can use riced cauliflower instead, making the recipe Paleo friendly and doubling up on your detoxifying crucifers.

1. Preheat the oven to 350°F.

2. In a large pot mix the Tomato Sauce with the Bone Broth, oregano, and paprika.

3. Cover, bring to a boil, and cook for about 5 minutes.

4. Add 1 teaspoon of arrowroot starch and boil until thick. Set aside.

5. Mix the cooked rice with the raw ground meat, salt, and pepper.

6. If you're using eggs, you can add them to the mixture to help bind it together, though they are not necessary.

7. Cut out the thick, tough core of the cabbage, and then place the head in a large pot of boiling water (cut side down).

8. Simmer for about 8 minutes on low until leaves become soft.

9. Drain, cool slightly, and gently unwrap the cabbage leaves from the cabbage head. Remove the thick stem from each leaf with a knife.

10. Place 2 tablespoons of meat filling into the center of each cabbage leaf, fold the sides over the meat, and roll into a little package.

11. Repeat until you've used up all of the meat filling.

12. Arrange the cabbage rolls seam side down in an 8 x 13-inch casserole dish, top with half of the sauce, and bake for 1 hour.

13. To serve, pour the remaining warmed sauce over the stuffed cabbages and enjoy!

Nutritional Analysis per Serving: Protein (g) 43.1; Fat (g) 25.49; Carbs (g) 39.74; B_{12} (mcg) 3.7; Iron (mg) 4.66; Iodine (mcg) 8; Magnesium (mg) 70.46; Potassium (mg) 1194.74; Selenium (mcg) 33.64; Sodium (mg) 514.69

Stuffed Portobello Mushrooms

Ⓟ PALEO

Prep time: 5 minutes

Cook time: 22 minutes

Serves: 4

4 large portobello mushrooms, washed

2 teaspoons avocado oil or coconut oil

1 small onion, finely diced

1 celery rib, finely diced

2 garlic cloves, diced

4 cups baby spinach, chopped

Sea salt or pink Himalayan sea salt to taste

Black pepper to taste (if tolerated)

1 cup Cashew Cream Cheese (p. 144)

2 tablespoons balsamic vinegar

2 tablespoons chopped walnuts (optional)

Stuffed mushrooms are always a great comfort food, but are often filled with cream cheese and breadcrumbs. My Stuffed Portobello Mushrooms are made with my Cashew Cream Cheese (p. 144), tons of veggies, and some walnuts for extra crunch. Portobello mushrooms have a meatlike texture and are chock full of the B-complex vitamins riboflavin, niacin, and pantothenic acid. Pairing this dish with a nice crisp salad, like my Apple-Carrot Salad (p. 293), creates a perfect light lunch.

1. Preheat the oven to 350°F.

2. Remove the stems from the mushrooms and scrape out the gills with a spoon to create a bowl in which to place the stuffing. Set aside.

3. In a medium-size skillet, heat the oil on medium and add the onion and celery. Cook until the onions are soft, about 5 minutes.

4. Add the garlic and spinach and cook until the spinach is wilted, about 2 minutes.

5. Place the spinach mixture in a bowl, season with salt and pepper, and mix in the cream cheese.

6. Place the mushrooms on a baking sheet and fill the mushrooms evenly with the spinach mixture. Top each mushroom with a drizzle of balsamic vinegar, and add ½ tablespoon of walnuts to the top of each mushroom, if using.

7. Bake for 15 minutes.

Nutritional Analysis per Serving: Protein (g) 14.01; Fat (g) 24.61; Carbs (g) 25; B_{12} (mcg) 0; Iron (mg) 5.47; Iodine (mcg) 0; Magnesium (mg) 185.5; Potassium (mg) 382.83; Selenium (mcg) 10.1; Sodium (mg) 256.53

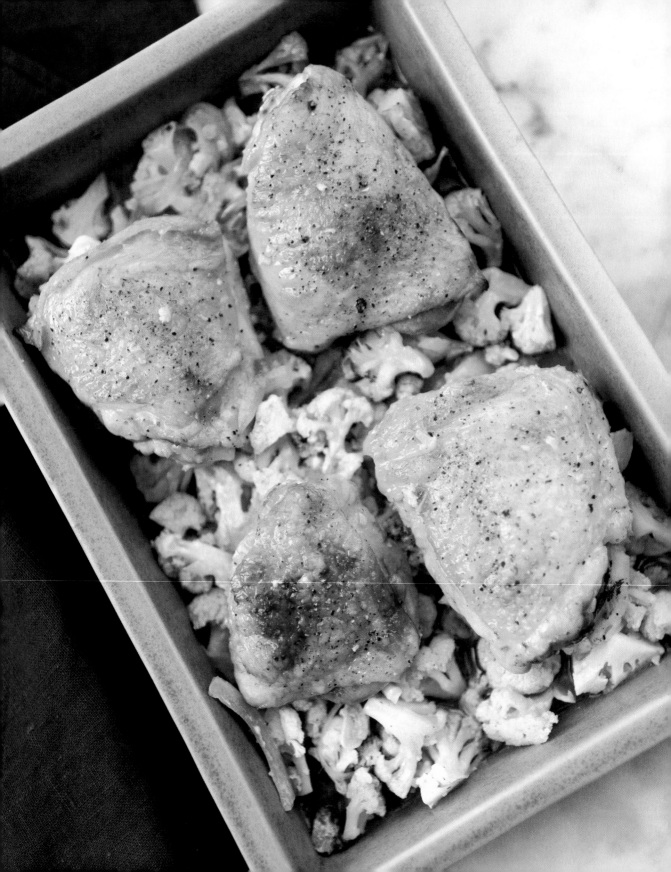

Baked Ginger-Lemon Chicken Thighs

Ⓐ AUTOIMMUNE

Prep time: 5 minutes

Cook time: 25 minutes

Serves: 4

2 teaspoons coconut oil

1 small onion, chopped

2 cloves garlic, minced

1 tablespoon grated fresh ginger

¼ cup lemon juice

2 teaspoons honey

4 bone-in chicken thighs

2 cups cauliflower florets
(about 1 medium head)

Sea salt or pink Himalayan sea salt
to taste

Black pepper to taste (if tolerated)

These savory Baked Ginger-Lemon Chicken Thighs are a rich source of protein with a lively flavor that is sure to please any palate. The cauliflower, ginger, and lemon make this dish one that will help reduce inflammation, aid in digestion, and boost the immune system.

1. Preheat the oven to 375°F.

2. In a small bowl, mix the oil, onion, garlic, ginger, lemon juice, and honey.

3. Place the chicken and cauliflower in a large bowl. Pour the onion mixture over them and mix well.

4. Spread the cauliflower in the bottom of a 12 x 12-inch baking dish and place the chicken on top, skin side up.

5. Cover and bake for 15 minutes. Then uncover and bake for an additional 10 minutes, until chicken is cooked through and cauliflower is tender.

6. Season to taste with salt and pepper. Serve warm.

Nutritional Analysis per Serving: Protein (g) 14.17; Fat (g) 45.47; Carbs (g) 11.38; B_{12} (mcg) 0.77; Iron (mg) 0.94; Iodine (mcg) 0; Magnesium (mg) 21.02; Potassium (mg) 347.72; Selenium (mcg) 13.01; Sodium (mg) 272.3

Sloppy Joes in a HeartBeet

Ⓐ AUTOIMMUNE

Prep time: 15 minutes

Cook time: 25 minutes

Serves: 6

SAUCE

3 beets

1½ cups cubed butternut squash

1½ cups cubed sweet potatoes

4 garlic cloves

¼ cup chopped onion

1 teaspoon dried oregano

1 teaspoon dried basil

1 teaspoon sea salt or pink Himalayan sea salt

1 tablespoon lemon juice

2 cups Bone Broth (p. 135)

MEAT

1 tablespoon coconut oil

1 pound ground beef

1 tablespoon garlic powder

1 teaspoon onion powder

1 teaspoon sea salt or pink Himalayan sea salt

Sloppy Joes in a HeartBeet is a family favorite that even the kids will love! An excellent source of iron as well as digestion-supporting betaine from the beets and loaded with vitamin-C-rich veggies, it also has a sweet, savory flavor that is irresistible. I was obsessed with this recipe when I was pregnant! You can serve these Sloppy Joes plain, in a lettuce wrap, with Biscuits (p. 315), or with Zucchini Bread (p. 313).

1. Place beets, butternut squash, sweet potatoes, garlic, onion, oregano, basil, salt, lemon juice, and bone broth in an electric pressure cooker and, on Manual, cook on high pressure for 15 minutes. Transfer contents of the pressure cooker in batches to a high-powered blender and blend on high until a saucelike consistency is reached. Take care when blending hot liquids and make sure the blender top is vented to let the steam escape.

2. Melt the coconut oil in a frying pan and add the beef, garlic powder, onion powder, and salt.

3. Cook until the meat is well browned, 5 to 10 minutes.

4. Combine the meat with the sauce and serve.

Nutritional Analysis per Serving: Protein (g) 17.53; Fat (g) 18.75; Carbs (g) 18.96; B$_{12}$ (mcg) 1.77; Iron (mg) 2.46; Iodine (mcg) 0; Magnesium (mg) 50.13; Potassium (mg) 698.42; Selenium (mcg) 13.33; Sodium (mg) 666.12

Chicken Burgers and Kale Chips

Ⓐ AUTOIMMUNE

Prep time: 10 minutes

Cook time: 29 minutes

Serves: 4

CHIPS

1 head kale leaves (ribs removed), torn

1 tablespoon avocado oil

Sea salt or pink Himalayan sea salt to taste

BURGERS

1 pound ground chicken

1 teaspoon sea salt or pink Himalayan sea salt

½ teaspoon dried parsley

½ teaspoon dried oregano

2 tablespoons avocado or coconut oil

Here is a super-quick meal that is nutritious and delicious: simple protein-rich Chicken Burgers, full of flavor, served with crunchy Kale Chips. If you don't want to make your own, you can also buy kale chips—just make sure you check the label to make sure they don't contain any ingredients you are sensitive to.

1. Preheat the oven to 350°F.

2. Place the torn kale pieces in a large bowl and massage the leaves with oil until they become soft.

3. Season to taste with salt.

4. Spread the leaves out flat in a single layer on baking sheets.

5. Bake for 10 to 15 minutes, or until the leaves are crispy and slightly brown.

6. Combine the chicken, salt, parsley, and oregano and form the mixture into 8 round, flat patties, about the size of your palm and 1 inch thick.

7. Heat the oil on medium in a cast-iron skillet. Add the patties and cook for approximately 7 minutes on each side, or until thoroughly cooked and lightly browned on the outside.

8. Serve alongside kale chips, and add any fixings you desire to the burger patty.

Nutritional Analysis per Serving: Protein (g) 22.65; Fat (g) 13.21; Carbs (g) 5.93; B_{12} (mcg) 0.64; Iron (mg) 1.92; Iodine (mcg) 0; Magnesium (mg) 55.46; Potassium (mg) 921.91; Selenium (mcg) 12.18; Sodium (mg) 288.67

Grilled Fish and Pineapple Salsa Packets with Green Beans

Ⓟ PALEO

Prep time: 15 minutes

Cook time: 20 minutes

Serves: 4

4 (6-ounce) cod fillets
(or other firm whitefish fillets)

1 cup diced pineapple

1 large tomato, diced

1 small shallot, chopped

4 tablespoons lime juice

Sea salt or pink Himalayan sea salt to taste

Black pepper to taste (if tolerated)

2 tablespoons chopped fresh cilantro

1 pound green beans, trimmed and cut in 2-inch pieces

Nutritional Analysis per Serving: Protein (g) 28.51; Fat (g) 0.69; Carbs (g) 16.14; B_{12} (mcg) 0; Iron (mg) 1.8; Iodine (mcg) 102; Magnesium (mg) 81.23; Potassium (mg) 898.79; Selenium (mcg) 0.87; Sodium (mg) 365.34

Fish fillets are smothered in fresh pineapple, tomato, and lime juice here to create a vibrant mix of sweet and tart. From grill to table, this recipe is not only supereasy but also healthy, as it provides omega-3s to promote heart health, antioxidants to support the immune system, and a wide range of vitamins and dietary fiber to improve digestion. To keep the iodine content low, I recommend using freshwater whitefish for this dish.

1. Preheat the grill to medium-high.

2. Place each fish fillet on a sheet of foil (you're going to create a "packet" for each fillet).

3. In large bowl, mix the pineapple, tomato, shallot, lime juice, salt, pepper, and cilantro and spoon over each fillet.

4. Cover the fish with a second sheet of foil and seal the edges.

5. Place the packets on the grill and cook for 15 to 20 minutes, until the fish flakes easily with a fork. (Alternatively, bake in the oven at 400°F for 15 to 20 minutes.)

6. While the fish is cooking, place the green beans in a steamer basket and steam for 8 to 10 minutes, or until tender and bright green.

7. Remove the fish packets from grill. Carefully (watch out for the steam!) open the packets and transfer the fish to plates for serving. Serve warm, alongside green beans.

Italian Meatza Pie

Ⓐ AUTOIMMUNE

Prep time: 15 minutes

Cook time: 20 minutes

Serves: 4

CRUST

1 tablespoon coconut oil

1 pound lean ground beef

1 tablespoon dried oregano

2 tablespoons chopped fresh basil

1 tablespoon chopped fresh parsley

2 cloves garlic, minced

Sea salt or pink Himalayan sea salt to taste

Black pepper to taste (if tolerated)

TOPPINGS

½ cup arugula leaves

½ cup canned artichoke heart halves

½ cup green olives, sliced

If you are a meat lover, then you will enjoy this meat-crust "pizza"! Feel free to change the fillings to suit your taste. I personally like the salty and bitter flavors of the arugula, olives, and artichoke hearts—and of course I love that they also add much-needed fiber and vitamins C, K, and E.

1. Preheat the oven to 400°F.

2. Grease an 8-inch round pie pan with coconut oil.

3. In a large bowl, combine the beef, oregano, basil, parsley, garlic, salt, and pepper until thoroughly mixed.

4. Press the meat mixture evenly on the bottom and up the sides of the greased pie pan.

5. Bake for 10 to 15 minutes, or until cooked throughout.

6. Remove and let cool for 5 minutes.

7. Spread the arugula over the meat crust and top with artichokes and olives. Bake for another 7 minutes.

8. Slice and serve warm.

Nutritional Analysis per Serving: Protein (g) 6.18; Fat (g) 12.25; Carbs (g) 4.91; B_{12} (mcg) 0.66; Iron (mg) 1.39; Iodine (mcg) 0; Magnesium (mg) 22.69; Potassium (mg) 184.97; Selenium (mcg) 4.95; Sodium (mg) 417.45

Kotlety (Polish Chicken Cutlets)

Ⓟ PALEO

Prep time: 5 minutes

Cook time: 6 to 10 minutes

Serves: 2

2 (4- to 6-ounce) boneless chicken breasts

1 egg

¼ cup shredded unsweetened coconut

***¼ cup almond flour**

2 tablespoons avocado oil

*Possible Modifications for Other Root Cause Diets: Replace the almond flour and egg with cassava flour for Autoimmune Diet.

When I was growing up in Poland, one of my favorite comfort foods was the breaded chicken cutlets known as Kotlety. I adjusted the recipe to make it gluten free, and it is still just as delicious as I remember! Serve with 2 cups of steamed mixed carrots and broccoli, topped with 2 tablespoons of extra-virgin olive oil and 2 tablespoons of lemon juice.

1. Place parchment paper over each chicken breast and pound with a meat-tenderizing hammer until the breasts are ⅓-inch thick.

2. Beat the egg in a shallow bowl.

3. Mix the coconut and almond flour together in another shallow bowl.

4. Coat both sides of each chicken breast in the egg mixture and dredge in the coconut-almond flour mixture.

5. Heat the avocado oil in a pan on medium-high. Add the coated chicken breasts and fry 3 to 5 minutes on each side until cooked through.

Nutritional Analysis per Serving: Protein (g) 32.83; Fat (g) 40.93; Carbs (g) 10.43; B_{12} (mcg) 0.52; Iron (mg) 1.79; Iodine (mcg) 12; Magnesium (mg) 74.75; Potassium (mg) 323.66; Selenium (mcg) 20.38; Sodium (mg) 109.21

Citrus Salmon

Ⓐ AUTOIMMUNE

Prep time: 5 minutes

Cook time: 35 minutes

Serves: 4

4 (4-ounce) salmon fillets

1 orange, sliced

¼ cup Everyday Dressing (p. 138)

Salmon is high in omega-3 fatty acids and a great source of protein and selenium. Choose wild-caught salmon for optimal nutrition. When it's paired with my Everyday Dressing and topped with orange slices, you also get a good burst of vitamin C!

1. Preheat the oven to 400°F.

2. Place salmon fillets next to each other on a pan lined with parchment paper and pour the dressing over them.

3. Top each fillet with 2 orange slices to cover the tops of the fillets.

4. Bake for 35 minutes, or until cooked through.

5. Before plating, press the orange slices lightly to release the juices on top of the salmon.

Nutritional Analysis per Serving: Protein (g) 23.12; Fat (g) 14.1; Carbs (g) 7.01; B_{12} (mcg) 3.61; Iron (mg) 1.49; Iodine (mcg) 14; Magnesium (mg) 41.12; Potassium (mg) 659.46; Selenium (mcg) 41.69; Sodium (mg) 51.08

Paleo Meatloaf

P PALEO

Prep time: 10 minutes

Cook time: 1 hour

Serves: 8

1 teaspoon dried oregano

1 teaspoon dried basil

1 teaspoon sea salt or pink Himalayan sea salt

1 teaspoon paprika (if tolerated)

1 teaspoon ground cumin (if tolerated)

½ teaspoon black pepper (if tolerated)

2 pounds ground pork, turkey, or beef (or a mixture)

1 cup fresh basil, chopped

1 cup fresh parsley, chopped

1 cup Tomato Sauce (p. 150)

Paleo Meatloaf is an easy, kid-approved meal. Combine all of the ingredients, mix, and bake! Pair it with mashed cauliflower, and you are sure to have everyone asking for seconds! I developed this recipe on a cold, rainy day in Amsterdam when I wanted some comfort food!

1. Preheat the oven to 350°F.

2. Mix all ingredients in a large bowl.

3. Press the mixture into a loaf pan, and bake for 1 hour.

Nutritional Analysis per Serving: Protein (g) 20.02; Fat (g) 24.26; Carbs (g) 3.75; B_{12} (mcg) 0.79; Iron (mg) 1.95; Iodine (mcg) 0; Magnesium (mg) 33.87; Potassium (mg) 507.18; Selenium (mcg) 28.22; Sodium (mg) 429.28

Poached Trout with Beets

Ⓐ AUTOIMMUNE

Prep time: 15 minutes

Cook time: 1 hour

Serves: 4

BEETS

4 large red beets, stemmed

2 large yellow or golden beets, stemmed

3 tablespoons coconut oil, melted

Sea salt or pink Himalayan sea salt to taste

Black pepper to taste (if tolerated)

FISH

6 cups Bone Broth (p. 135)

4 (6-ounce) trout fillets

Sea salt or pink Himalayan sea salt to taste

Black pepper to taste (if tolerated)

Lemon wedges, for garnish

4 tablespoons chopped fresh parsley, for garnish

Nutritional Analysis per Serving: Protein (g) 44.29; Fat (g) 22.3; Carbs (g) 11.55; B_{12} (mcg) 8.51; Iron (mg) 1.62; Iodine (mcg) 68.04; Magnesium (mg) 71.99; Potassium (mg) 1345.46; Selenium (mcg) 31.4; Sodium (mg) 530.96

In Poached Trout with Beets, the combination of trout and beets delivers a healthy, flavorful alternative to ordinary meat and potatoes. Trout, which has lower levels of iodine, is poached in gut-healing Bone Broth (p. 135) and served with folate-rich beets; together they support your immune system and heart health while delivering a rich and satisfying meal. Garnish with lemon and parsley for a vibrant finish!

1. Preheat the oven to 400°F.

2. On a large cutting board, place beets individually on sheets of aluminum foil, drizzle oil on top of each beet, and pull the foil closed to wrap each beet.

3. Place wrapped beets in a large baking dish and bake for 1 hour.

4. Remove the beets from the oven and let cool for 15 minutes.

5. Remove skins, season to taste with salt and pepper, and set aside.

6. In large skillet over medium-high heat, bring the broth to a simmer.

7. Add 1 trout fillet to the simmering liquid and poach for 7 to 9 minutes, or until the fish is opaque.

8. Remove from the skillet, season to taste with salt and pepper, and keep warm.

9. Serve the fish alongside the roasted beets and garnish with parsley and lemon wedges.

Pork Chops with Balsamic Glazed Onions

Ⓐ AUTOIMMUNE

Prep time: 5 minutes

Cook time: 30 minutes

Serves: 4

CHOPS

1½ pounds bone-in pork chops (about 2 large)

1 teaspoon dried rosemary

Sea salt or pink Himalayan sea salt to taste

Black pepper to taste (if tolerated)

2 tablespoons avocado oil

ONIONS

1 large onion, sliced ¼-inch thick

1 teaspoon dried oregano

Sea salt or pink Himalayan sea salt to taste

Black pepper to taste (if tolerated)

2 tablespoons balsamic vinegar

1 teaspoon maple syrup

These chops are sure to impress guests and won't keep you in the kitchen for hours! The lean, iron-rich pork chops have a simple, inflammation-reducing seasoning, and the sauce provides a burst of robust flavor. If possible, choose pasture-raised pork to ensure optimal nutrition.

1. Heat a large cast-iron skillet on medium. Season pork chops with rosemary, salt, and pepper.

2. Add the avocado oil and swirl to coat the bottom of the skillet. Add the pork chops and cook on each side for 12 minutes, or until no longer pink in the middle.

3. Remove the pork chops, set aside, and keep warm.

4. To the same pan, add the onions and sauté for 5 to 7 minutes, or until softened.

5. Add the oregano, salt, and pepper to the onions and stir to combine. Add the balsamic vinegar and maple syrup and cook down until thick, about 1 minute.

6. Serve onions over the top of the pork chops.

Nutritional Analysis per Serving: Protein (g) 27.45; Fat (g) 37.89; Carbs (g) 8.38; B$_{12}$ (mcg) 1.7; Iron (mg) 1.08; Iodine (mcg) 11.9; Magnesium (mg) 35.84; Potassium (mg) 528.2; Selenium (mcg) 15.67; Sodium (mg) 371.95

Pulled Cherry Pork

Ⓐ AUTOIMMUNE

Prep time: 10 minutes

Cook time: 5 to 6 hours on high or 10 to 12 hours on low in a slow cooker

Serves: 8

3 to 4 pounds boneless pork ribs or dark-meat chicken

1 cup pitted frozen tart cherries

6 cloves garlic

½ cup coconut aminos

½ cup apple cider vinegar

1 cup cherry juice

⅓ cup maple syrup

Pulled Cherry Pork is slow-cooked to perfection in antioxidant-rich, inflammation-fighting tart cherry juice. Add a side of steamed broccoli, cauliflower, or a salad, and you have the ultimate gourmet meal with very little effort.

1. Place the meat, cherries, and garlic in a slow cooker.

2. In a bowl mix the coconut aminos, vinegar, cherry juice, and maple syrup and pour over the meat.

3. Cover and cook on high for 5 to 6 hours or on low for 10 to 12 hours.

Nutritional Analysis per Serving: Protein (g) 45.73; Fat (g) 31.83; Carbs (g) 19.87; B$_{12}$ (mcg) 1.13; Iron (mg) 1.87; Iodine (mcg) 0; Magnesium (mg) 50.77; Potassium (mg) 1017.71; Selenium (mcg) 72.97; Sodium (mg) 418.79

Quail with Grapes

Ⓐ AUTOIMMUNE

Prep time: 10 minutes

Cook time: 25 to 30 minutes

Serves: 4

1 tablespoon coconut oil

4 flattened quails (or 4 boneless chicken breasts)

1 cup red seedless grapes, halved

½ cup balsamic vinegar (if tolerated)

4 slices bacon, cooked and chopped

¼ cup fresh mint, chopped

This recipe was inspired by my lifelong love of quail and a trip to Italy, where I had a dish similar to this one at a charming restaurant in Tuscany! Quail has a rich, distinctive flavor that pairs well with the savory goodness of bacon and a refreshing hint of mint. Adding grapes provides just the right amount of sweetness, while also boosting heart health.

1. Melt the coconut oil in a large frying pan, add the flattened quails, sauté until both sides are browned and the meat is cooked through, about 15 to 20 minutes, and set aside.

2. While the pan is still hot, add the grapes and balsamic vinegar and simmer until reduced by half for 5 to 10 minutes.

3. Add the bacon and quail to the pan and swirl around until the sauce is covering the quail.

4. Pour onto a serving plate, top with mint, and serve.

Nutritional Analysis per Serving: Protein (g) 26.68; Fat (g) 31.69; Carbs (g) 12.98; B_{12} (mcg) 0.66; Iron (mg) 4.93; Iodine (mcg) 0; Magnesium (mg) 37.37; Potassium (mg) 427.5; Selenium (mcg) 25.77; Sodium (mg) 317.9

Gnocchi with Peas and Pancetta

❶ INTRO

Prep time: 20 minutes

Cook time: 20 minutes

Serves: 6

GNOCCHI

3 cups peeled, steamed, mashed Russet or white sweet potatoes

½ cup arrowroot flour

1½ cups sweet potato starch

Salted water

SAUCE

2 tablespoons avocado oil

1 small onion, sliced

¼ cup chopped (uncooked) pancetta or bacon

1 teaspoon minced garlic

1 batch Tomato Sauce (p. 150)

¼ cup green peas

2 tablespoons minced fresh parsley

Sea salt or pink Himalayan sea salt to taste

Black pepper to taste (if tolerated)

Olive oil, for garnish

Don't be intimidated by making your own gluten-free pasta! Gnocchi with Peas and Pancetta comes together lightning fast. In fact, it takes longer to steam the potatoes than to cook the entire meal! My gnocchi are gluten and dairy free, but do contain white potatoes. If you are sensitive to white potatoes, you can use white sweet potatoes instead.

1. Place the mashed potatoes in a large bowl. Add the arrowroot flour and sweet potato starch and mix by hand, about 2 minutes, until the dough combines and forms a sticky ball.

2. Place the dough on an arrowroot-floured surface and divide into 8 equal parts.

3. Roll each portion of dough into a rope about 9 inches long and ½-inch wide.

4. Cut each rope into ½- to 1-inch pieces resembling little pillows and lightly indent the tops with a fork. Set aside.

5. Heat the avocado oil on medium in a large saucepan. Add the onion and pancetta or bacon and cook until the bacon is crisp and onions are translucent, about 5 minutes (do not allow the pancetta to burn).

6. Add the garlic and cook for 1 minute, ensuring it does not burn.

7. Add the tomato sauce, peas, parsley, salt, and pepper and cook until heated through, about 10 minutes.

8. Set aside.

9. Bring a pot of salted water to a boil. Add the gnocchi and cook until they float to the top, about 4 minutes.

10. Remove the gnocchi immediately and divide into four bowls.

11. Ladle the sauce over the top, drizzle with olive oil, and serve immediately.

Nutritional Analysis per Serving: Protein (g) 8.61; Fat (g) 13.87; Carbs (g) 47.17; B$_{12}$ (mcg) 0; Iron (mg) 2.51; Iodine (mcg) 40.85; Magnesium (mg) 55.39; Potassium (mg) 925.42; Selenium (mcg) 1.86; Sodium (mg) 615.92

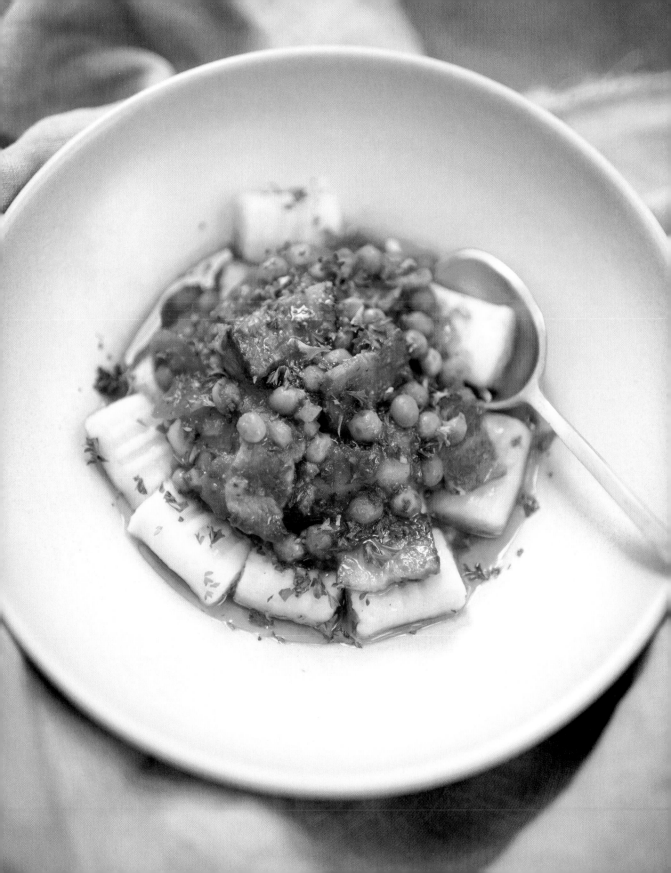

Slow-Cooked Chicken

(A) AUTOIMMUNE

Prep time: 20 minutes

Cook time: 6 hours in a slow cooker

Serves: 4

1 (4- to 5-pound) whole chicken, interior organ packet removed

2 tablespoons coconut oil

2 cloves garlic, minced

Sea salt or pink Himalayan sea salt to taste

Black pepper to taste (if tolerated)

2 tablespoons chopped fresh rosemary

Did I mention I love my slow cooker? As the chicken slowly cooks to the perfect tenderness, an appetizing aroma from the rub of coconut oil, garlic, and earthy rosemary will fill your kitchen—this is a sign that delicious nourishment is on its way!

1. Place the chicken on a large cutting board.

2. Use your fingers to loosen the skin away from the chicken meat.

3. In a small bowl, mix the coconut oil, garlic, salt, pepper, and rosemary to form a paste.

4. Rub the paste under the skin of the chicken.

5. Place chicken in a large slow cooker, cover, and cook on low for 6 hours, or until the chicken is falling off the bone.

6. Let cool slightly, remove the chicken from the bones, and serve.

Nutritional Analysis per Serving: Protein (g) 52.01; Fat (g) 8.65; Carbs (g) 0.42; B_{12} (mcg) 1.63; Iron (mg) 2.1; Iodine (mcg) 0; Magnesium (mg) 62.13; Potassium (mg) 867.56; Selenium (mcg) 0.1; Sodium (mg) 330.89

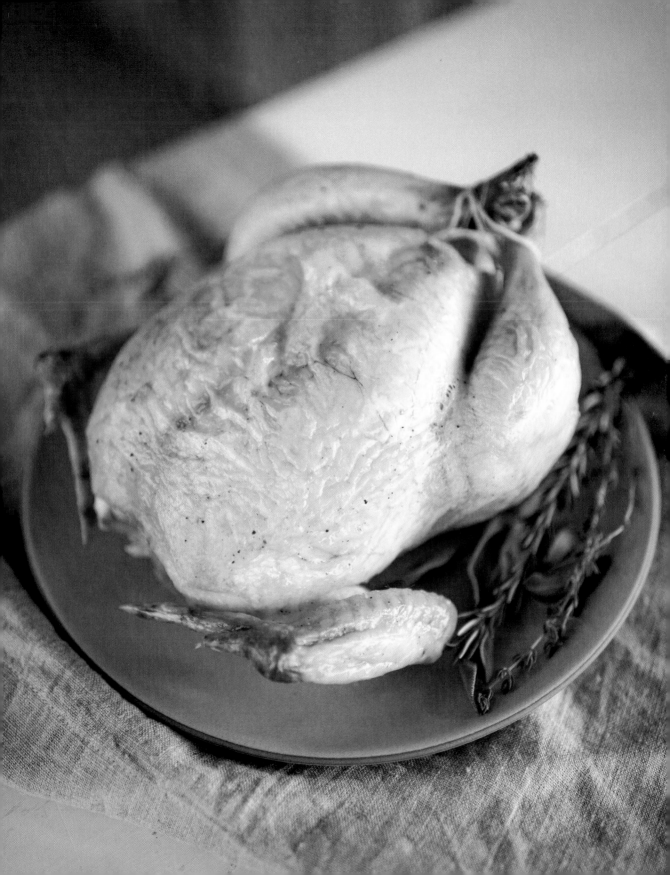

Ginger-Peach Pork Tenderloin

Ⓐ AUTOIMMUNE

Prep time: 10 minutes

Cook time: 25 minutes

Serves: 6

PORK

1 tablespoon coconut oil, melted

1 (2-pound) pork tenderloin

2 teaspoons minced fresh rosemary

2 teaspoons minced garlic

Sea salt or pink Himalayan sea salt to taste

Black pepper to taste (if tolerated)

SAUCE

½ cup water

2 cups sliced peaches

1 tablespoon balsamic vinegar

1 teaspoon grated fresh ginger

1 tablespoon honey

2 tablespoons canned full-fat coconut milk

In Ginger-Peach Pork Tenderloin, the pork and peach sauce go great together, but the peach sauce can also be used separately as a side dish. The rosemary creates an earthy, fresh flavor, while the peaches bring some bright sweetness to the dish.

1. Preheat the oven to 400°F.

2. Rub the coconut oil all over the tenderloin and set aside.

3. Mix together the rosemary and garlic and rub on top of the tenderloin.

4. Season with salt and pepper (if tolerated), and roast in the oven, covered, for 15 to 20 minutes, or until the internal temperature reaches 145°F.

5. Meanwhile, simmer the peaches in the water until softened, about 5 minutes.

6. Add the vinegar, ginger, honey, and coconut milk and remove from the heat.

7. In a high-speed blender, puree the peach mixture.

8. Slice the tenderloin and serve with the sauce.

Nutritional Analysis per Serving: Protein (g) 32.44; Fat (g) 8.4; Carbs (g) 9.39; B_{12} (mcg) 0.77; Iron (mg) 1.8; Iodine (mcg) 0; Magnesium (mg) 48.84; Potassium (mg) 732.05; Selenium (mcg) 47.25; Sodium (mg) 212.14

Eggplant Lasagna Stacks

Ⓟ PALEO

Prep time: 1 hour draining, 30 minutes

Cook time: 15 minutes

Serves: 6

EGGPLANT

2 medium-size eggplants, sliced into ⅛-inch rounds

Sea salt or pink Himalayan sea salt

½ cup almond flour

½ teaspoon onion powder

½ teaspoon garlic powder

½ teaspoon sea salt or pink Himalayan sea salt

½ teaspoon black pepper (if tolerated)

1 tablespoon avocado oil

FILLING

1 tablespoon avocado oil

4 mushrooms, finely chopped

½ small onion, finely diced

1 garlic clove, minced

1 cup spinach, chopped

1 cup Cashew Cream Cheese (p. 144)

¼ teaspoon sea salt or pink Himalayan sea salt

¼ teaspoon black pepper (if tolerated)

SAUCE

1 batch Tomato Sauce (p. 150) or Bolognese Sauce (p. 151)

If you are looking to make an elegant meal, look no further. In Eggplant Lasagna Stacks, eggplant "noodles" are surrounded by a luscious filling made with my Cashew Cream Cheese (p. 144), spinach, and mushrooms. It's topped off with my homemade Tomato Sauce (p. 150). This recipe takes more time than most of the others in this cookbook, but I promise it will be well worth it. Enjoy!

1. Spread the eggplant slices out in a single layer on baking sheets and generously salt the tops of the slices.

2. Let the eggplant slices sit for 1 hour to draw out the moisture.

3. Rinse each slice under cool running water and pat dry with a clean kitchen towel.

4. Preheat the oven to 400°F.

5. Meanwhile, for the filling, heat 1 tablespoon avocado oil in a pan on medium, add the mushrooms and onions, and cook until the mushrooms are soft and the onion is translucent, about 8 minutes. Add the chopped garlic and spinach and cook for 1 minute longer, until the garlic is soft and the spinach is wilted.

6. Remove from the heat and let cool slightly. Fold the spinach mixture into the Cashew Cream Cheese and season with salt and pepper. Set aside.

7. In a separate dish, mix the almond flour, onion powder, garlic powder, ½ teaspoon salt, and pepper. Reserve ¼ cup and set aside.

8. Heat a large skillet on medium and add 1 tablespoon avocado oil. Lightly dip each eggplant slice in the coating and then fry until golden, about 1 minute per side. If necessary, fry in batches.

9. In a large (13 × 9-inch) baking dish, lay out 6 eggplant slices in a single layer. Top each with 1 tablespoon of filling and 1 tablespoon of Tomato Sauce. Place a second eggplant slice on top of each stack. Top those with 1 tablespoon of filling and 1 tablespoon of sauce, a third eggplant slice, more filling and sauce, and the fourth and final eggplant slice (there should be 4 eggplant slices in each stack). Finish off the very top with 1 tablespoon of sauce and a sprinkle of the reserved breading.

10. Cover, place in the oven, and bake for 15 minutes.

Nutritional Analysis per Serving: Protein (g) 10.95; Fat (g) 21.46; Carbs (g) 30.14; B_{12} (mcg) 0; Iron (mg) 3.74; Iodine (mcg) 0; Magnesium (mg) 160.64; Potassium (mg) 967.14; Selenium (mcg) 7.81; Sodium (mg) 341.63

Truffled Veggies

Ⓐ AUTOIMMUNE

Prep time: 10 minutes

Cook time: 10 minutes

Serves: 4

1 tablespoon coconut oil

1 onion, diced

12 medium mushrooms, diced

1 pound asparagus, finely diced

1 pound green beans, finely diced

1 tablespoon truffle olive oil (or plain olive oil if using truffle salt), for garnish

Sea salt, pink Himalayan sea salt, or truffle salt to taste

This fast and easy recipe is a tasty way to increase your veggie intake. I love to use truffle salt or truffle olive oil to make this side dish feel a little decadent. A truffle is the fruiting body of a subterranean ascomycete fungus and is praised for its rich flavor and healing benefits. Its flavor pairs well with most meats!

1. Heat the coconut oil in a large pan on medium until melted. Add the diced onion, mushrooms, asparagus, and green beans and cook until fragrant and cooked through, approximately 7 to 10 minutes.

2. Season with salt and toss with olive oil.

Nutritional Analysis per Serving: Protein (g) 7.33; Fat (g) 7.91; Carbs (g) 12.23; B_{12} (mcg) 0.02; Iron (mg) 2.31; Iodine (mcg) 0; Magnesium (mg) 50.70; Potassium (mg) 746; Selenium (mcg) 6.97; Sodium (mg) 109.31

Cowboy Caviar

① INTRO

Prep time: 20 minutes

Serves: 6

2 cups cooked black beans

1 cup chopped tomato

½ cup fresh cilantro, chopped

¼ cup chopped green bell pepper

¼ red onion, chopped

½ teaspoon sea salt or pink Himalayan sea salt

½ teaspoon garlic powder

½ teaspoon dried oregano

½ teaspoon dried basil

Juice of 1 lime

2 tablespoons olive oil

2 tablespoons apple cider vinegar

I modified the classic take on Southwest Cowboy Caviar for my sweet hubby, Michael, who grew up in Texas. This versatile dish can very well serve as a main meal and pairs well with pulled pork. I like cooking the beans in a pressure cooker. Black beans are full of fiber and phytonutrients and, combined with the tomato and spices, create an irresistible combination.

1. Place all ingredients in a large bowl and mix.

Nutritional Analysis per Serving: Protein (g) 5.63; Fat (g) 4.93; Carbs (g) 16.19; B_{12} (mcg) 0; Iron (mg) 1.62; Iodine (mcg) 2.67; Magnesium (mg) 47.64; Potassium (mg) 333.34; Selenium (mcg) 0.82; Sodium (mg) 136.2

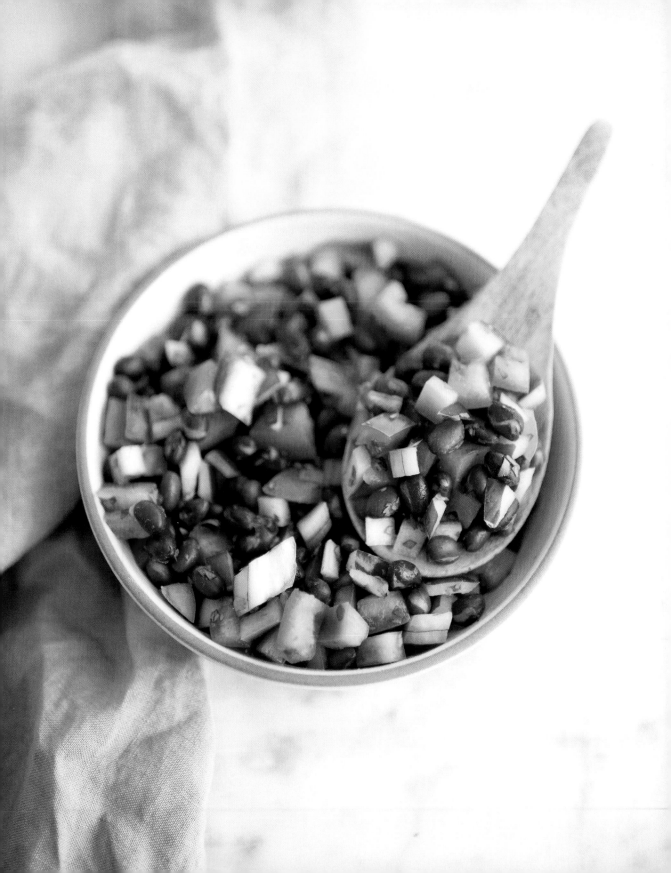

Bacon and Chive Scalloped Potatoes

Ⓐ AUTOIMMUNE

Prep time: 10 minutes

Cook time: 35 minutes

Serves: 6

8 ounces bacon, chopped

2 large sweet potatoes, thinly sliced

½ small onion, halved and thinly sliced

2 tablespoons coconut oil, melted

Sea salt or pink Himalayan sea salt to taste

Black pepper to taste (if tolerated)

1 teaspoon minced fresh thyme

1 cup canned full-fat coconut milk

2 tablespoons chopped chives, for garnish

Nothing quite compares to the luscious aroma and tasty crunch of crispy bacon. Despite its reputation as an unhealthy food, bacon is actually packed with heart-benefiting omega-3 fatty acids and can be eaten in reasonable quantities. Choose a bacon that is free of nitrates and additives. Adding onions, chives, and coconut oil to the sweet potatoes and bacon produces a savory dish that is hard to resist.

1. Preheat the oven to 375°F.

2. In a large skillet over medium heat, cook the bacon for 10 minutes until crispy.

3. Using a slotted spoon, transfer the bacon to a paper towel–lined plate. Cool slightly and chop.

4. In a large bowl, mix the bacon with sweet potatoes, onion, coconut oil, salt, pepper, and thyme.

5. Pour the contents of the bowl into a 12 x 12-inch baking dish.

6. Pour coconut milk over the potato mixture.

7. Cover and bake for 25 minutes, or until the potatoes are tender.

8. Serve warm and garnish with chopped chives.

Nutritional Analysis per Serving: Protein (g) 6.57; Fat (g) 29.12; Carbs (g) 12.85; B$_{12}$ (mcg) 0.19; Iron (mg) 1.16; Iodine (mcg) 0; Magnesium (mg) 32.44; Potassium (mg) 351.64; Selenium (mcg) 10.42; Sodium (mg) 345.68

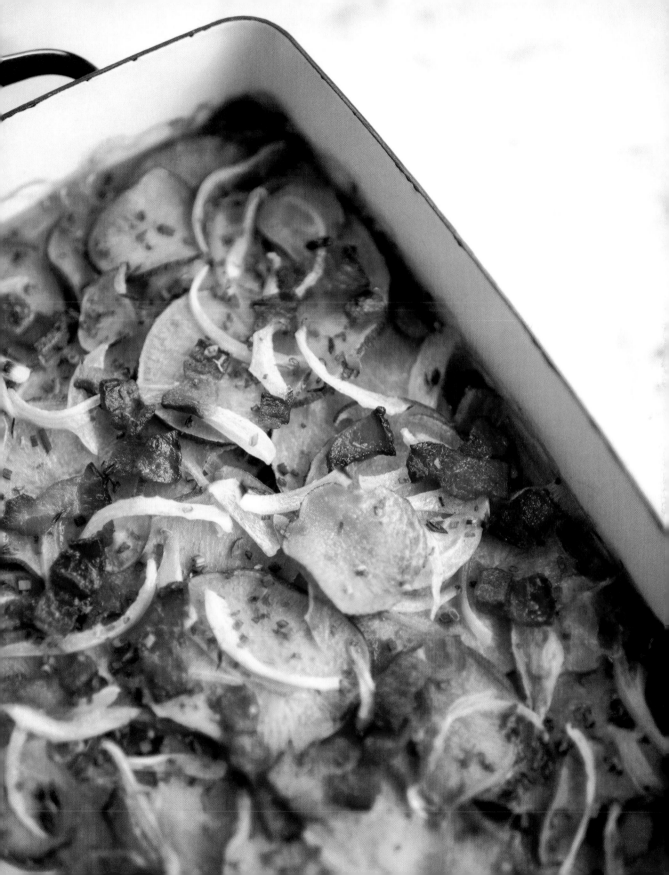

Chicken Spring Rolls with Almond Dipping Sauce

1 INTRO

Prep time: 12 minutes,
plus 10 minutes assembly

Serves: 6

ROLLS

¾ cup thinly sliced red cabbage, *divided*

6 rice paper wrappers

Hot water

½ cup cooked rice noodles, prepared according to package directions

¼ cup thinly sliced carrots

¼ cup cucumber matchsticks

1 avocado, thinly sliced

1 (6-ounce) boneless chicken breast, cooked and thinly sliced

3 tablespoons cilantro leaves, *divided*

1 lime, sliced into 6 wedges

SAUCE

¼ cup almond butter

Juice of ½ lime

1 teaspoon coconut aminos

1 teaspoon honey

3 tablespoons water

Nutritional Analysis per Serving: Protein (g) 6.45; Fat (g) 14.44; Carbs (g) 24.9; B_{12} (mcg) 0.06; Iron (mg) 1.29; Iodine (mcg) 3.78; Magnesium (mg) 45.56; Potassium (mg) 275.29; Selenium (mcg) 5.32; Sodium (mg) 278.88

Here is my take on Asian spring rolls. The crunch from the gut-healing vegetables makes these rolls extra satisfying. If you don't want to use rice wraps, replace them with romaine lettuce. Have fun with these—the rice paper is virtually tasteless, so any flavor combination you choose as a filling will be the predominant taste! If using rice paper, be sure it's gluten-free.

1. Spread ½ cup of the sliced red cabbage on a serving plate and sprinkle with 1 tablespoon of cilantro. Set aside.

2. Place the hot water in a shallow dish and immerse a rice paper wrapper for 10 seconds. The wrapper should be firm but pliable.

3. Lay the wrapper on a clean, moist dish towel and place a sixth of the noodles about ⅓ away from the edge of the wrapper closest to you. Top with a sixth of the remaining red cabbage, a sixth of the carrots, and so on, ending with a sixth of the remaining cilantro.

4. To wrap, bring the bottom edge of the wrapper over the top the vegetables and roll over once. Fold in the sides and then continue rolling up until the spring roll is sealed. Set aside.

5. Continue filling and wrapping the remaining rolls.

6. To make the almond dipping sauce, place almond butter in a small bowl, add the remaining ingredients and whisk until a smooth sauce forms. It should be slightly thick.

7. Slice the spring rolls in half and place them on the prepared serving plate with the lime wedges and almond dipping sauce.

Chicken Plantain "Nachos"

Ⓐ AUTOIMMUNE

Prep time: 15 minutes

Cook time: 35 minutes

Serves: 4

2 cups ¼-inch sliced plantains

¼ cup olive oil

Sea salt or pink Himalayan sea salt to taste

Black pepper to taste (if tolerated)

2 tablespoons chopped green onion

2 tablespoons lime juice

1 large avocado, peeled, pitted, and mashed

½ cup shredded cooked chicken breast

Who says you can't have nachos? Nachos that aren't full of preservatives, corn, and other Hashimoto's-unfriendly ingredients, that is. Try my Chicken Plantain "Nachos" with my favorite toppings or get creative and add your own Hashimoto's-approved accompaniments. Plantains are an excellent source of fiber, vitamins A, C, and B$_6$, and the minerals magnesium and potassium.

1. Preheat the oven to 350°F.

2. Line two baking sheets with foil or parchment paper.

3. In a medium bowl, toss the sliced plantains with oil. Season with salt and pepper and then toss again.

4. Arrange the plantain slices on the baking sheets in a single layer.

5. Bake for around 15 to 17 minutes; then turn the plantains over and rotate baking sheets. Bake for an additional 15 to 17 minutes, or until golden and crisp.

6. Remove the plantain chips from the oven and let cool slightly. Spread them on a large plate.

7. In a medium bowl, mix the green onion, lime juice, and avocado with salt and pepper to taste.

8. Top the chips with the avocado mixture and chicken and serve.

Nutritional Analysis per Serving: Protein (g) 7.12; Fat (g) 8.32; Carbs (g) 28.3; B$_{12}$ (mcg) 0.57; Iron (mg) 0.96; Iodine (mcg) 0; Magnesium (mg) 46.11; Potassium (mg) 650.79; Selenium (mcg) 5.64; Sodium (mg) 117.03

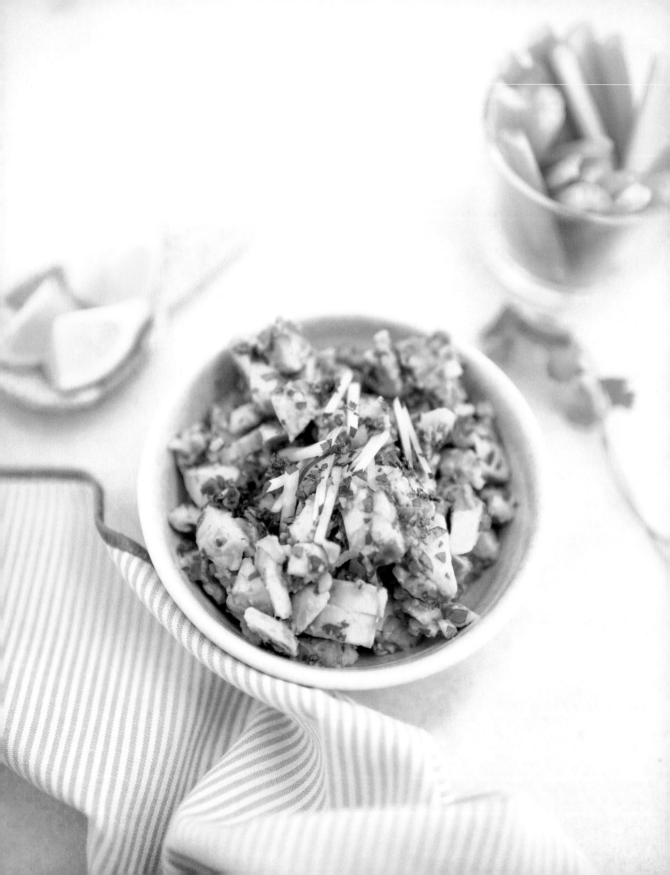

Cilantro-Lime Guacamole

Ⓐ AUTOIMMUNE

Prep time: 15 minutes

Serves: 4

2 large avocados, peeled, pitted, and cubed (about 3½ cups)

1 large radish, chopped

Sea salt or pink Himalayan sea salt to taste

Black pepper to taste (if tolerated)

1 tablespoon chopped leek

2 tablespoons chopped fresh cilantro

2 tablespoons lime juice

3 large stalks celery, cut into 3- to 4-inch sticks (about 3 cups)

Nutrient-dense Cilantro-Lime Guacamole offers a smooth texture with a delicate mix of fresh, fragrant cilantro and zingy citrus (thanks to the lime). Celery sticks easily replace traditional chips for a satisfying crunch, so you don't miss out on any of the good guacamole flavor!

1. In a large bowl, mix the avocado, radish, salt, pepper, leek, cilantro, and lime juice.

2. Serve the guacamole with celery for dipping.

Nutritional Analysis per Serving: Protein (g) 1.66; Fat (g) 10.38; Carbs (g) 7.81; B_{12} (mcg) 0; Iron (mg) 0.58; Iodine (mcg) 0; Magnesium (mg) 24.97; Potassium (mg) 451.7; Selenium (mcg) 0.46; Sodium (mg) 129.91

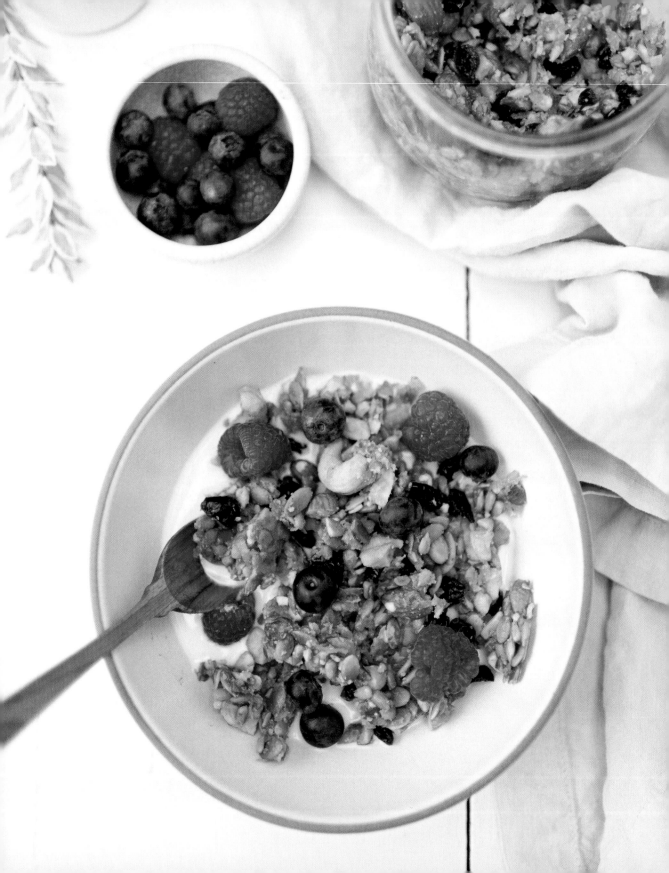

Sweet and Salty "Granola"

ⓟ PALEO

Prep time: 10 minutes

Cook time: 45 minutes

Serves: 12

1 cup unsalted cashews

¾ cup unsalted almonds

½ cup unsweetened coconut flakes

¼ cup shelled unsalted pumpkin seeds

¼ cup coconut oil

1 teaspoon pure vanilla extract

¼ cup honey

¼ cup shelled unsalted sunflower seeds

1 cup dried cranberries

1 teaspoon sea salt or pink Himalayan sea salt

Coconut Yogurt (p. 131, optional)

Sweet and Salty "Granola," a combination of nutrient-dense nuts and seeds and immune-supporting honey, delivers a healthy, yet simple Paleo-approved snack. The addition of antioxidant-rich dried cranberries adds a little sweetness to the salty flavor of the nuts and seeds. Serve over Coconut Yogurt (p. 131) if you wish.

1. Preheat the oven to 300°F.

2. Line a baking sheet with parchment paper.

3. Place the cashews, almonds, coconut flakes, and pumpkin seeds in a blender and pulse to break the large nuts into smaller pieces.

4. In a medium saucepan, heat the coconut oil, vanilla, and honey for 5 minutes, until melted.

5. Into the saucepan, pour the mixture from the blender, add the sunflower seeds, and stir to coat.

6. Spread the mixture out on the prepared baking sheet and bake for 20 minutes, stirring once, until the mixture is lightly browned.

7. Remove from oven, and stir in the dried cranberries and salt.

8. Press the granola mixture together to form a flat, even surface.

9. Cool for about 15 minutes, break into chunks, and store in an airtight container or resealable bag.

Nutritional Analysis per Serving: Protein (g) 5.22; Fat (g) 13.04; Carbs (g) 22.03; B_{12} (mcg) 0; Iron (mg) 1.67; Iodine (mcg) 0; Magnesium (mg) 79.39; Potassium (mg) 185.87; Selenium (mcg) 3.59; Sodium (mg) 143.06

Liver Pâté

Ⓐ AUTOIMMUNE

Prep time: 10 minutes

Cook time: 5 to 7 minutes

Serves: 8

Note: It is helpful to eat a serving with a cup of hot lemon water to improve digestion.

1 pound beef, chicken, or pork liver, cut into chunks

1 onion, chopped

1 tablespoon duck fat or coconut oil

1 tablespoon coconut fat from coconut milk

1 garlic clove, crushed

¼ cup chopped fresh basil

4 teaspoons apple cider vinegar

Juice from ½ lemon

1 tablespoon ground cinnamon

Sea salt or pink Himalayan sea salt to taste

Black pepper to taste (if tolerated)

Pickles, for garnish

Hashimoto's patients are often deficient in ferritin, which may result in residual symptoms like fatigue and hair loss. Liver is one of the richest sources of iron and may be helpful in restoring iron and ferritin levels, but it is not most people's favorite. Even if you haven't liked liver in the past, I hope you'll try this Liver Pâté recipe I make at home—it's full of other bold flavors that help balance out the richness of the liver.

1. Fry the liver and onion in a pan with the duck fat or coconut oil until cooked through, about 5 to 7 minutes.

2. Place the liver and onion along with the coconut fat, garlic, basil, vinegar, lemon juice, and cinnamon in food processor and blend until smooth. Season with salt and pepper to taste.

3. Form the mixture into a ball and chill for 1 hour.

4. To serve, place in a bowl or slice in thick slices and garnish with pickles.

Nutritional Analysis per Serving: Protein (g) 11.88; Fat (g) 4.35; Carbs (g) 4.71; B_{12} (mcg) 33.62; Iron (mg) 2.98; Iodine (mcg) 0; Magnesium (mg) 13.85; Potassium (mg) 216.66; Selenium (mcg) 22.67; Sodium (mg) 88.74

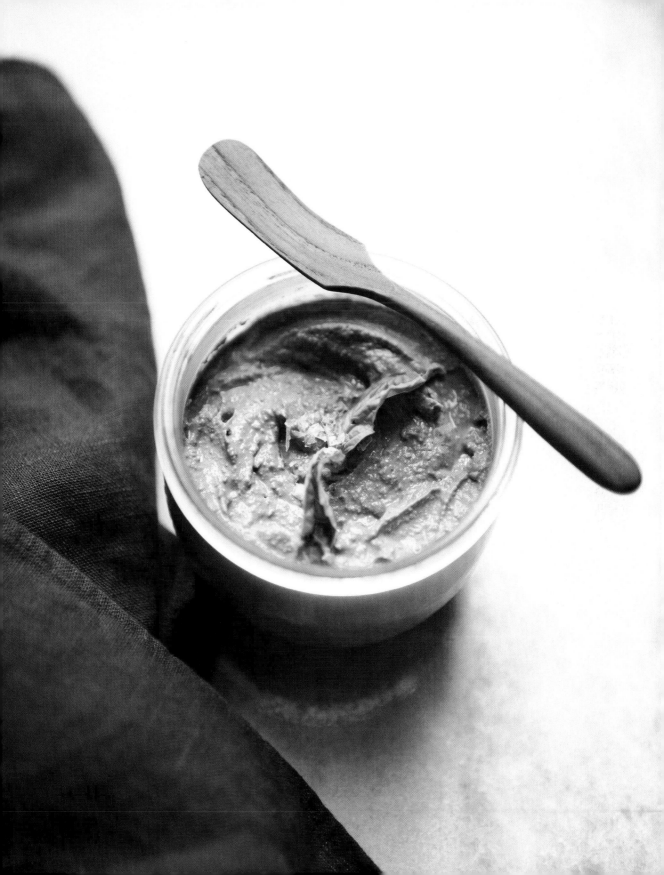

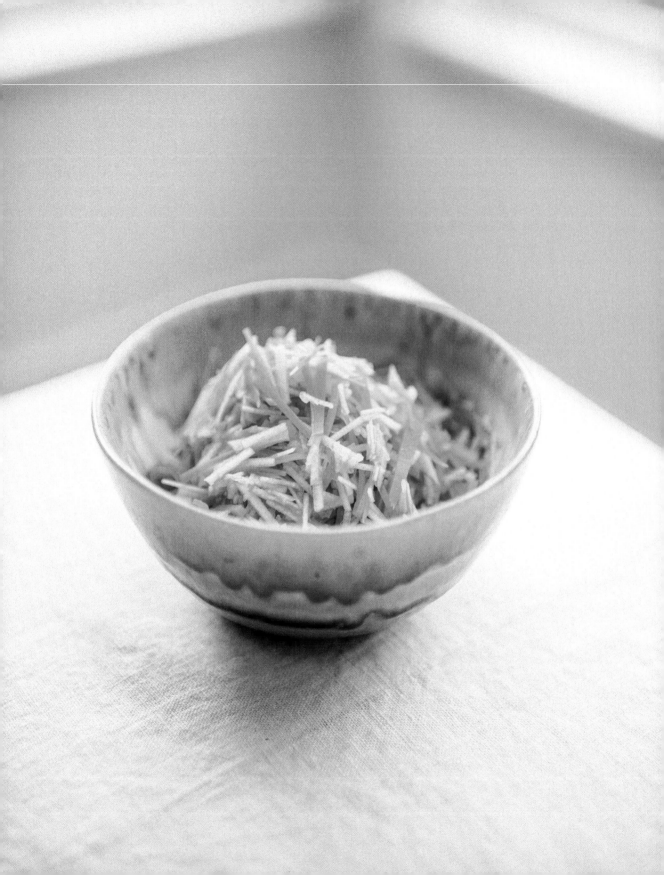

Apple-Carrot Salad

Ⓐ AUTOIMMUNE

Prep time: 15 minutes

Serves: 2

2 medium green apples, peeled and coarsely chopped (about 2 cups)

1 cup baby carrots

Juice of ½ lemon

This dish is known as a traditional Polish surówka, or "raw salad." Apple-Carrot Salad is one of the easiest recipes you can make, yet it's surprisingly refreshing. It's fantastic for digestive distress and makes a great side for hot dishes and meats. An extra bonus is that kids love this dish!

1. Place apples, carrots, and lemon juice in a food processor. Process on high for 1 to 2 minutes, until the carrots and apples are finely chopped.

2. Refrigerate until ready to serve.

Nutritional Analysis per Serving: Protein (g) 1.13; Fat (g) 0.31; Carbs (g) 26.99; B_{12} (mcg) 0; Iron (mg) 1.11; Iodine (mcg) 0; Magnesium (mg) 17.38; Potassium (mg) 402.86; Selenium (mcg) 1.04; Sodium (mg) 88.6

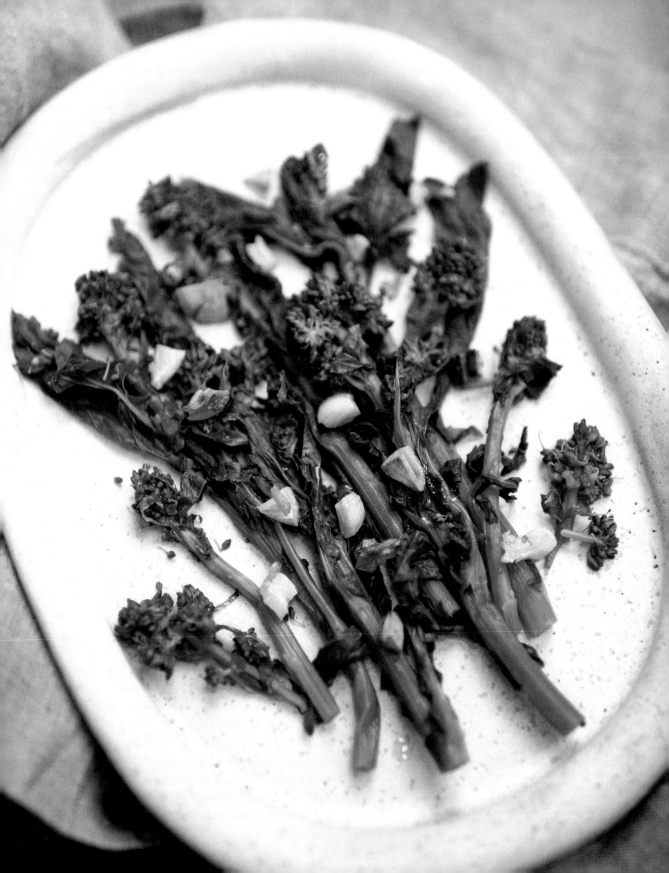

Sautéed Rapini

A AUTOIMMUNE

Prep time: 5 minutes

Cook time: 30 minutes

Serves: 6

3 cloves garlic

2 bunches rapini, ends trimmed and washed

2 tablespoons olive oil

Apple cider vinegar or lemon wedges, for garnish (optional)

Sea salt or pink Himalayan sea salt to taste

Black pepper to taste (if tolerated)

Rapini, also known as broccoli rabe, a member of the brassica family, is chock full of nutrients, including calcium, magnesium, zinc, and indole-3-carbinol, a cancer-fighting phytochemical! Rapini also contains sulfur, which can help support the detoxification process in the liver (apple cider vinegar and lemon juice offer detox aid too!). By cutting the garlic first and letting it sit out for about 10 minutes, you will increase its allicin content. Allicin is the compound responsible for garlic's antiviral, antibacterial, and healing properties.

1. Cut the garlic cloves in quarters, and set aside.

2. In a large pot with a steamer basket, steam the rapini until soft, tender, and bright green, about 12 minutes. To decrease bitterness, steam for 20 minutes.

3. Remove the basket from the pot and let rest for 10 minutes so excess moisture evaporates.

4. Place the garlic and olive oil in a large saucepan and heat on medium-low. Add the rapini and sauté for 15 minutes.

5. Remove from the heat and drizzle with apple cider vinegar or lemon juice for a burst of flavor.

6. Season with salt and black pepper, and serve warm.

Nutritional Analysis per Serving: Protein (g) 1.09; Fat (g) 4.66; Carbs (g) 1.39; B$_{12}$ (mcg) 0; Iron (mg) 0.72; Iodine (mcg) 0; Magnesium (mg) 7.27; Potassium (mg) 67.46; Selenium (mcg) 0.53; Sodium (mg) 10.68

Mango Salsa

Ⓐ AUTOIMMUNE

Prep time: 15 minutes

Cook time: 15 minutes marinating

Serves: 6

Note: If you want a milder ginger flavor, grate the ginger; if you like the peppery bite of ginger, then chopping is a better option.

¼ cup coconut milk

Juice of 2 fresh limes

1 cup peeled and diced mango

¾ cup diced cucumber

2 tablespoons diced red onion

1 tablespoon chopped fresh cilantro

1 teaspoon grated or chopped fresh ginger

Romaine lettuce leaves (optional)

*Possible Modifications for Other Root Cause Diets: For Intro and Paleo versions, add ⅓ cup diced red bell pepper.

I've always loved Mango Salsa! It's refreshing as a side dish and is an all-around tasty treat. When I became dairy free in 2011, I modified my favorite mango salsa recipe by swapping coconut milk for dairy, and I have to say—the result is even tastier. I eat this salsa at least once a month! Mangoes are little powerhouses of vitamin C and carotenoids and have a great fiber content.

1. In a small bowl, whisk together the coconut milk and lime juice.

2. Place the mango, cucumber, onion, cilantro, and ginger in a medium-size bowl and mix thoroughly.

3. Pour the coconut mixture over the mango and vegetable mixture and let sit for at least 15 minutes.

4. Enjoy over chicken or fish or in romaine lettuce-leaf wrappers.

Nutritional Analysis per Serving: Protein (g) 0.74; Fat (g) 2.55; Carbs (g) 6.98; B$_{12}$ (mcg) 0; Iron (mg) 0.32; Iodine (mcg) 0; Magnesium (mg) 10.94; Potassium (mg) 135.08; Selenium (mcg) 0.87; Sodium (mg) 3.27

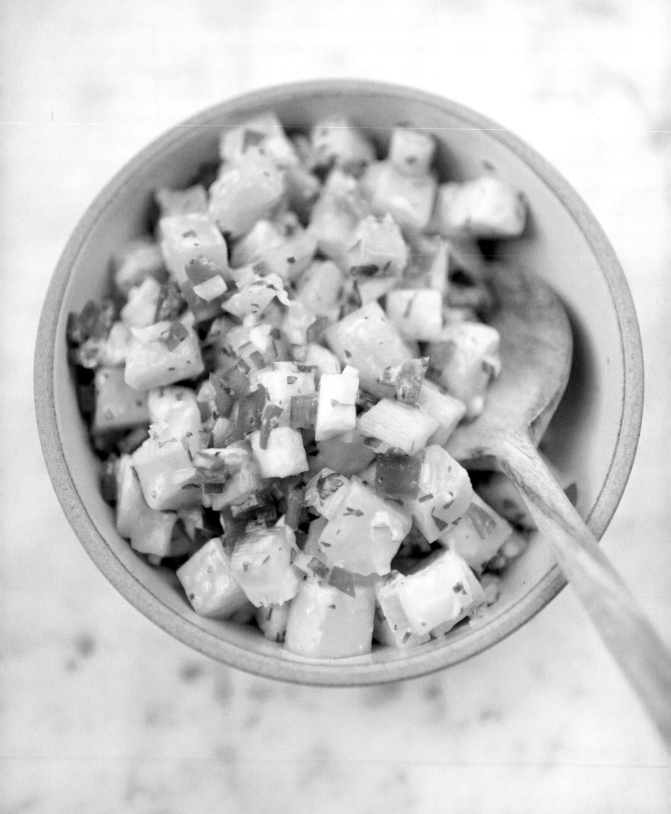

Mizeria (Polish Cucumber Salad)

Ⓐ AUTOIMMUNE

Prep time: 15 minutes

Serves: 2

4 medium cucumbers, peeled and thinly sliced (about 1½ cups)

1 tablespoon finely chopped dill

⅓ cup coconut milk or ½ cup plain Coconut Yogurt (p. 131)

1 tablespoon apple cider vinegar or freshly squeezed lemon juice

Sea salt or pink Himalayan sea salt to taste (I usually add ½ teaspoon)

A refreshing cucumber salad, in Poland Mizeria is often paired with hot dishes, such as Kotlety (p. 264) and various roasts. You can also experiment with this dish by adding other ingredients, such as onions, peppers, lemon juice, dill, chives, mint, or parsley.

1. Mix all ingredients together in a large bowl.

2. Refrigerate until ready to use.

3. Serve with hot meals.

Nutritional Analysis per Serving: Protein (g) 4.26; Fat (g) 3; Carbs (g) 27.21; B_{12} (mcg) 0.7; Iron (mg) 2.07; Iodine (mcg) 0; Magnesium (mg) 118.44; Potassium (mg) 887.01; Selenium (mcg) 1.81; Sodium (mg) 405.55

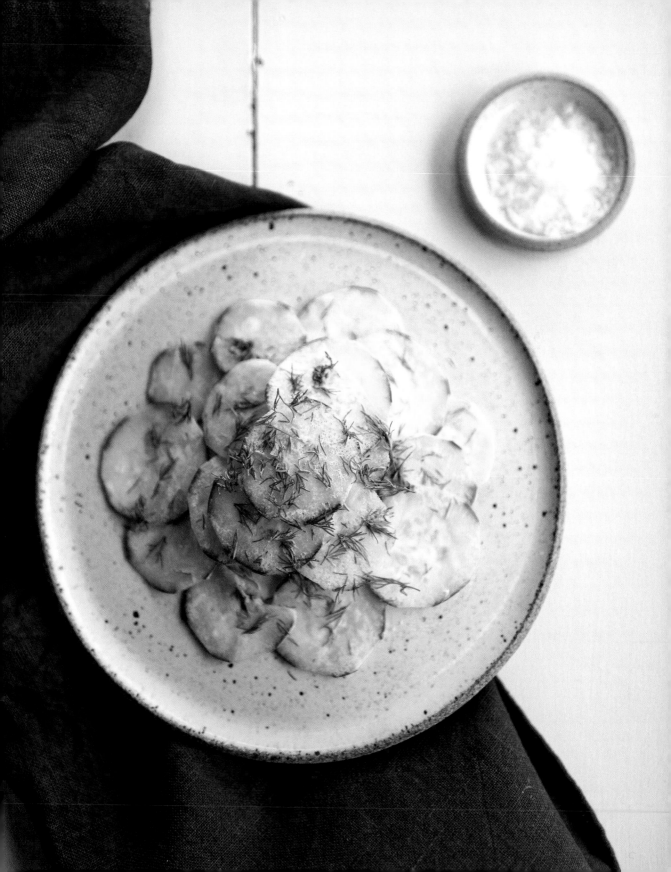

Twice-Baked Sweet Potatoes

Ⓐ AUTOIMMUNE

Prep time: 5 minutes

Cook time: 1 hour, 20 minutes

Serves: 8

4 large sweet potatoes, cut lengthwise in half

½ cup coconut milk

½ cup Coconut Yogurt (p. 131)

Sea salt or pink Himalayan sea salt to taste

⅓ cup cooked and chopped bacon

3 tablespoons chopped chives or green onion tops, for garnish

Sweet potatoes are one of my go-to starchy side dishes. Coconut Yogurt (p. 131) adds a creaminess to Twice-Baked Sweet Potatoes, and also a slight tang. The bacon provides a punch of protein and fat to help balance out the insulin response to potatoes. If you like, you can substitute butternut squash for the sweet potatoes.

1. Preheat the oven to 400°F.

2. Scrub and dry the potatoes. Bake for 45 minutes, or until the potatoes can be pierced easily with a fork.

3. Remove the baked potatoes, and scoop the flesh out with a spoon.

4. Place the potatoes, coconut milk, coconut yogurt, and salt in a high-speed blender and blend until ingredients achieve a whipped consistency.

5. Spread the potatoes in a 12 x 12-inch baking dish and top with bacon.

6. Bake for 15 to 20 minutes.

7. Remove, let cool slightly, and top with chopped chives.

Nutritional Analysis per Serving: Protein (g) 3.94; Fat (g) 11.75; Carbs (g) 15.62; B_{12} (mcg) 0.27; Iron (mg) 0.86; Iodine (mcg) 0; Magnesium (mg) 35.35; Potassium (mg) 305; Selenium (mcg) 5.17; Sodium (mg) 213.45

Spaghetti Squash Sauté

Ⓐ AUTOIMMUNE

Prep time: 8 minutes

Cook time: 1 hour

Serves: 4

1 spaghetti squash

2 tablespoons olive oil

½ teaspoon dried basil

½ teaspoon dried parsley

Sea salt or pink Himalayan sea salt to taste

Black pepper to taste (if tolerated)

Spaghetti squash is such a versatile vegetable. You can use it as a base for tomato and other types of sauces or as a side dish. Spaghetti squash is also hailed for its nutritional value, which includes the essential minerals calcium, iron, phosphorus, and zinc. I've used olive oil in this recipe to give the squash an extra layer of flavor.

1. Preheat the oven to 425°F.

2. Cut the spaghetti squash in half and remove the seeds and stringy stuff.

3. Place the squash cut-side down on a baking sheet and cover with foil. Bake for 1 hour or until the flesh can be easily pierced with a fork.

4. Remove from the oven and let cool.

5. When cool, scrape the flesh out with a spoon.

6. Heat the olive oil in a pan on medium-low. Add the squash, basil, parsley, salt, and pepper and sauté until warmed through, about 2 minutes.

Nutritional Analysis per Serving: Protein (g) 0.68; Fat (g) 7.34; Carbs (g) 7.14; B_{12} (mcg) 0; Iron (mg) 0.41; Iodine (mcg) 0; Magnesium (mg) 12.86; Potassium (mg) 114.9; Selenium (mcg) 0.32; Sodium (mg) 212.53

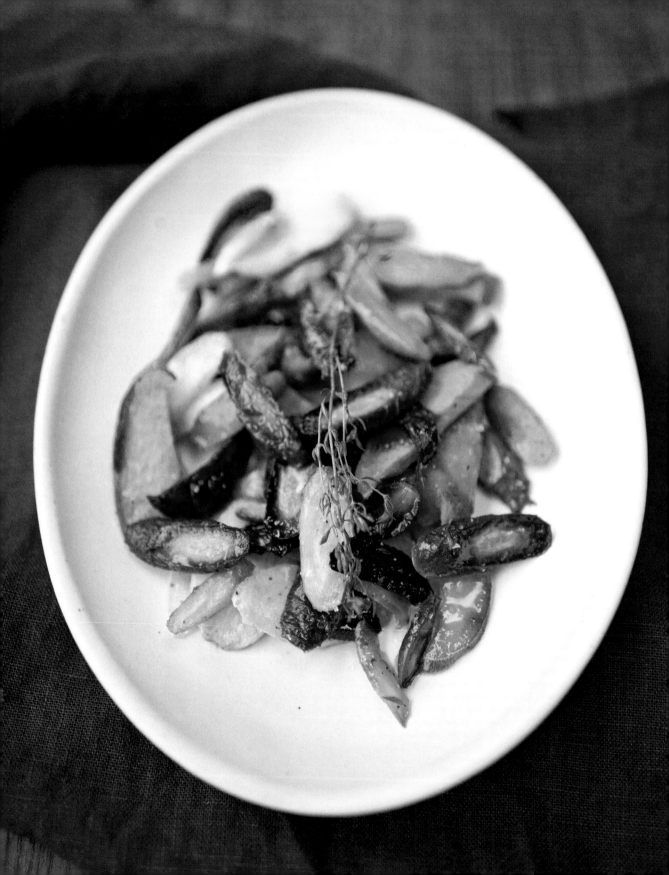

Root Veggie Bake

Ⓐ AUTOIMMUNE

Prep time: 20 minutes

Cook time: 1 hour

Serves: 6

5 to 6 cups cut-up root veggies (parsnips, turnips, sweet potatoes, daikon radishes, beets, black radishes, or carrots)

1 diced apple (optional)

¼ cup olive oil, duck fat, or other oil

½ teaspoon dried thyme

½ teaspoon dried basil

½ teaspoon sea salt or pink Himalayan sea salt

Honey, maple syrup, or extra-virgin olive oil, for drizzling

What better way to get some comfort food into your day than to make and enjoy a Root Veggie Bake! Not only will this dish provide comfort and warmth; it's also highly nutritious thanks to the vitamin A, vitamin C, and fiber it contains. This bake keeps and reheats well, so make it a day ahead or serve it as a side with your lunches during the week.

1. Preheat the oven to 350°F.

2. Mix the root vegetables, apple, oil, thyme, basil, and salt in a Dutch oven or 9 x 13-inch baking dish.

3. Cover and bake until vegetables are tender, about 1 hour.

4. Drizzle the vegetables with honey, maple syrup, and/or olive oil if desired.

Nutritional Analysis per Serving: Protein (g) 1.4; Fat (g) 9.2; Carbs (g) 14.06; B_{12} (mcg) 0; Iron (mg) 0.87; Iodine (mcg) 0; Magnesium (mg) 23.06; Potassium (mg) 341.55; Selenium (mcg) 0.87; Sodium (mg) 190.94

Parsnip-Carrot Mash

Ⓐ AUTOIMMUNE

Prep time: 5 minutes

Cook time: 30 to 40 minutes

Serves: 4

8 large carrots

2 large parsnips

2 tablespoons coconut oil

½ teaspoon sea salt or pink Himalayan sea salt

¼ cup water

If you're looking for a healthier alternative to mashed potatoes, this mix of parsnips and carrots really hits the spot! Parsnip-Carrot Mash is slightly sweet, with a delicate licorice taste coming from the parsnips.

1. Peel and chop the carrots and parsnips into uniform pieces.

2. Steam the vegetables for 15 to 25 minutes, until they are fork tender. (Alternatively, the vegetables can be steamed in an electric pressure cooker on Manual on high for 3 minutes.)

3. Place the carrots and parsnips in a high-speed blender with the coconut oil, salt, and water. Blend on low, increasing to high for 30 seconds, or until the mixture reaches the desired consistency.

4. Alternatively, mash the vegetables in a bowl with a potato masher.

Nutritional Analysis per Serving: Protein (g) 1.64; Fat (g) 7.22; Carbs (g) 19.29; B_{12} (mcg) 0; Iron (mg) 0.62; Iodine (mcg) 0; Magnesium (mg) 26.9; Potassium (mg) 548.95; Selenium (mcg) 0.88; Sodium (mg) 283.41

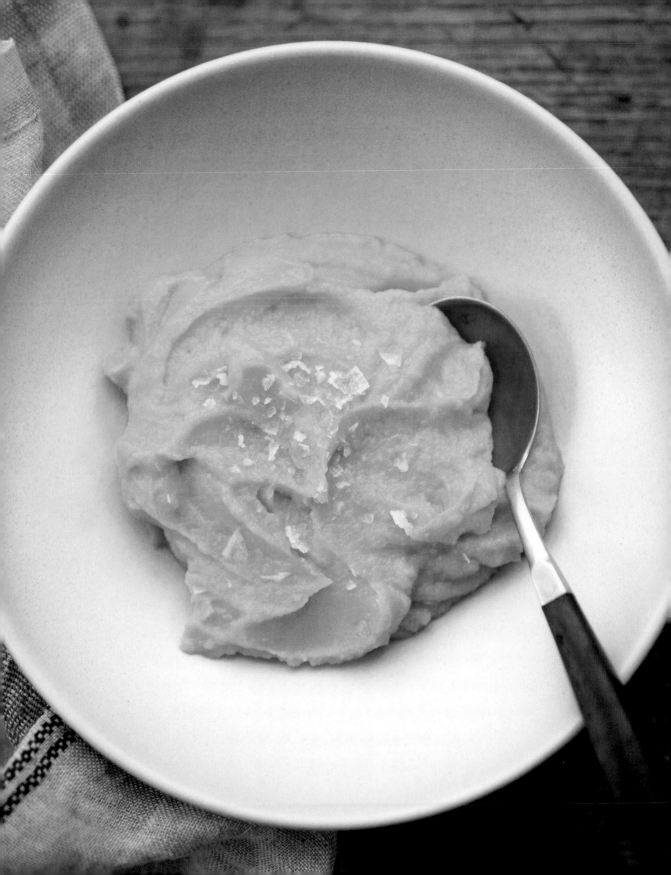

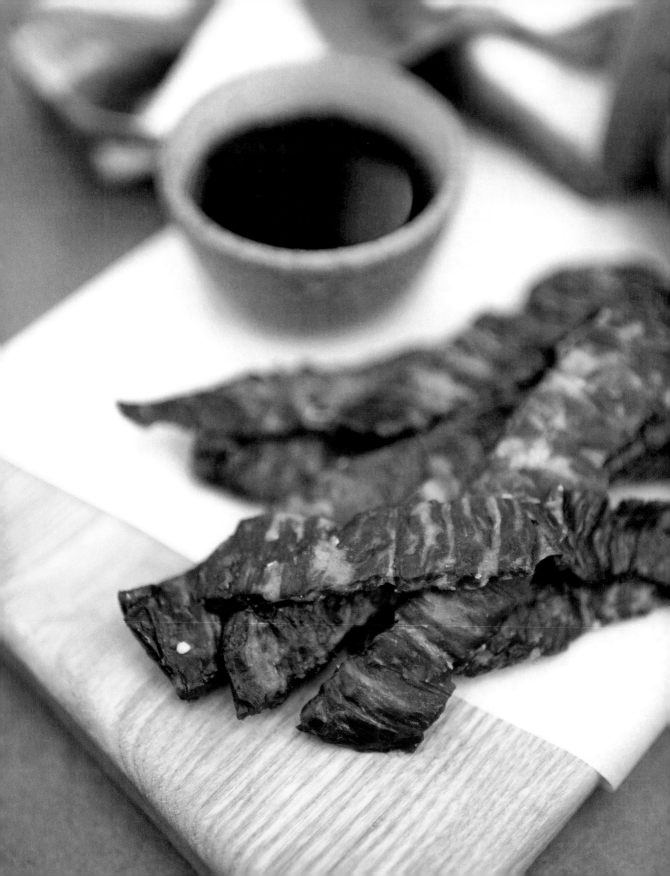

Beef Jerky

Ⓐ AUTOIMMUNE

Prep time: 2 hours, 10 minutes

Cook time: 2 hours

Serves: 6

1 pound top sirloin, trimmed, cut in thinly sliced small pieces

½ cup coconut aminos

1 tablespoon sea salt or pink Himalayan sea salt

*Possible Modifications for Other Root Cause Diets: See variation (p. 308).

This is my sweet take on beef jerky, thanks to the coconut-aminos marinade. The gluten-free, soy-free coconut aminos provide just enough sweetness to balance the salt in my Beef Jerky. Protein-rich top sirloin is also high in immune-boosting zinc. To make cutting the sirloin easier, I recommend placing the meat in the freezer for 30 to 45 minutes before slicing.

1. Place all ingredients in a resealable bag and refrigerate for 2 hours.

2. Line two large baking sheets with parchment paper and set aside.

3. Preheat the oven to 200°F.

4. Spread the jerky out in a single layer on the baking sheets, leaving a little space between pieces.

5. Bake for 2 hours, flipping halfway, or until dry.

6. Serve immediately or store in an airtight container.

Nutritional Analysis per Serving: Protein (g) 20.86; Fat (g) 12.64; Carbs (g) 3.78; B_{12} (mcg) 2.03; Iron (mg) 2.28; Iodine (mcg) 0; Magnesium (mg) 21.16; Potassium (mg) 274.27; Selenium (mcg) 20.17; Sodium (mg) 1253.97

Variation: Thai Beef Jerky

P PALEO

Prep time: 2 hours, 10 minutes

Cook time: 2 hours

Serves: 6

1 pound top sirloin, trimmed, cut in thinly sliced small pieces

2 teaspoons garlic powder

1 teaspoon sea salt or pink Himalayan sea salt

1 cup pineapple juice

1 teaspoon sesame oil

2 tablespoons coconut aminos

1. Place all ingredients in a resealable plastic bag and refrigerate for 2 hours.

2. Line two large baking sheets with parchment paper and set aside.

3. Preheat the oven to 200°F.

4. Spread the jerky out in a single layer on the baking sheets, leaving a little space between pieces.

5. Bake for 2 hours, flipping halfway, or until dry.

6. Serve immediately or store in an airtight container.

Nutritional Analysis per Serving: Protein (g) 14.65; Fat (g) 12.16; Carbs 6.52; B_{12} (mcg) 2.19; Iron (mg) 1.92; Iodine (mcg) 0; Magnesium (mg) 21.69; Potassium (mg) 288.01; Selenium (mcg) 14.08; Sodium (mg) 300.52

Red Pepper Turkey Dip

⓿ PALEO

Prep time: 10 minutes

Cook time: 40 minutes

Serves: 4

1 cup ground turkey

1 large tomato, chopped

2 tablespoons chopped red onion

1 large red bell pepper, chopped

3 tablespoons lemon juice

2 tablespoons chopped fresh basil

Sea salt or pink Himalayan sea salt to taste

Black pepper to taste (if tolerated)

2 tablespoons melted coconut oil (for greasing baking dish)

1 large cucumber, sliced (for dipping)

A succulent combination of turkey, sweet bell peppers, onions, and herbs delivers a savory dip perfect for snacks and parties. In addition to tissue-repairing protein, Red Pepper Turkey Dip is loaded with antioxidants and immune-boosting vitamins. Serve with toxin-reducing cucumber slices for a tasty snack.

1. Preheat the oven to 350°F.

2. In a large bowl, mix the turkey, tomato, onion, bell pepper, lemon juice, basil, salt, and pepper until combined.

3. Pour the mixture into a greased 12 x 12-inch baking dish or 10- to 12-inch cast-iron skillet.

4. Bake for 40 minutes, or until cooked through and bubbling.

5. Remove from oven, cool slightly, and pulse in a blender or food processor until the mixture forms a "dip" consistency.

6. Serve warm or at room temperature with cucumber slices.

Nutritional Analysis per Serving: Protein (g) 16.82; Fat (g) 5.18; Carbs (g) 6.55; B_{12} (mcg) 1.82; Iron (mg) 1.08; Iodine (mcg) 0; Magnesium (mg) 29.17; Potassium (mg) 447.08; Selenium (mcg) 4.49; Sodium (mg) 149.42

Almond and Date Snack Bars

ⓟ PALEO

Prep time: 7 minutes

Cook time: 15 minutes

Serves: 8

½ cup almond butter

¼ cup chopped unsalted almonds

⅓ cup unsweetened coconut flakes (about 1 ounce)

4 large eggs, beaten

¼ cup shelled unsalted sunflower seeds

8 large dates, pitted and chopped (about 1 cup)

Sea salt or pink Himalayan sea salt to taste

2 tablespoons melted coconut oil (for greasing baking dish)

Almond and Date Snack Bars make great breakfast bars because they are packed with nutrients to help stabilize blood-sugar levels and get your day off to a great start! The satisfying, salty crunch of the almonds and sunflower seeds paired with the natural sweetness of the fiber-rich dates provides a simple yet healthy snack the entire family is sure to love. These bars keep well in the fridge for 1 week.

1. Preheat the oven to 350°F.

2. Place all ingredients in a food processor and pulse until the mixture sticks together.

3. Press the mixture into a greased 12 x 12-inch baking dish.

4. Bake for 15 minutes, until the top is golden brown and a toothpick inserted into the middle comes out clean.

5. Allow baking dish to cool.

6. Slice and serve.

> Nutritional Analysis per Serving: Protein (g) 8.72; Fat (g) 15.95; Carbs (g) 23.46; B_{12} (mcg) 0.22; Iron (mg) 1.57; Iodine (mcg) 12; Magnesium (mg) 79.6; Potassium (mg) 350.24; Selenium (mcg) 11.23; Sodium (mg) 86.25

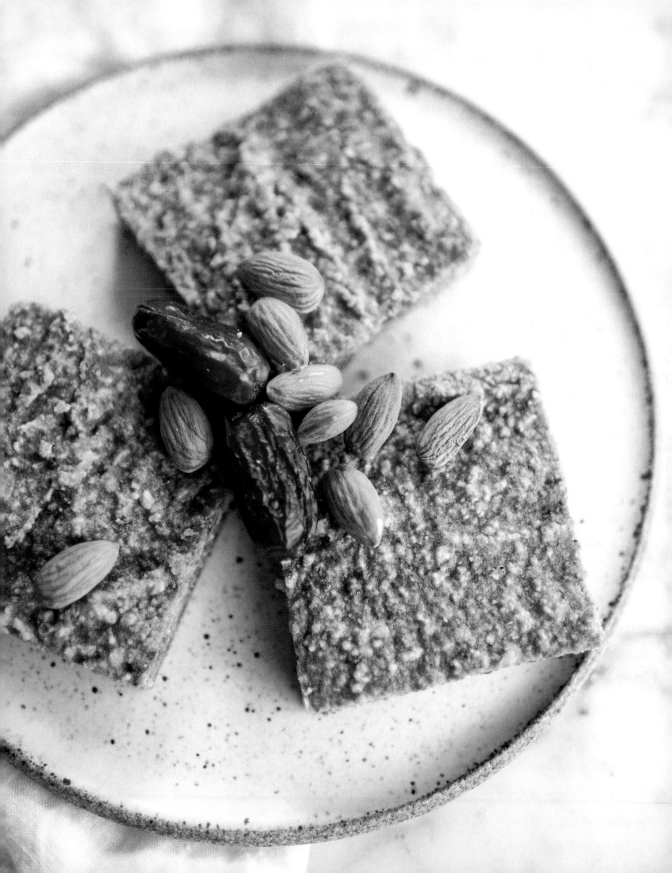

Carrot Fries

Ⓐ AUTOIMMUNE

Prep time: 15 minutes

Cook time: 30 minutes

Serves: 4

1 teaspoon sea salt or pink Himalayan sea salt to taste

Black pepper to taste (if tolerated)

½ teaspoon garlic powder

½ teaspoon dried thyme

12 medium-size carrots, cut into sticks 4 inches long and ½-inch thick

1½ tablespoons coconut oil

Looking for the perfect side dish or snack? Look no further! The mouthwatering combination of carrots, garlic, and thyme creates a flavorful dish that packs a nutritious punch by boosting the immune system, improving heart health, and reducing cancer risks.

1. Preheat the oven to 400°F.

2. Line a large baking sheet with parchment paper and set aside.

3. In a small bowl, mix the salt, pepper, garlic powder, and thyme.

4. In a large bowl, combine the carrots and oil and mix thoroughly to ensure an even coating. Sprinkle the spice mixture over the carrots and mix again until well distributed.

5. Spread the carrots out evenly on the prepared baking sheet.

6. Bake for 25 to 30 minutes, flipping halfway, or until the carrots have softened slightly and are tender.

7. Allow to cool for a few minutes and serve warm.

> Nutritional Analysis per Serving: Protein (g) 1.23; Fat (g) 3.7; Carbs (g) 12.14; B_{12} (mcg) 0; Iron (mg) 0.41; Iodine (mcg) 0; Magnesium (mg) 15.3; Potassium (mg) 398.3; Selenium (mcg) 0.24; Sodium (mg) 344.5

Zucchini Bread

ⓟ PALEO

Prep time: 10 minutes

Cook time: 45 to 60 minutes

Serves: 8

2 cups chopped zucchini

4 eggs

¼ cup maple syrup

¼ cup palm oil–based vegetable shortening

1 teaspoon vanilla

½ cup coconut milk

½ cup coconut flour

½ cup cassava flour

½ teaspoon baking soda

½ teaspoon (cornstarch-free) baking powder

1 teaspoon sea salt or pink Himalayan sea salt

½ teaspoon ground cinnamon

2 tablespoons melted coconut oil (for greasing loaf pan)

This Paleo Zucchini Bread is a delicious choice if you're looking for a side or a breakfast dish, or you want to make a sandwich with the Sloppy Joes in a HeartBeet (p. 260) or Maple Meatloaf Muffins (p. 233). Alternatively, you can use ripe bananas or pumpkin puree for variety as well as make zucchini muffins by placing the mixture into a muffin pan and reducing the baking time by about half.

1. Preheat the oven to 375°F.

2. Mix all ingredients in a stand mixer.

3. Pour into a 5 × 9-inch greased loaf pan and bake for 45 to 55 minutes, or until browned and a toothpick comes out clean when inserted into the middle.

4. Let cool completely before cutting.

Nutritional Analysis per Serving: Protein (g) 5.67; Fat (g) 6.97; Carbs (g) 37.08; B_{12} (mcg) 0.22; Iron (mg) 1.18; Iodine (mcg) 12; Magnesium (mg) 28.77; Potassium (mg) 367.12; Selenium (mcg) 9.16; Sodium (mg) 323.75

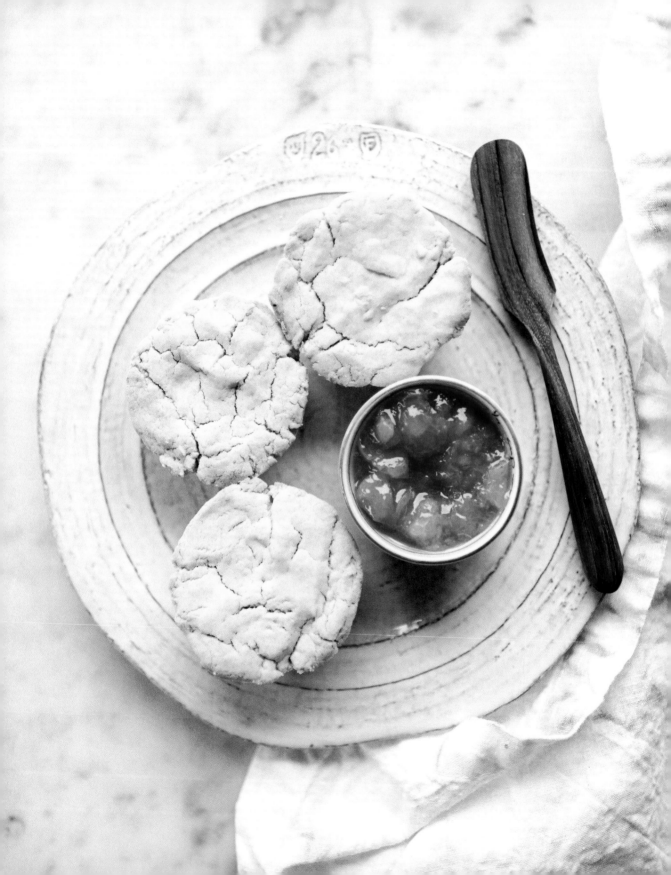

Biscuits

Ⓐ AUTOIMMUNE

Prep time: 20 minutes

Cook time: 8 to 10 minutes

Serves: 8

2 cups cassava flour

¼ teaspoon sea salt or pink Himalayan sea salt

1 tablespoon (cornstarch-free) baking powder

¼ cup palm oil–based vegetable shortening

1 tablespoon maple syrup

1 to 1½ cups coconut milk

These autoimmune biscuits are an easy side to many dishes and have just the right flaky texture, thanks to the palm shortening.

1. Preheat the oven to 450°F.

2. Place the first 5 ingredients in a stand mixer and blend until well mixed.

3. Add ½ cup of coconut milk at a time and continue blending until the batter becomes smooth, with a doughlike consistency.

4. Spoon the mixture into 8 muffin cups.

5. Bake for 8 to 10 minutes or until lightly browned.

Nutritional Analysis per Serving: Protein (g) 1.34; Fat (g) 11.3; Carbs (g) 28.15; B_{12} (mcg) 0; Iron (mg) 0.59; Iodine (mcg) 0; Magnesium (mg) 21.97; Potassium (mg) 238.13; Selenium (mcg) 1.7; Sodium (mg) 158.38

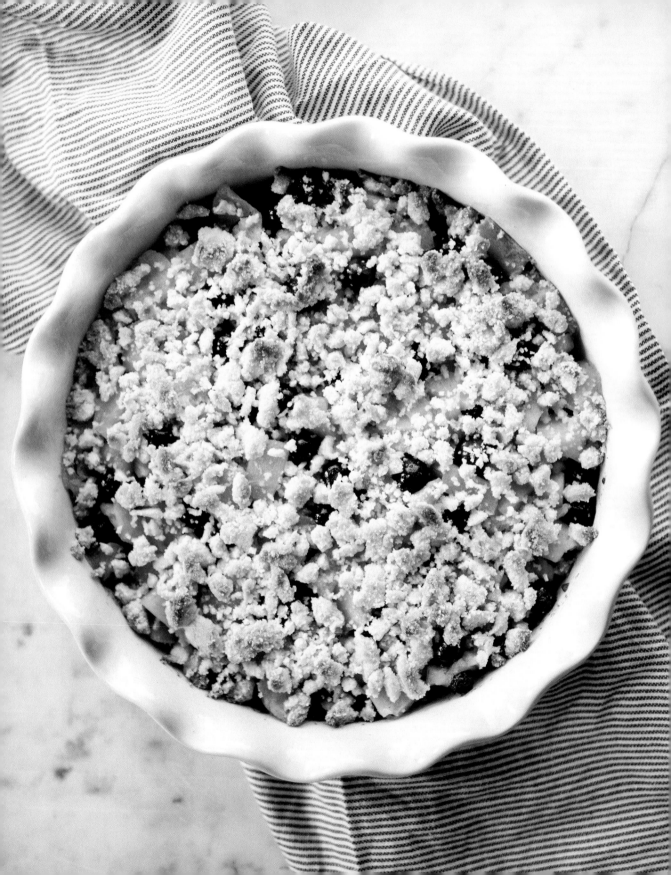

Apple-Blueberry Crumble

Ⓟ PALEO

Prep time: 10 minutes

Cook time: 35 to 45 minutes

Serves: 10

CRUST

3 cups almond flour, *divided*

½ cup melted coconut oil

4 tablespoons honey

1 teaspoon vanilla extract

FILLING

3 cups stewed apple chunks and slices (see Chunky Applesauce, p. 146. When the apples are cooked, do not mash them; instead add them to the pie without the liquid.)

1 cup fresh blueberries

Nutritional Analysis per Serving: Protein (g) 6.4; Fat (g) 25.12; Carbs (g) 16.81; B_{12} (mcg) 0; Iron (mg) 1.19; Iodine (mcg) 0.59; Magnesium (mg) 81.03; Potassium (mg) 283.16; Selenium (mcg) 1.19; Sodium (mg) 1.22

There's something soothing about baking! Growing up in Poland, I loved eating my mom's apple pie szarlotka on Sunday mornings. As an adult, I decided to apply my extensive training in chemistry to my own baking. I love the precision and detail it takes to make a baked good that is just right! Before my gluten-free journey started, I used to make homemade treats for family, friends, and coworkers and have since found a way to modify my favorites and create delicious healthier versions. This Apple-Blueberry Crumble is gluten free, dairy free, and Paleo friendly, includes protein, and is 100 percent delicious! Enjoy!

1. Preheat the oven to 350°F.

2. Mix 2 cups of the almond flour, coconut oil, honey, and vanilla in a stand mixer until smooth.

3. Remove one quarter of the almond-flour mixture and set aside. Then, by hand or using the low speed on the mixer, add the remaining 1 cup of almond flour to create a dough with a crumblike consistency.

4. Press the mixture onto the bottom and up the sides of a 9-inch round pie dish.

5. Bake the crust for 10 minutes, or until lightly browned.

6. Once browned, remove the crust from the oven and let rest for 5 minutes.

7. Gently mix the apples and blueberries and pour into the pie crust.

8. Add the reserved crumble to the top and bake for 35 to 45 minutes, until the blueberries are soft and the crumble topping is golden brown.

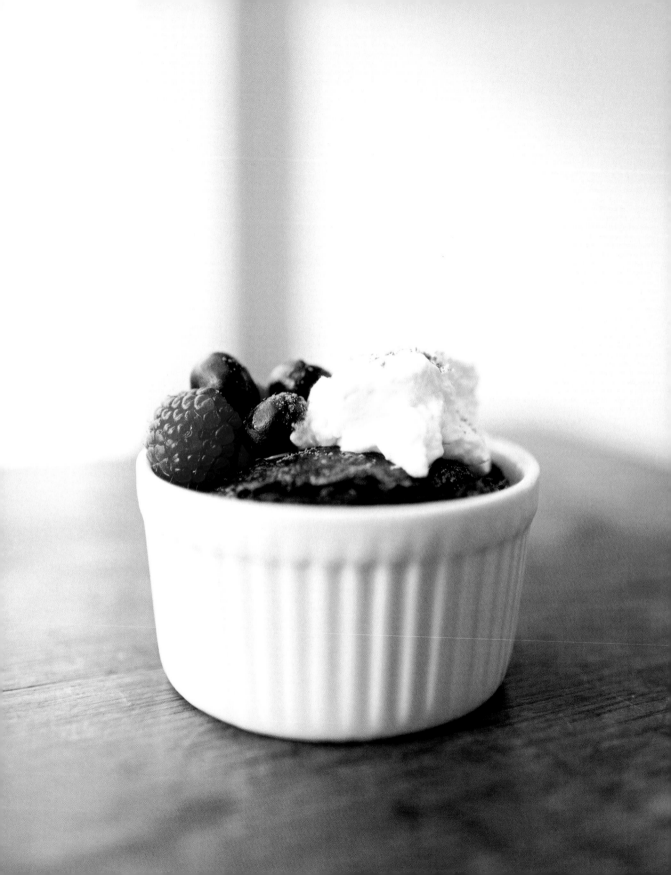

Carob Lava Cakes

A AUTOIMMUNE

Prep time: 15 minutes

Cook time: 30 minutes

Serves: 6

4 tablespoons of coconut oil, melted, *divided*

1½ cups frozen blueberries, thawed

1 cup unsweetened carob powder

½ cup maple syrup

2 teaspoons cream of tartar

1 teaspoon baking soda

Pinch sea salt or pink Himalayan sea salt to taste

2 tablespoons gelatin

4 tablespoons boiling water

¼ cup hot water

6 tablespoons of coconut cream or whipped coconut cream (optional)

Although chocolate is not on the Autoimmune Diet menu, delicious carob can be used for this tasty dessert! Carob Lava Cakes have a soft texture and a rich flavor. I use 4-ounce ramekins. Serve with berries!

1. Preheat the oven to 350°F.

2. Grease six 4-ounce ramekins with 2 tablespoons melted coconut oil.

3. In a food processor or blender, place the remaining 2 tablespoons coconut oil, blueberries, carob powder, maple syrup, cream of tartar, baking soda, and salt and blend until smooth.

4. In a small bowl, vigorously whisk together the gelatin and boiling water until the gelatin dissolves.

5. Pour the gelatin into the food processor or blender with the other ingredients and blend until well combined.

6. Add the ¼ cup hot water and briefly blend.

7. Spoon the mixture into the prepared ramekins.

8. Bake for 30 minutes, or until the tops of the cakes have formed a light crust and feel slightly firm.

9. Let cool slightly and serve warm.

10. Optional: Top each lava cake with 1 tablespoon of coconut cream or whipped coconut cream.

Nutritional Analysis per Serving: Protein (g) 2.79; Fat (g) 9.28; Carbs (g) 20.63; B$_{12}$ (mcg) 0; Iron (mg) 0.1; Iodine (mcg) 0; Magnesium (mg) 14.85; Potassium (mg) 368.12; Selenium (mcg) 1.83; Sodium (mg) 223.59

Chocolate Avocado Pudding

P PALEO

Prep time: 15 minutes

Serves: 4

1½ cups coconut milk

*¼ cup Rootcology Paleo Protein

1 avocado

*1 tablespoon cocoa powder

1 tablespoon maple syrup to taste

*Possible Modifications for Other Root Cause Diets: This recipe can be made Autoimmune friendly by replacing carob for cocoa powder and AI Paleo Protein for Rootcology Protein.

Desserts! Sometimes we just want a sweet treat, but in the early stages of the healing journey, blood-sugar swings can lead to imbalanced moods and energy crashes and place stress on our adrenals. One way to offset the effects of sugar is to be sure you mix chocolate with good fats and protein, which in Chocolate Avocado Pudding are found in the coconut milk and Rootcology protein powder. I recommend this pudding with fresh berries or shaved coconut on top!

1. Place all ingredients in a high-powered blender and blend until smooth.

2. Refrigerate until ready to serve.

Nutritional Analysis per Serving: Protein (g) 7.88; Fat (g) 23.66; Carbs (g) 6.05; B_{12} (mcg) 0; Iron (mg) 3.19; Iodine (mcg) 0; Magnesium (mg) 55.41; Potassium (mg) 376.47; Selenium (mcg) 0.33; Sodium (mg) 51.47

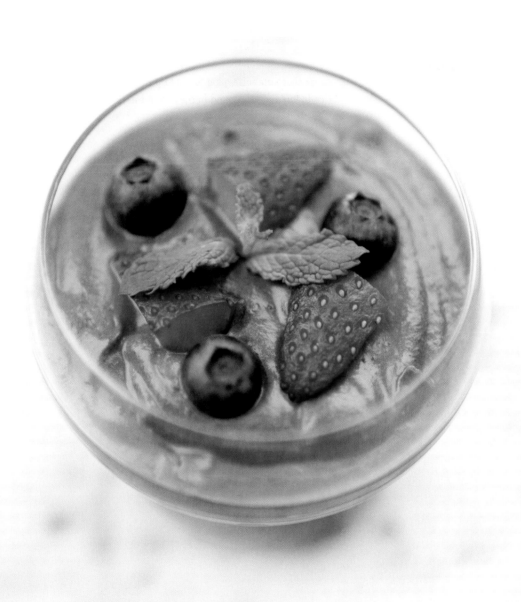

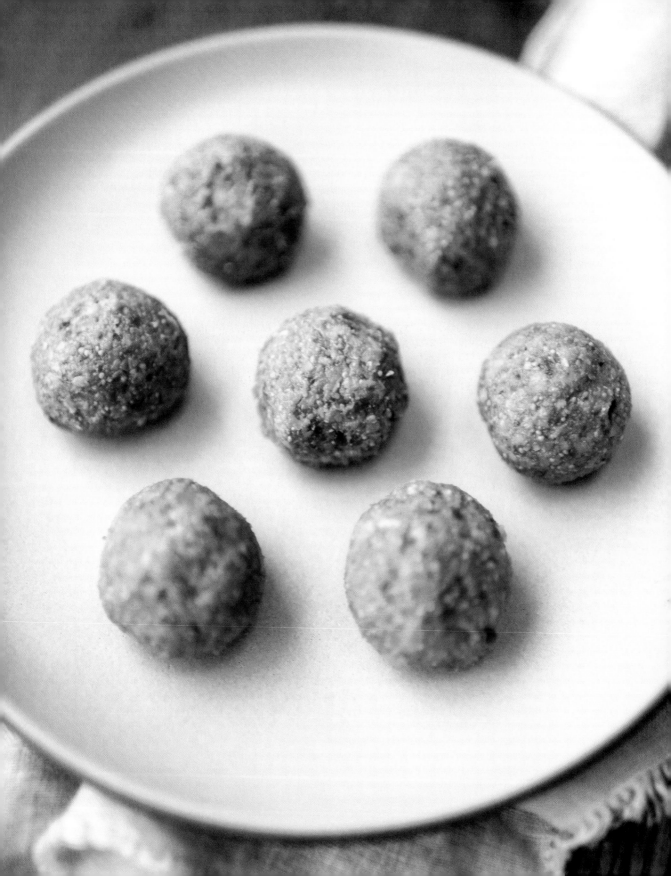

Coconut-Fig Energy Balls

Ⓐ AUTOIMMUNE

Prep time: 20 minutes

Cook time: 30 minutes chilling

Serves: 10

30 dried unsweetened Turkish figs

2 cups unsweetened shredded coconut, *divided*

⅓ cup coconut oil, melted

¼ teaspoon ground cinnamon

Sea salt or pink Himalayan sea salt to taste

When we're eating for healing, it can be challenging to find a treat that meets your dietary needs and delights your taste buds. Store-bought gluten-free and Paleo snacks aren't always safe, since they can contain nuts, which are not autoimmune friendly. I'm excited to tell you that Coconut-Fig Energy Balls will hit the spot for you; plus they are high in fiber and iron. This is also a kid-approved recipe! But be warned. I often make these for my brother, Robert, and he swears they're addictive! You can easily switch out the figs for dates for a variation.

1. Line a large baking sheet with parchment paper and set aside.

2. In a food processor or blender, place the figs, 1½ cups coconut, coconut oil, cinnamon, and salt and blend until a smooth paste forms. It will have the consistency of brown sugar.

3. Form the dough into 1-inch balls, about 1 tablespoon of batter for each, and then roll the balls in the remaining shredded coconut.

4. Refrigerate for 30 minutes and serve.

Nutritional Analysis per Serving: Protein (g) 1.62; Fat (g) 12.95; Carbs (g) 2.48; B_{12} (mcg) 0; Iron (mg) 1.25; Iodine (mcg) 1.36; Magnesium (mg) 26.25; Potassium (mg) 319.16; Selenium (mcg) 1.62; Sodium (mg) 46.97

Paleo Banana-Almond Muffins

℗ PALEO

Prep time: 10 minutes

Cook time: 45 to 60 minutes

Serves: 12

1¼ cups almond flour

2 teaspoons baking powder

¼ teaspoon baking soda

1 teaspoon ground cinnamon

½ cup unsweetened applesauce
(see Chunky Applesauce, p. 146)

2 eggs

3 ripe mashed bananas

OPTIONAL ADDITIONS

½ cup shaved unsweetened coconut

½ cup blueberries

½ cup walnuts

¼ cup poppy seeds

1 tablespoon unsweetened cocoa
powder plus ¼ cup honey

*Possible Modifications for Other Root
Cause Diets: If avoiding eggs, substitute
1 tablespoon of apple cider vinegar for
each egg.

Paleo Banana-Almond Muffins, which are not only delicious but gluten free and sugar free, can help stabilize your blood sugar while providing a delicious dose of antioxidants! When you add the coconut and walnuts, these make a great addition to a kid's breakfast, providing slow-burning fat that will help keep them energized throughout the school morning. This recipe was inspired by the Specific Carbohydrate Diet.

1. Preheat the oven to 350°F.

2. Place paper liners in a 12-cup muffin tin.

3. In a medium-size bowl, mix the almond flour, baking powder, baking soda, and cinnamon until combined.

4. Make a well in the center and add the applesauce, eggs, and mashed banana; mix the wet with the dry ingredients until combined.

5. Fold in the optional ingredients, if using.

6. Pour the batter evenly into the 12 paper-lined cups.

7. Bake for 45 to 60 minutes or until tops of muffins are lightly browned and a toothpick inserted comes out clean. (Alternatively, grease a 5 × 9-inch loaf pan with coconut oil and pour in the batter. Bake 1 hour or until the top is browned and a toothpick inserted into the center comes out clean.)

Nutritional Analysis per Serving: Protein (g) 3.47; Fat (g) 5.84; Carbs (g) 10.27; B_{12} (mcg) 0.07; Iron (mg) 0.67; Iodine (mcg) 4.75; Magnesium (mg) 36.05; Potassium (mg) 196.41; Selenium (mcg) 3.29; Sodium (mg) 83.06

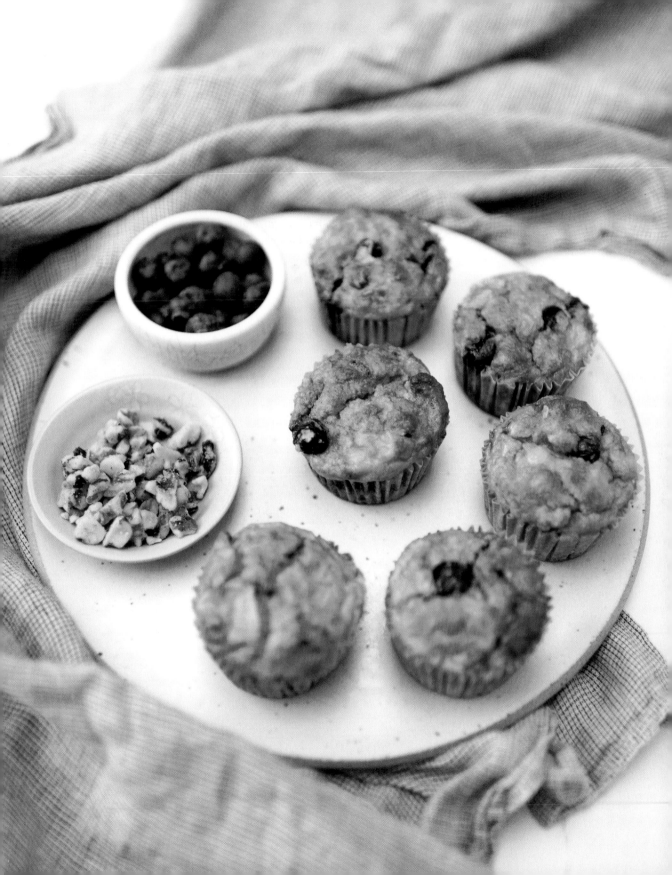

Cherry Berry Gelatin Snacks

Ⓐ AUTOIMMUNE

Prep time: 5 minutes

Cook time: 15 minutes, 2 hours chilling

Serves: 6

4 cups tart cherry juice, *divided*

4 tablespoons gelatin

1 cup chopped strawberries

Nutritional Analysis per Serving: Protein (g) 5.52; Fat (g) 0.71; Carbs (g) 1.84; B_{12} (mcg) 0; Iron (mg) 0.15; Iodine (mcg) 2.13; Magnesium (mg) 4.15; Potassium (mg) 37.45; Selenium (mcg) 1.94; Sodium (mg) 9.39

Gelatin is an excellent source of gut-healing glycine and, like its cousin collagen, can also help with preventing wrinkles and improving joint pain. You can make your own gelatin-based snacks and desserts with a few simple ingredients. I like to make gelatin desserts in multiple small containers to have as desserts and snacks throughout the week. For parties, I'll occasionally make gelatin in a big bowl.

Cherry Berry Gelatin Snacks combines the healing power of gelatin with tart cherry juice, which is known for its anti-inflammatory and pain-relieving qualities, and strawberries, which are high in antioxidants and offer additional anti-inflammatory benefits. For the cherry juice, I recommend purchasing one that's made from ripe whole cherries instead of from concentrate.

1. Pour 2 cups of cold cherry juice into a glass container.

2. Add gelatin to the cold juice, mix, and let sit for 1 minute.

3. In a small pan on medium-low, heat the 2 remaining cups of juice for 5 minutes.

4. Slowly pour the hot juice into the gelatin mixture while whisking until fully incorporated.

5. Add 1 cup of chopped strawberries.

6. Pour the mixture into a 2-quart baking dish and refrigerate for 2 hours.

7. Cut into desired size pieces and serve.

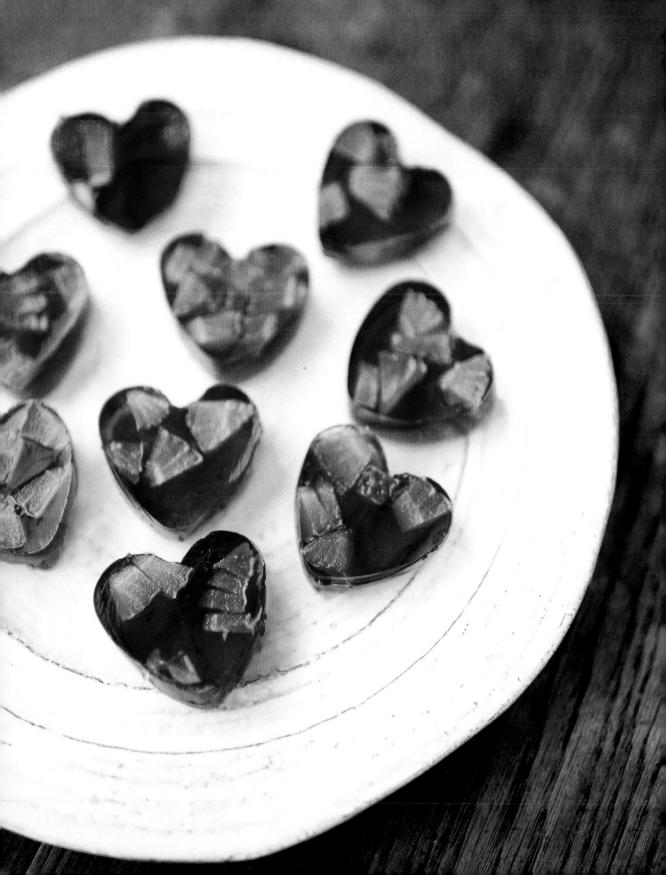

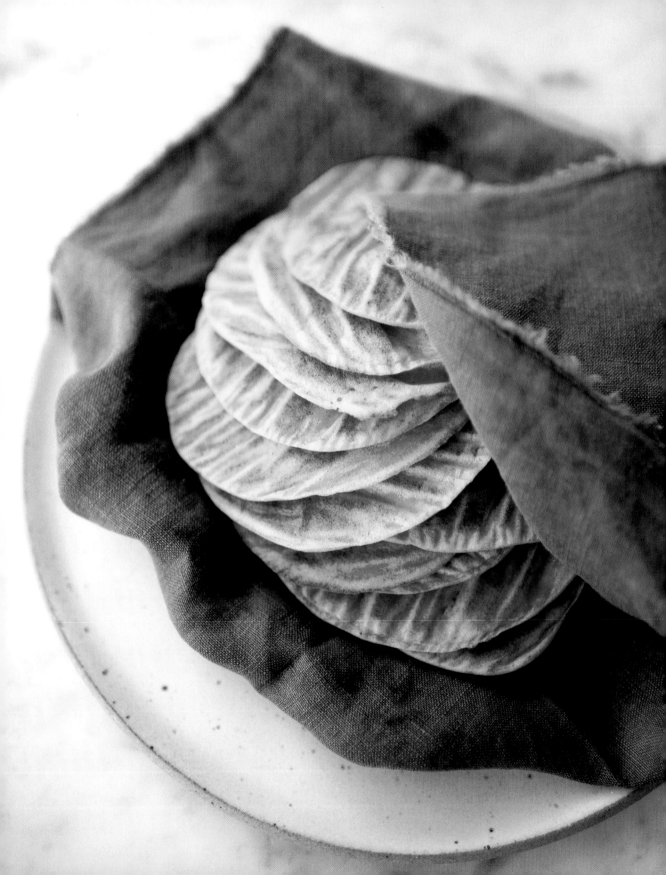

Plantain Crepes

P PALEO

Prep time: 15 minutes

Cook time: 15 minutes

Serves: 4

3 ripe plantains
(soft and black in color)

¼ cup coconut oil

1 teaspoon tapioca starch

½ tablespoon balsamic vinegar

¼ cup water

½ tablespoon lemon juice

1 egg

Coconut whipped cream (optional)

Crepes are very thin pancakes typically made from wheat flour. These Paleo Plantain Crepes use tapioca starch and pureed plantains to create a delicious crepe (you can substitute cassava flour for tapioca starch). Top them with fresh antioxidant-loaded berries and coconut whipped cream for an extraordinary dessert, or have them with shredded pork and avocadoes for a savory lunch.

1. Preheat the oven to 400°F.

2. Line two baking sheets with parchment paper and set aside.

3. Place all ingredients in a high-speed blender and blend until smooth.

4. Pour ¼ to ⅓ cup of the mixture for each of four crepes onto the parchment paper. You will get 4 to 6 crepes, depending on the size of the plantains.

5. Bake for 15 minutes.

6. Serve plain and hot or, for a sweet treat, add some fresh berries and coconut whipped cream (mix 1 cup heavy coconut milk or coconut cream with 1 teaspoon vanilla and 1 tablespoon maple syrup in a blender on high for 30 seconds, until fluffy).

Nutritional Analysis per Serving: Protein (g) 3.34; Fat (g) 15.29; Carbs (g) 43.93; B_{12} (mcg) 0.11; Iron (mg) 1.05; Iodine (mcg) 6; Magnesium (mg) 51.53; Potassium (mg) 691.39; Selenium (mcg) 5.85; Sodium (mg) 23.6

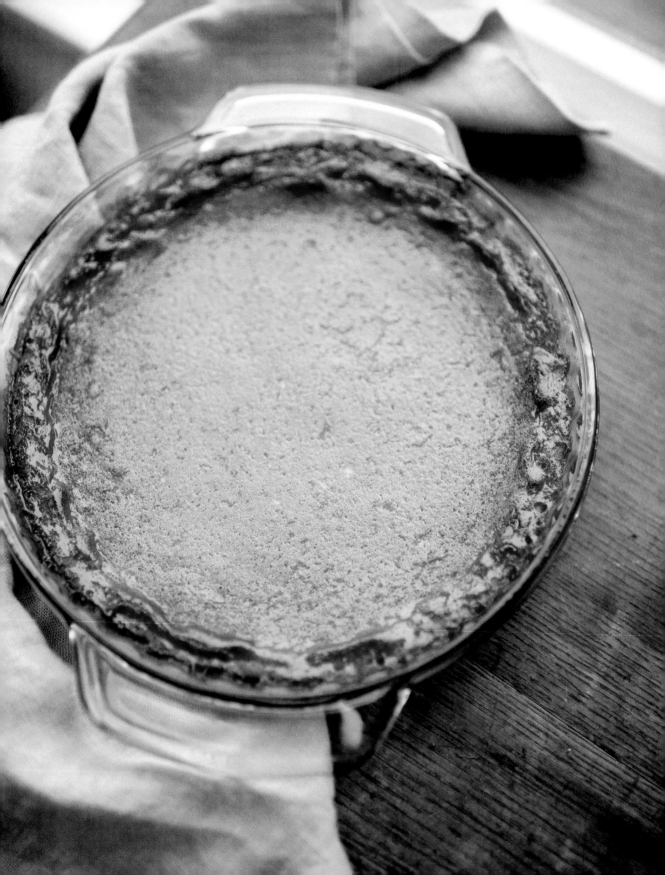

Pumpkin Pie

Ⓟ PALEO

Prep time: 10 minutes

Cook time: 60 to 70 minutes

Serves: 8

Coconut oil

15 ounces canned pumpkin puree

½ cup honey or pureed dates

3 eggs

1¼ cups coconut milk

2 tablespoons Pumpkin Pie Spice

¼ teaspoon sea salt or pink Himalayan sea salt

Coconut whipped cream (optional), for garnish

You won't even miss the crust after making this Pumpkin Pie! This pie is rich in pumpkin spice flavor and holds up very well when slicing. And even better, all of the spices used in the pumpkin pie spice—typically cinnamon, ginger, cloves, and others—are very warming to the body, which is perfect on a cool fall day. Garnish with coconut whipped cream! This recipe is great in the fall, or any time of year!

1. Preheat the oven to 350°F.

2. Grease a 9-inch round baking dish with coconut oil.

3. In a large bowl, mix the pumpkin, dates, eggs, coconut milk, pumpkin pie spice, and salt until thoroughly combined.

4. Pour the batter into the prepared dish.

5. Bake for 1 hour. Check to see if the middle jiggles. If it does, bake for another 10 minutes and check again.

6. Cool completely before serving.

7. Optional: Garnish with coconut whipped cream (mix 1 cup heavy coconut milk or coconut cream with 1 tablespoon vanilla and 1 tablespoon maple syrup in a high-speed blender on high for 30 seconds, until fluffy).

Nutritional Analysis per Serving: Protein (g) 3.94; Fat (g) 11.32; Carbs (g) 24.7; B$_{12}$ (mcg) 0.167; Iron (mg) 2.02; Iodine (mcg) 9; Magnesium (mg) 30.51; Potassium (mg) 253.37; Selenium (mcg) 8.58; Sodium (mg) 85.16

Sweet Potato Pistachio Pudding

P PALEO

Prep time: 5 minutes

Cook time: 2 hours chilling

Serves: 6

1 cup fresh or canned pureed sweet potato

2 cups unsweetened almond milk or alternate nut milk

⅓ cup chia seeds

½ cup chopped pistachios

4 tablespoons honey

Sea salt or pink Himalayan sea salt to taste

Sweet Potato Pistachio Pudding is a healthy pudding that is full of fiber from the chia seeds with a nice hint of sweetness from the sweet potatoes and honey—what better way to get your vegetables in than with a sweet-tasting dessert!

1. In a large bowl, mix all ingredients well.

2. Cover the bowl and refrigerate for at least 2 hours, until the pudding is set. Alternatively, pour the pudding mixture into six small serving bowls and refrigerate until set.

3. Serve chilled.

Nutritional Analysis per Serving: Protein (g) 8.6; Fat (g) 10.2; Carbs (g) 30.28; B$_{12}$ (mcg) 0; Iron (mg) 2.27; Iodine (mcg) 0; Magnesium (mg) 22.88; Potassium (mg) 310.39; Selenium (mcg) 1.17; Sodium (mg) 107.54

Baked Coconut Bananas

Ⓐ AUTOIMMUNE

Prep time: 10 minutes

Cook time: 25 minutes

Serves: 4

½ cup unsweetened shredded coconut

3 tablespoons coconut oil, melted

Juice of ½ lemon

2 teaspoons maple syrup

½ teaspoon pure vanilla extract

*½ teaspoon AI Pumpkin Pie Spice, p. 95)

¼ teaspoon allspice (if tolerated)

¼ teaspoon ground cloves

Sea salt or pink Himalayan sea salt to taste

3 medium ripe bananas (about 2 cups), peeled and sliced

*Possible Modifications for Other Root Cause Diets: If using storebought pumpkin pie spice, this recipe will become Paleo, not Autoimmune.

In the 1930s, bananas were thought to be a cure for celiac disease in children. Dr. Sydney Haas recommended a special diet that included eating up to seven bananas a day for hundreds of children who presented with symptoms of celiac disease. This diet, which was later described and named as the Specific Carbohydrate Diet by Elaine Gottschall, also eliminated most starches and was so effective for these children that many then transitioned to the Standard American Diet without obvious digestive concerns.

Unfortunately, we have since learned that bananas won't reverse celiac disease or gluten sensitivity, but they are still one of the safer starchy foods for people with digestive issues. They can also provide healing benefits to the digestive tract. Bananas are also packed with a satisfying sweetness that you'll get to enjoy in Baked Coconut Bananas, a truly crave-worthy dessert!

1. Preheat the oven to 350°F.

2. In a small bowl, mix the coconut, coconut oil, lemon juice, maple syrup, vanilla extract, pumpkin pie spice, allspice, cloves, and salt.

3. Place the sliced bananas in a small baking dish and cover with the coconut mixture.

4. Bake for 25 minutes or until lightly golden brown.

5. Serve warm.

Nutritional Analysis per Serving: Protein (g) 1.27; Fat (g) 12.08; Carbs (g) 26.68; B_{12} (mcg) 0; Iron (mg) 0.34; Iodine (mcg) 2.25; Magnesium (mg) 25.05; Potassium (mg) 325.09; Selenium (mcg) 0.92; Sodium (mg) 1.8

Strawberries and Cream Dream

Ⓐ AUTOIMMUNE

Prep time: 7 minutes

Serves: 2

1½ cups strawberries (6 ounces),
at room temperature

1 cup Coconut Yogurt (p. 131)
or coconut milk

1 scoop Rootcology AI Paleo Protein

Juice of ½ lemon

*Up to 2 tablespoons maple syrup to
taste (optional)

*Possible Modifications for Other
Root Cause Diets: If you're following
the Paleo protocol, you can use the
Rootcology Paleo Protein (Vanilla) for
sweetness.

One of my favorite summer treats growing up in Poland was strawberries mashed with sour cream and sprinkled with sugar. My dad would often make this treat for me when strawberries were in season. A couple of months after I started my gluten- and dairy-free journey, I was visiting my parents when my dad brought home some fresh strawberries! I was determined to make a healthier version of my favorite snack that was just as yummy as the original—and Strawberries and Cream Dream is it! This version includes protein powder, which will help balance out the sugar from the strawberries.

1. In a mixing bowl, mash strawberries with a fork or potato masher.

2. Add Coconut Yogurt (p. 131) or coconut milk and mix.

3. Sprinkle with Rootcology protein and mix well.

4. Add lemon juice and any optional sweetener and mix again.

5. Alternatively, for a smooth consistency place all ingredients in a high-powered blender and blend.

Nutritional Analysis per Serving: Protein (g) 14.43; Fat (g) 5.32; Carbs (g) 32.76; B_{12} (mcg) 1.40; Iron (mg) 1.41; Iodine (mcg) 9.61; Magnesium (mg) 98.85; Potassium (mg) 220.96; Selenium (mcg) 0.56; Sodium (mg) 97.12

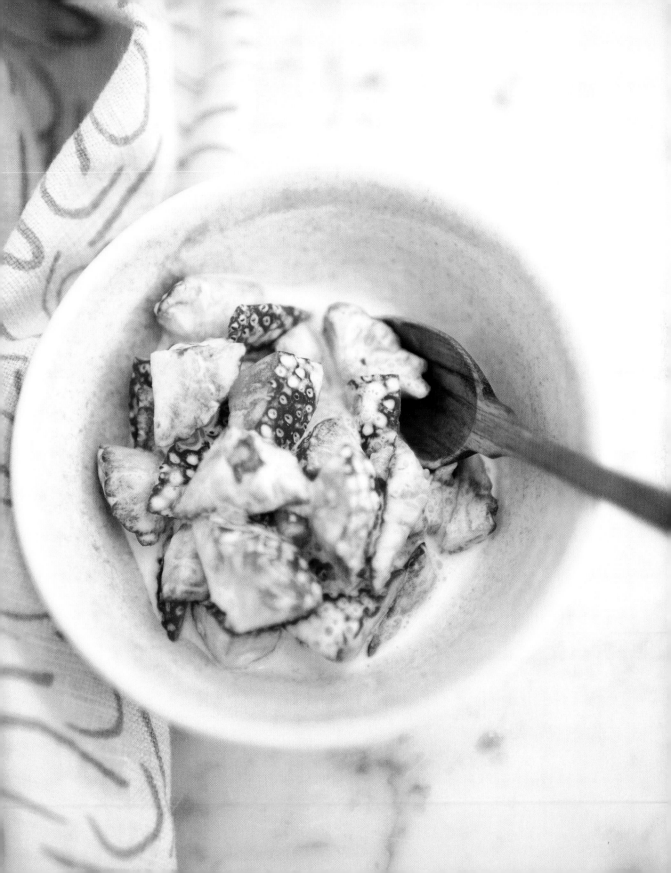

Waffles

① INTRO

Prep time: 10 minutes mixing

Cook time: 5 minutes

Serves: 1

Note: This amount of batter will make 1 large waffle. Simply increase the ingredient amounts to make additional waffles. The batter will stiffen if not used up within an hour, so plan your batch size accordingly.

½ cup garbanzo-bean flour

½ cup cassava flour
(I like Otto's Naturals brand)

1 egg

1 teaspoon vanilla extract

1 teaspoon maple syrup (optional)

Up to 2 cups coconut milk

¼ cup olive oil, melted coconut oil, or pure sprayable oil

Nutritional Analysis per Serving: Protein (g) 7.8; Fat (g) 44.5; Carbs (g) 30.49; B_{12} (mcg) 0.11; Iron (mg) 3.19; Iodine (mcg) 6; Magnesium (mg) 53.82; Potassium (mg) 434.05; Selenium (mcg) 11.54; Sodium (mg) 43.51

I love making these Waffles on a weekend morning! Compared to traditional waffles and even waffles made with most gluten-free flours, these waffles, made with garbanzo-bean flour, are lower in carbohydrates and higher in protein and fiber and thus easier on blood-sugar levels! That said, I recommend eating these with a good side of bacon or sausage as well. These waffles are delicious with pure maple syrup, fresh strawberries, whipped coconut cream, chunky applesauce, or preserves. They can be modified to a Paleo version by taking out the garbanzo-bean flour and doubling the cassava flour. However, removing the garbanzo flour will reduce the protein and fiber content.

1. Preheat the waffle iron.

2. Place the garbanzo-bean flour, cassava flour, egg, vanilla extract, and optional maple syrup into the bowl of a stand mixer. Add ½ cup coconut milk and mix for 2 to 4 minutes.

3. Continue to add the coconut milk, ½ cup at a time, mixing for 1 to 2 minutes after each addition, until the batter reaches a smooth, slightly runny consistency.

4. Using a silicone brush, brush the waffle grid with the oil. Occasionally, you may find coconut oil or olive oil in spray bottles, but be sure to check the ingredients.

5. Pour the waffle batter onto the oiled hot waffle-iron grid and close the lid. Let cook for 5 minutes or until the waffle is a golden color.

6. Use tongs to remove the waffle and serve with maple syrup, berries, whipped coconut cream, chunky applesauce, and/or preserves—and don't forget the side of protein!

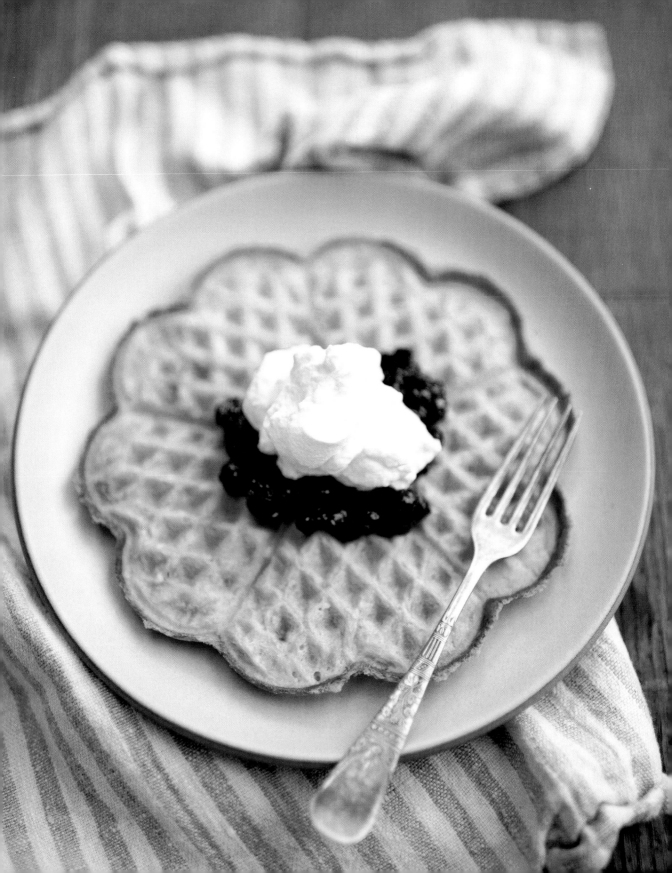

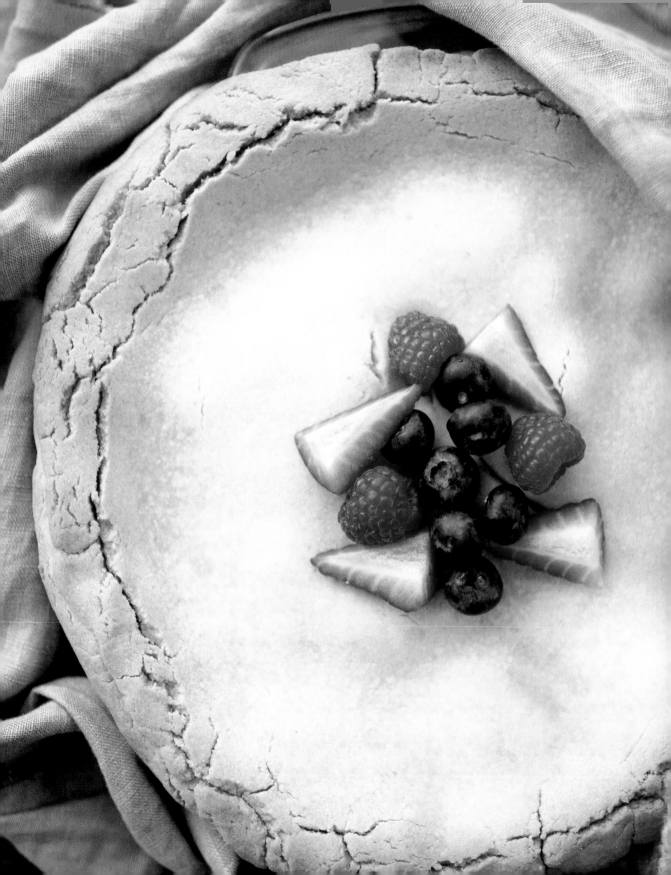

AI Very Berry Pie

Ⓐ AUTOIMMUNE

Prep time: 30 minutes

Cook time: 15 to 20 minutes

Serves: 10

CRUST

3 cups cassava flour

1 teaspoon sea salt or pink Himalayan sea salt

1 teaspoon baking soda

1 tablespoon vanilla

½ cup maple syrup

1⅓ cup palm shortening

FILLING

5 cups mixed berries (halved strawberries, blueberries, blackberries, and raspberries)

¼ cup maple syrup (optional)

Nutritional Analysis per Serving: Protein (g) 1.81; Fat (g) 29.49; Carbs (g) 54.72; B_{12} (mcg) 0; Iron (mg) 0.59; Iodine (mcg) 1.6; Magnesium (mg) 32.71; Potassium (mg) 367.62; Selenium (mcg) 0.91; Sodium (mg) 299.53

AI Very Berry Pie has the texture of a crumbly shortcake and even browns like a traditional pie. The secret to the yummy texture is the palm shortening, which can be used in Paleo baking instead of butter, while the maple syrup allows for a nice light brown color. Cassava flour is a fantastic gluten-free substitute for this kind of baking! I chose a mix of berries to include in this pie because of their antioxidant status; however, you can replace the fruit in the filling with apples, cherries, plums, peaches, or any other type of fruit you like. This pie is sure to be a hit with friends and family members!

1. Preheat the oven to 400°F.

2. In a stand mixer, mix the cassava flour, salt, and baking soda.

3. Add the maple syrup, vanilla, and mix until the texture becomes crumbly.

4. Add the palm shortening, ⅓ cup at a time, until the crust reaches a pliable texture.

5. Divide the dough in thirds; reserve two-thirds for the base, and one-third for the pie top.

6. Roll out the dough with a rolling pin (I recommend having one that is used specifically for gluten-free baking).

7. Gently press one-third of the dough into the bottom of a 9-inch round pie pan to create the pie base and another third of the pie dough onto the sides of the pie pan.

8. Toss the berries with maple syrup if added sweetness is desired and place into the crust.

9. Roll out the remaining third of the crust and place on top.

10. Bake for 15 to 20 minutes until the fruit is cooked through and the top is lightly browned.

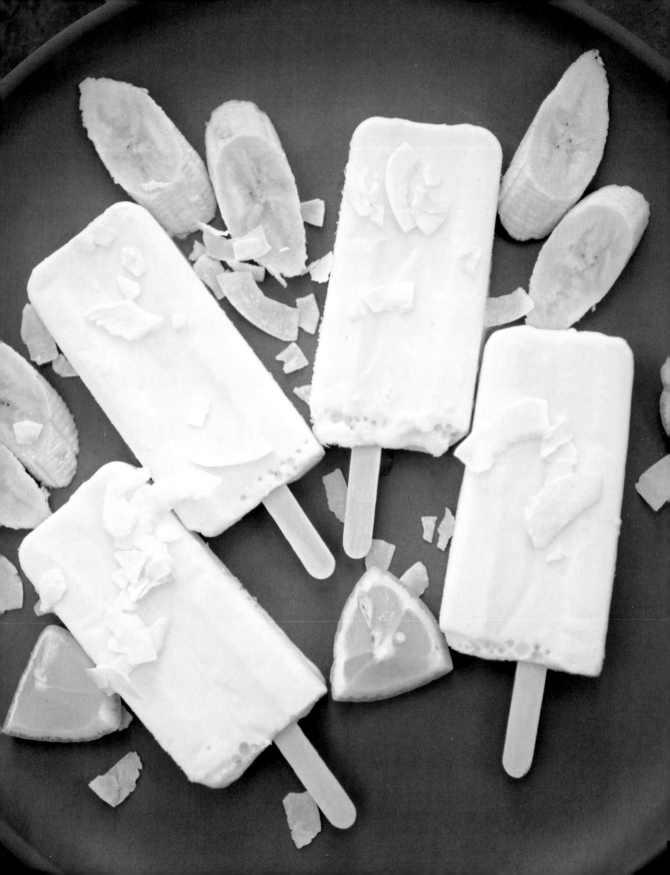

Lemon–Banana Cream Ice Pops

P PALEO

Prep time: 5 minutes

Cook time: 4 hours freezing

Serves: 6

1 large banana

1 cup coconut milk

1 scoop Rootcology AI Paleo Protein

Juice of 2 lemons

What's better than a tasty ice pop on a hot day? An ice pop that will help your digestion and keep your blood sugar balanced! Lemon–Banana Cream Ice Pops are not just delicious, but also contain lemon juice to help with digestion and good fat and protein to keep your blood sugar from crashing. I created this recipe when I was pregnant with my son, Dimitry, and wanted a sweet but healthy snack. You can also add strawberries or blueberries to this recipe to vary up the flavor. You'll love the taste and so will your whole family!

1. Place all ingredients in a high-powered blender and blend until smooth.

2. Pour the mixture into ice-pop molds (or ice cube trays with sticks) and freeze for at least 4 hours or overnight.

3. To remove the ice pops from the molds, fill a container as tall as the molds with hot water, and dip the ice pop-containing molds for 30 seconds. The ice pops should slide right out!

4. Eat immediately, or wrap in wax paper and place in freezer.

Nutritional Analysis per Serving: Protein (g) 4.63; Fat (g) 9.77; Carbs (g) 6.76; B_{12} (mcg) 0; Iron (mg) 0.71; Iodine (mcg) 0.5; Magnesium (mg) 20.11; Potassium (mg) 176.21; Selenium (mcg) 2.67; Sodium (mg) 31.22

Gratitude

This book is truly a community effort! I am so grateful to the wonderful people in my life who helped me create this healing resource.

My family: Michael—I'm so lucky to have you as my soulmate and I love growing with you. Thank you for dreaming with me, for believing in me and most of all, for loving me. You are my world!

My mama, Marta—I can't thank you enough! Thank you for moving into our house with your little dog to take care of our family and helping me finish this cookbook when I was too pregnant, tired, and wobbly to cook! My dad, Adam—for all of your support and for always providing honest feedback on each recipe! My brother and sister in love, Robert and Amanda Nowosadzki—thank you for letting us use your gorgeous kitchen for photos and for talking me out of hiding my pregnant belly behind a roast for the book cover! My son, Dimitry—for inspiring most of the sweet recipes and iron-rich foods you'll find in the cookbook section :-) My dog, Boomer—for being my constant companion and licking up the crumbs and plates from all of the recipe tests.

My dear Boulder sisters: Leanne Ely, my dear friend and fabulous cook and hostess who constantly inspires me—thank you for generously sharing some of your own healing recipes that have become family favorites for this cookbook!! Magdalena Wszelaki, my Polish sister and phenomenal cookbook author—thank you for cookbook publishing coaching and encouragement throughout the process. Debbie Steinbock, my lovely friend and fellow nutrition nerd—thank you for the constant inspiration, support, and fun conversations.

Mary Sullivan, our talented chef—thank you for testing and creating some delicious recipes for us! You are truly a gem!

My Thyroid Pharmacist team: Stephanie DuFour, our wonderful nutritionist—thank you for tirelessly testing and developing recipes, meal plans, and creating the nutritional analysis while meeting some crazy deadlines—all with a smile on your face! Brittany Moore, our project manager ninja—you are an amazing, capable, and gifted person! Thank you for tackling each project big or small with such grace, courage, and determination! Tina Chan,

343

our content editor—thank you for your creative wordsmithery and the fun recipe names! Katie Stehura, our operations manager ninja—you are a force to be reckoned with; we are so grateful for your dedication and brilliance! Whitey Guerin, our sweet assistant—thank you for helping to keep us organized! Anna Amorim and Robin Baker—thank you for taking such great care of our readers and clients and gathering insights for the cookbook. Mary Agnes Antonopoulos, Christin Eastman, and Courtney Kenney—thank you for your dedication and expertise! Laurie Roman—thank you for being a wonderful COO with such great strategy, leadership, and suggestions.

My publishing team: Celeste Fine and John Maas—I am so lucky to have you two powerhouses as my literary agents. Thank you for your constant support, advocacy, and for believing in my vision! The entire team of rock stars at HarperOne, especially Gideon Weil, Julia Kent, Sydney Rogers, Melinda Mullin, Laina Adler, and Lisa Zuniga—thank you for your guidance and trust and partnership.

Charlotte DuPont, our talented and lovely photographer—thank you for making our recipes shine!

My fellow thyroid advocate, functional medicine, health, and Paleo friends: My mentor JJ Virgin for your constant support, encouragement, inspiration, and guidance. Sarah Ballantyne, Mickey Trescott, Robb Wolf, Carrie Vitt, Diane Sanfilippo, Michele Tam, Carol Lovett, and Sophie Van Tiggelen for paving the way for healing with food with your delicious cookbooks! Alan Christianson, Andrea Nakayama, Hashimoto's 411, Dana Trentini, Stacey Robbins, Danna Bowman, Mary Shomon, Christa Orecchio, Carter Black, Katie Wells, Pedram Shojai, Datis Kharrazian, Shannon Garrett, Eric Osansky, Kelly Brogan, James Maskell, Kirk Gair, Michelle Corey, Donna Gates, Dave Asprey, Nik Hedberg, Steve Wright, Trudy Scott, Jolene Brighten, Amy Medling, Brian Mowll, Robyn Openshaw, Kellyann Petrucci, Trevor Cates, Tom Malterre, Emily Rosen, Mark David, Mariza Snyder, Amber Spears, Karl Krummenacher, Tom O'Bryan, Kevin Gianni, Chris Kresser, Ben Lynch, Mark Hyman, the entire faculty of the Institute of Functional Medicine and many others—thank you for all you do to help move self-healing forward. I am proud to be a part of this effort with you!

My clients and readers—for being my greatest teachers and inspiration. I'm so proud to be a part of your healing journeys and still get tears in my eyes with every success story! You can do it!

References

CHAPTER 2

Messina G, Esposito T, Lobaccaro J et al. Effects of low-carbohydrate diet therapy in overweight subject with autoimmune thyroiditis: possible synergism with ChREBP. *Drug Des Devel Ther*. 2016; Volume 10:2939-2946. doi:10.2147/dddt.s106440.

Xu J, Liu X, Yang X, Guo H, Zhao L, Sun X. Supplemental selenium alleviates the toxic effects of excessive iodine on thyroid. *Biol Trace Elem Res*. 2010; 141(1-3):110-118. doi:10.1007/s12011-010-8728-8.

Tonstad S, Nathan E, Oda K, Fraser G. Vegan diets and hypothyroidism. *Nutrients*. 2013;5(11): 4642-4652. doi:10.3390/nu5114642.

Eleftheriou P, Kynigopoulos S, Giovou A et al. Prevalence of anti-neu5Gc antibodies in patients with hypothyroidism. *Biomed Res Int*. 2014;2014:1-9. doi:10.1155/2014/963230.

Small G, Siddarth P, Li Z et al. Memory and Brain Amyloid and Tau Effects of a Bioavailable Form of Curcumin in Non-Demented Adults: A Double-Blind, Placebo-Controlled 18-Month Trial. *The American Journal of Geriatric Psychiatry*. 2018;26(3):266-277. doi:10.1016/j.jagp.2017.10.010.

Krysiak R, Szkróbka W, Okopień B. The effect of vitamin D on thyroid autoimmunity in levothyroxine-treated women with Hashimoto's thyroiditis and normal vitamin D status. *Experimental and Clinical Endocrinology & Diabetes*. 2017; 125(04):229-233. doi:10.1055/s-0042-123038.

Tamer G, Arik S, Tamer I, Coksert D. Relative vitamin D insufficiency in Hashimoto's thyroiditis. *Thyroid*. 2011;21(8):891-896. doi:10.1089/thy.2009.0200.

Ucan B, Sahin M, Sayki Arslan M et al. Vitamin D treatment in patients with Hashimoto's thyroiditis may decrease the development of hypothyroidism. *International Journal for Vitamin and Nutrition Research*. 2016;86(1-2):9-17. doi:10.1024/0300-9831/a000269.

Baker H, Meawed T. Relevance of 25 (OH) vitamin D deficiency on Hashimoto's thyroiditis. *Egyptian Journal of Immunology*. 2017;24(2):53-62.

CHAPTER 3

Collins J, Robinson C, Danhof H et al. Dietary trehalose enhances virulence of epidemic Clostridium difficile. *Nature*. 2018;553(7688):291-294. doi:10.1038/nature25178.

Kyantchakhadze R. Wobenzym in the complex treatment of autoimmune thyroiditis. *International Journal on Immunorehabilitation*. 2002;4(1):114 [Czech abstract, Russian abstract, *Research and Therapeutic Center of Rheumatology* (Tbilisi, Gruzia), VIII International Congress on Immunorehabilitation: Allergy, Immunology, and Global Network, April 21–24, 2002, Cannes, France.]

CHAPTER 4

Barański M, Średnicka-Tober D, Volakakis N et al. Higher antioxidant and lower cadmium concentrations and lower incidence of pesticide residues in organically grown crops: a systematic literature review and meta-analyses. *British Journal of Nutrition*. 2014;112(05):794-811. doi:10.1017/s0007114514001366.

Benzie I, Wachtel-Galor S. *Herbal Medicine*. 2nd ed. Boca Raton: Taylor & Francis; 2011.

Lee B, Yang A, Kim M, McCurdy S, Boisvert W. Natural sea salt consumption confers protection against hypertension and kidney damage in Dahl salt-sensitive rats. *Food Nutr Res*.

2016;61(1):1264713. doi:10.1080/16546628.2017.12
64713.

Benzie I, Wachtel-Galor S. *Herbal Medicine.* 2nd
ed. Boca Raton: Taylor & Francis; 2011:Chapter 2,
Antioxidants in Herbs and Spices: Roles in Oxidative Stress and Redox Signaling.

Rao P, Gan S. Cinnamon: A multifaceted medicinal plant. *Evidence-Based Complementary and Alternative Medicine.* 2014;2014:1-12. doi:10.1155/2014
/642942

Sharma R. Cardamom comfort. *Dent Res J
(Isfahan).* 2012;9(2):237. doi:10.4103/1735-3327.95243.

Środnicka-Tober D, Barański M, Seal C et
al. Higher PUFA and n-3 PUFA, conjugated
linoleic acid, α-tocopherol and iron, but
lower iodine and selenium concentrations in
organic milk: a systematic literature review
and meta- and redundancy analyses. *British Journal
of Nutrition.* 2016;115(06):1043-1060. doi:10.1017
/s0007114516000349.

Index

fructose malabsorption, 78

fruit: apples, 88, 103, 146–47, 292–93, 316–17; bananas, 92, 101, 103, 324–25, 333, 340–41; berries, 42, 316–19, 338–39; cantaloupes, 88; cherries, 40, 88, 102, 269, 326–27; Cilantro-Citrus Cooler recipe, 164–65; Clean Fifteen list, 88; Crunchy Arugula Salad recipe, 206–7; Dirty Dozen Plus list, 88; Ginger-Peach Pork Tenderloin recipe, 276; grapes, 88, 270; mangoes, 88, 101, 296–97; Orange Cream Smoothie recipe, 101, 162–63; papayas, 88; Peaches and Steak recipe, 204–5; pears, 88, 106, 186–87; pineapples, 75, 88, 103, 236–37, 262; plantains, 101, 113, 250–51, 285–86, 328–29; Quail with Grapes recipe, 270; SAM Salad recipe, 106, 113, 212–13; strawberries, 63, 88, 168–69, 334–35, 338–39. *See also* avocados; produce

Galaretka (Polish Gelatin Broth) recipe, 40, 188–89

gallbladder issues: common causes and solutions, 81; gallstones, 75

gallbladder removal, 75

GAPS (Gut and Psychology Syndrome) diet, 36

garlic powder, 94

gelatin: Cherry Berry Gelatin Snacks recipe, 40, 326–27; Galaretka (Polish Gelatin Broth), 40, 188–89; healing benefits of, 40

genetic predisposition, 18, 19

gene triggers, 18

GERD, 81

Gi MAP stool test, 37

ginger: Ginger-Peach Pork Tenderloin recipe, 276; healing benefits of, 94

glass baking dishes, 85

glucosinolates, 31

gluten/dairy digestive enzymes: supplements to support, 79; take when traveling, 111; understanding healing power of, 72, 77–78

gluten-free diet: avoiding hidden gluten, 109; cheating on your, 111; eating out suggestions, 105–8; Find Me Gluten Free app on restaurants, 105; getting family members to support your, 103–4; healing benefits of, 29, 34, 37; substitutions for gluten-containing products, 90. *See also* food sensitivities

gluten sensitivity testing, 60

gluteomorphins, 61

GMO seeds, 89

Gnocchi with Peas and Pancetta recipe, 271–72

Goddess of Detox Dressing, 148–49, 213

goitrogens: interference with thyroid function by, 31; Root Cause Approach to, 31

Gołąbki (Polish Stuffed Cabbage Rolls) recipe, 254–56

Golden Raisin Chicken Salad recipe, 103, 195

grain-free diet, 29, 65–66

grapes: Dirty Dozen list, 88; Quail with Grapes recipe, 270

grass-fed beef, 67

Graves' disease, 15, 49

green beans: Grilled Fish and Pineapple Salsa Packets with Green Beans recipe, 103, 262; Truffled Veggies recipe, 80, 279; well tolerated by people with Hashimoto's, 67. *See also* beans; vegetables

greening your kitchen, 84

green juices: Green Juice recipe, 42, 152–53; healing benefits of chlorophyll and, 41–42

green smoothies: healing benefits of, 39; how they can help your thyroid, 39; Root Cause Original Smoothie recipe, 39, 101, 107, 112–13, 166–67

Grilled Fish and Pineapple Salsa Packets with Green Beans recipe, 103, 262

hair loss: common causes and solutions, 81; as Hashimoto's symptom, 4, 15; how carbohydrates can increase, 43

ham (Frittata with Ham and White Sweet Potato recipe), 113, 216

Hashi Hash Hash recipe, 103, 113, 230–31

Hashi-Mayo recipe, 142

Hashi-Mojito recipe, 63, 154–55

Hashi-Mojito Smoothie recipe, 170

Hashimoto's Protocol: A 90-Day Plan for Reversing Thyroid Symptoms and Getting Your Life Back (Wentz): on ferritin information, 55; healing journey leading to the, 3–4, 8; on iodine supplementation, 50; Liver Support Protocol of the, 59; on the Root Cause Approach to Hashimoto's, 25; success studies from people who have implemented approach in, 23, 59–60

Hashimoto's Thyroiditis: Lifestyle Interventions for Finding and Treating the Root Cause (Wentz), 3, 7, 8, 19, 23, 25

Hashimoto's thyroiditis: author's personal journey toward healing, 3–7, 11; as autoimmune condition, 12; description of, 2; the five stages of, 19; hypothyroidism due to, 2, 4; testing for, 14–18; 2015 diet survey of

2,232 people with, 29; understanding causes of, 12; "Vicious Cycle of Hashimoto's," 20–23; what it feels like to have, 13–14. *See also* Safety Theory of Hashimoto's; thyroid disorders; thyroid function

Hashimoto's treatment: continuing symptoms with pharmacological, 5, 12–13; multifaceted approach to, 6–7; pharmacological, 4, 5, 12–13; understanding limitations of diet for, 24, 26. *See also* lifestyle interventions; Root Cause Approach

headaches, 51

healing diets: "Also Try" strategy, 80; healing enzymes to support, 72–79; nourishment knowledge to help you heal, 71–78; Root Cause Autoimmune Diet, 57–58, 67–68; Root Cause Intro Diet, 57–63; Root Cause Paleo Diet, 57–58, 64–67; where to start and which diet to implement next, 71

healing foods: beets, 41; berries, 42; bone broth, 40; cilantro, 41; cruciferous veggies, 41; fiber, 41; gelatin, 40; green juices and chlorophyll, 41–42; green smoothies, 39; hot lemon water, 40–41; turmeric, 42. *See also specific food*

health-food stores, 91

heat intolerance, 15

Heirloom Tomato and Beet Salad recipe, 198–99

hemp protein powder, 46

Herbes de Provence, 95

hidden gluten, 109

high-powered blender, 85

Hippocrates, 71, 72

histamine intolerance, 112

histamine reactions, 112

homocysteine (amino acid), 41

honeydew melons, Clean Fifteen list, 88

Hot Chocolate recipe, 172–73

hot lemon water, 40–41

hot peppers: Dirty Dozen list, 88; Root Cause Paleo Diet exclusion of, 66. *See also* bell peppers

H. pylori infection, 54, 81, 113

Hubby's Carnitas recipe, 85, 103, 228–29

Hummus recipe, 92

hydrochloric acid deficiency, 21

hydrolyzed beef protein, 91

hydrolyzed beef protein powder, 46, 67

hyperthyroidism symptoms, 15

hypoallergenic protein powders, 45

hypothyroidism: Hashimoto's symptoms of, 15; Hashimoto's thyroiditis as leading cause of, 2, 4, 12; hydrochloric acid deficiency due to, 21; iodine deficiency cause of, 12, 32. *See also* thyroid disorders

IgE antibodies, 22, 64

IgG antibodies, 22

immune system: connection between the thyroid gland and, 2; Hashimoto's thyroiditis and the, 12

impaired detoxification, 78

impaired protein digestion, 21

infections: *Candida,* 63, 78; *H. pylori,* 54, 81, 113; as intestinal permeability ("leaky gut") factor, 23

inflammation–meat debate, 35

ingredients: additional tips for choosing, 89; choosing quality, 86–93; EWG's 2018 Shopper's Guide to Pesticides in Produce, 88; organic produce, 86, 88–89; stocking up on safe, 91; substitutions for traditional, 90, 113; where to shop for quality, 91–92. *See also* foods

insomnia, 51

intermittent fasting, 113

intestinal permeability ("leaky gut"). *See* leaky gut

iodine deficiency: glucosinolates causing, 31; hypothyroidism caused by, 12, 32

iodine-free diet, 38

iodine-rich foods, 67

iodine supplementation, 50

iodine supplements debate, 32–33

irritability: as Hashimoto's symptom, 15; how carbohydrates can increase, 43

irritable bowel syndrome (IBS): common causes and solutions, 81; grain-free diet in case of, 65; Hashimoto's thyroiditis symptom of, 4; risk of selenium deficiency associated with, 49

Italian Meatza Pie recipe, 114, 263

Jar Salad recipe, 196–97

joint pain, 15, 51

kale: Chicken Burgers and Kale Chips recipe, 261; healing benefits of, 41; Lentil Shepherd's Pie recipe, 224–25. *See also* vegetables

Katy's Greek Salad recipe, 101, 200–201

keto-friendly recipes, 114

ketogenic diet, 114

kitchens: greening your, 84; recommended tools to have in your, 42, 85–86

kitchen tools: masticating juicer, 42; recommendations on, 42, 85–86; simplify your life with great, 85

kiwis (Clean Fifteen list), 88
Kotlety (Polish Chicken Cutlets) recipe, 264

labels on canned foods, 89
lab tests. *See* tests
lamb: as blood sugar-stabilizing food, 67; Moroccan
    Lamb Stew recipe, 184–85; Shepherd's Pie
    recipe, 240–41; US Wellness Meats, 91–92
leaky gut: autoimmunity and, 18; description
    and symptoms associated with, 20, 22–23;
    factors that can contribute to, 23; histamine
    intolerance due to, 112; *H. pylori* infection
    that can trigger a, 54, 81, 113; vegetarian diet
    prevents healing from, 35
legumes: green beans, 67, 80, 103, 262, 279;
    pea protein, 46, 67; Root Cause Paleo Diet
    eliminating, 66
Lemon-Banana Cream Ice Pops recipe, 92, 101,
    103, 340–41
Lentil Shepherd's Pie recipe, 224–25
Levothyroxine, 25
L-glutamine, 21
lifestyle interventions: author's journey to
    seek out, 5–7; author's personal journey to
    healing through, 3–7, 11; diet as central to
    successful, 7–9; healing Hashimoto's patterns
    with nutrition, 20–23; readers looking for
    "Done-for-You Guide" on, 7–8; to reduce
    autoimmunity, 18, 20; the *Root Cause* and
    Hashimoto's Protocol strategies for, 3, 7–8, 19;
    understanding limitations of diet and, 24, 26.
    See also Hashimoto's treatment; nourishment
    knowledge; Root Cause Approach
Liver and Gallbladder Support, 76, 81
Liver Pâté recipe, 290–91
low blood sugar, 63
Low FODMAP diet, 29
low-histamine diet, 112
low stomach acid, 21
L-tyrosine, 21
lupus, 19
Lyme disease, 63
lysozyme complex, 68

Maca Latte recipe, 158–59
macronutrients: deficiencies in, 20–21; as
    more important to body health than calories,
    43–45, 47
magnesium, 51–52
magnesium citrate, 52
magnesium glycinate, 52

main dish recipes. *See* Cookbook recipes
mangoes: Clean Fifteen list, 88; Mango Salsa
    recipe, 101, 296–97
Maple Meatloaf Muffins recipe, 101, 103, 232–33
Mason Jar Hack recipe, 102
Mason jars, 85, 102
Massachusetts General Hospital, 18
masticating juicer, 42, 85
Meal Plans: AI (Autoimmune) Diet Week 1, 124–25;
    AI (Autoimmune) Diet Week 2, 126–27; Intro
    Diet Week 1, 116–17; Intro Diet Week 2, 118–19;
    Paleo Diet Week 1, 120–21; Paleo Week 2, 122–23
meats: debate over inflammatory impact of, 35;
    tips for saving money on, 93; US Wellness
    Meats, 91–92. *See also specific type of meat*
medications: NSAIDS (nonsteroidal anti-
    inflammatory drugs), 23, 74; synthetic thyroid,
    4, 5, 12–13, 25
memory loss, 4
menstrual irregularities, 15, 51
mercury toxicity: customized dietary
    modifications to avoid, 78; in different fish
    species, 87; eating fish low in, 86
metabolism: responding to "famine" signal, 2, 3,
    44; thyroid gland's regulation of, 2, 3
Mexican Quiche recipe, 85, 114, 244–45
micronutrients: deficiencies in, 20; importance
    to Hashimoto's recovery, 47; as required
    nutrient, 43
migraines, 51, 78, 81
Mint Tea recipe, 62, 156–57
Mizeria (Polish Cucumber Salad) recipe, 298–99
molecular mimicry, 2
Mom's Dill Pickles recipe, 133–34
Moroccan Lamb Stew recipe, 184–85
MSG (monosodium glutamate), 89
MTHFR gene mutation, 41
mushrooms: Broccoli and Chicken Quiche recipe,
    85, 103, 113, 114, 246–47; Hashi Hash Hash
    recipe, 103, 113, 230–31; Lentil Shepherd's
    Pie recipe, 224–25; Shepherd's Pie recipe, 103,
    240–41; Stuffed Portobello Mushrooms recipe,
    257; Tropical Grilled Chicken Skewers recipe,
    103, 236–37; Truffled Veggies recipe, 80, 279.
    See also vegetables
My Duck Salad recipe, 101
MyMedLab, 65
Myo-inositol (sugar alcohol), 63

National Academy of Clinical Biochemists, 16
natural carbohydrates, 47